ANNALS OF THE NEW YORK ACADEMY OF SCIENCES
Volume 562

PRENATAL ABUSE OF LICIT AND ILLICIT DRUGS

Edited by Donald E. Hutchings

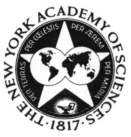

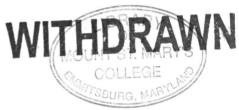

D1481577

The New York Academy of Sciences
New York, New York
1989

Cover (paper edition): *Logo of the Behavioral Teratology Society (drawn by Barbara Cummings).*

Library of Congress Cataloging-in-Publication Data

Prenatal abuse of licit and illicit drugs.

(Annals of the New York Academy of Sciences, ISSN 0077-8923 ; v. 562)
Contains papers from a conference held by the Behavioral Teratology Society, the National Institute on Drug Abuse (National Institutes of Health), and the New York Academy of Sciences in Bethesda, Maryland, Sept. 7–9, 1988.
Includes bibliographies and index.
1. Fetus—Effect of drugs on—Congresses.
2. Drug abuse in pregnancy—Congresses. 3. Pregnant women—Drug use—Congresses. I. Hutchings, Donald E. II. Behavioral Teratology Society. III. National Institute on Drug Abuse. IV. New York Academy of Sciences. V. Series. [DNLM: 1. Fetus—drug effects— congresses. 2. Prenatal Exposure Delayed Effects— congresses. 3. Substance Abuse—in pregnancy— congresses. W1 AN626YL v.562 / WQ 210 P9232 1988] Q11.N5 vol. 562 [RG627.6.D79] 500s 89-12279 ISBN 0-89766-521-X (alk. paper) [618.3′2] ISBN 0-89766-522-8 (pbk. : alk. paper)

PCP

Printed in the United States of America

ISBN 0-89766-521-X (cloth)

ISBN 0-89766-522-8 (paper)

ISSN 0077-8923

ANNALS OF THE NEW YORK ACADEMY OF SCIENCES

Volume 562
June 30, 1989

PRENATAL ABUSE OF LICIT AND ILLICIT DRUGS [a]

Editor and Conference Chair
DONALD E. HUTCHINGS

CONTENTS

[a] The papers in this volume were presented at a conference entitled Prenatal Abuse of Licit
and Illicit Drugs, which was held by the Behavioral Teratology Society, the National Institute
on Drug Abuse (National Institutes of Health), and the New York Academy of Sciences in
Bethesda, Maryland on September 7-9, 1988.

Major funding was provided by:

- NATIONAL INSTITUTE ON DRUG ABUSE/NATIONAL INSTITUTES OF HEALTH

Financial assistance was also received from:

- BEHAVIORAL TERATOLOGY SOCIETY
- E. I. DU PONT DE NEMOURS & COMPANY
- SCHERING LABORATORIES
- E. R. SQUIBB & SONS

Preface

To the best of my knowledge, this is the first meeting on prenatal drug use that brings together basic and clinical researchers, epidemiologists, healthcare providers, those concerned with legal and ethical issues, and policy makers. But what makes this conference especially unique is the unusually broad range of drugs that will be discussed. These include major licit substances—alcohol, nicotine and caffeine, as well as the major illicit drugs—opioids, cannabinoids, central nervous system (CNS) stimulants and phencylidine. Traditionally, the public health aspects of these compounds have been assigned to and administratively sequestered in various governmental agencies. The National Institute on Alcohol Abuse and Alcoholism has been concerned exclusively with alcohol. Illicit drugs fall under the purview of the National Institute on Drug Abuse, although this agency also funds basic research on nicotine in both adult and immature organism. At the same time, the National Institute on Child Health and Human Development has a long history of interest in the effects of smoking on human pregnancy.

One result of this compartmentalization is that it has, in part, given rise to increasingly specialized and narrowly focused scientific disciplines, meetings, societies and journals. And while this is all quite understandable as the natural evolution of scientific activity, information has become widely scattered yet, at the same time, isolated in scientific minicommunities. This clearly serves the interests of the specialized practitioners and scientists, enabling them to interact and share mutual technical and scientific problems unique to their endeavors. But inevitably, boundaries have become more rigid and these specialty groups more insular and self-directed with the result that communication between groups has been impeded.

For example, clinicians concerned with drug-exposed infants often view the basic researcher as reducing whole organisms to neurochemical systems, receptors and binding sites, and their mechanistic findings may be dismissed as either tortuously arcane or of ambiguous relevance to their clinical problems. And, indeed, the daily world of the perinatal treatment staff and the one that they publish papers about, consists of women in a compulsive pattern of drug abuse who also happen to be pregnant and are likely to give birth to very sick, at-risk babies that will require highly specialized medical management. Their major concern is to utilize their medical skills to provide increasingly improved healthcare and treatment to these infants to ensure as optimum an outcome as possible.

On the other hand, clinical researchers may not be as well informed about pharmacokinetics or the fundamental pharmacological processes of tolerance, physical dependence and abstinence. To cite an example from the mid-1970s, at that time pediatric lore suggested that the prolonged or subacute abstinence lasting some 4-6 months in infants that had been prenatally exposed to methadone, was the likely result of the persistence and slow clearance of methadone from the babies' CNS. But opioid pharmacologists knew that human adults in withdrawal from either morphine or methadone similarly show a prolonged abstinence. Although the adult symptoms have a different temporal pattern compared with infants, their symptoms do persist for six months or longer and are not associated with the persistence of the drug in the CNS. Thus, what was thought by some pediatricians to be pharmacologically unique to the neonate would have been viewed by an opioid pharmacologist as possibly a minor variation on the adult phenomenon of prolonged abstinence.

Likewise, basic researchers, in their quest to develop animal models, assess risk, and discover mechanisms underlying toxic outcomes while grappling with the intractable problem of extrapolation to humans, may suffer from a certain amount of clinical illiteracy. The clinical perinatal abuse literature may be viewed somewhat opportunistically and exploited as a bountiful reservoir that holds the rationale and scientific justification for a basic research grant proposal. Clinical papers may be eagerly scoured for epidemiological excesses and horrific clinical outcomes, all the better to add spice to significance sections of grant applications. But some of these researchers may have no more than a lay understanding of the etiology and psychobiology of drug abuse, and only a superficial appreciation of issues of medical management of the pregnant drug user and care and assessment of drug-exposed neonates. Thus, some attempts to develop animal models may miss fundamental elements of the clinical problem so that the significance of the research findings may be obscure.

So as not to sound unreasonably harsh, I do acknowledge that given such a vast literature and the enormous complexity of the phenomena that we study, it is often difficult to judge appropriately the proper emphasis that should be given specific information. Clearly, we cannot know and be expert at everything, and primary care physicians and clinical and basic researchers each have a different set of goals and priorities. But we must not lose sight of the fact that together, we make up a larger scientific community that shares a common goal: first, to understand the disease mechanisms associated with prenatal exposure to particular classes of drugs; second, to describe the short- and long-term clinical, biochemical and neurobehavioral manifestations that result from such exposure; and third, through the means by which we understand the mechanisms of such drug exposure, to develop specific treatments, management and prevention.

We come together at a time of gloomy foreboding, when some are saying that the country is in the midst of a national tragedy; our neonatal mortality rate is one of the worst of all of the industrial nations, and the poor and disadvantaged have severe economic barriers, not just to advanced medical technology but, shamefully, to the minimum of prenatal care. Drug use in no small way contributes to this overall grim problem. Let us hope that in this conference, as we learn new information and enlarge our conceptual vocabulary, that we may strike a fresh alliance of understanding and ideas so that for each of us and our respective disciplines, our ignorance of these urgent problems may be palpably diminished.

We are grateful to the New York Academy of Sciences for sponsoring this conference. I want to extend special thanks to Drs. Roger Brown and Marvin Snyder and their able staff at the National Institute on Drug Abuse for their efforts in ensuring the funding for it. I must also express my profound appreciation both to the Conference Committee of the New York Academy of Sciences for their help and encouragement in organizing the program, and to Ellen Marks, the Conference Director, and her outstanding staff, for their skillful and efficient labors in stewarding this meeting into reality. Without the finely tuned organizational process that so swiftly and surely goes into motion once a conference is approved, none of us would have found ourselves at this meeting so expeditiously.

Donald E. Hutchings

Perspectives on the Concern for and Management of Prenatal Chemical Exposure and Postnatal Effects[a]

CAROLE A. KIMMEL

Reproductive and Developmental Toxicology Branch (RD-689)
Office of Health and Environmental Assessment
Office of Research and Development
United States Environmental Protection Agency
401 M Street, S.W.
Washington, DC 20460

Although teratology and developmental toxicology had their experimental beginnings in the early part of this century, the potential for human developmental toxicity due to chemical exposure was not generally recognized until the thalidomide tragedy of the early 1960s.[1] Furthermore, the fact that exposure to chemicals during development might have subtle and long-lasting postnatal consequences in humans was not generally recognized until the late 1960s and early 1970s.[2] Thus, the last 20 years have seen a remarkable increase in the number of reports of chemical effects on development, particularly on the function of the neonate and young child, reflecting in part the heightened awareness by researchers of the potential for such effects.

A number of agents have been reported to have adverse consequences on the neonate and on later development in both humans and animals. At present, at least nine of these agents have sufficient evidence to confirm that they can cause developmental neurotoxic effects in humans.[3] Of these, several are substances of abuse (heroin, methadone, alcohol, cocaine). At least one therapeutic agent (diphenylhydantoin) and one physical agent (x-irradiation) are also documented human developmental neurotoxicants. In addition, there are three environmental chemicals (lead, methylmercury and polychlorinated biphenyls) for which evidence is sufficient to indicate the unique susceptibility of the developing organism to the developmental neurotoxic effects of these agents. Thus, a variety of agents are capable of affecting the unborn child and neonate in devastating and often irreversible ways.

When one evaluates the available data on the developmental toxicity of chemicals, the types of evidence required to indicate that an agent is a developmental toxicant are similar, whether the agent is a therapeutic agent, an abused substance or a physical or environmental agent.[4] The data available are usually most extensive for therapeutic agents or environmental chemicals for which standard testing is required prior to marketing or release into the environment. In fact, testing of certain chemicals specifically for developmental neurotoxicity has recently been added to the overall developmental toxicity testing battery.[5] For substances of abuse, on the other hand, there is no standard testing (unless the drug is a therapeutic agent), and data may be sketchy

---

[a]Disclaimer. The views in this paper are those of the author and do not necessarily reflect the views or policies of the U.S. Environmental Protection Agency.

1

or nonexistent until a problem is recognized in humans. Even then, data are gathered primarily by basic science researchers through grant-funded research, and are not necessarily focused to provide a comprehensive evaluation of the developmental toxicity of an agent.

The management and control of exposure to different chemical agents also varies tremendously. For example, therapeutic agents can be carefully controlled via the federal government and the medical community, and are marketed to be prescribed for certain uses, although misuse does occur. Environmental agents are also regulated by the federal government, and their release into the environment can be controlled to some extent. However, with them there is a much greater potential for misuse and exposure of unsuspecting individuals.

Unfortunately, the management and control of exposure to substances of abuse is much more difficult or impossible. Thus, the contribution by substances of abuse to the overall incidence of developmental toxicity is significant, and may be increasing. In the growing and changing environment of drug abuse in which we live, it is important to educate the general public about the drastic consequences of such abuse during pregnancy. This conference comes as an appropriate step in heightening that awareness among researchers, clinicians, and government officials. I only hope that it will stimulate health care and public health organizations, as well the media, to communicate these concerns and problems to the public, and to provide appropriate education concerning the use of drugs and chemicals during pregnancy.

REFERENCES

1. WILSON, J. G. 1979. The evolution of teratological testing. Teratology **20:** 205-212.
2. VORHEES, C. V. 1986. Origins of behavioral teratology. *In* Handbook of Behavioral Teratology. E. P. Riley & C. V. Vorhees, Eds. 3-22. Plenum Press. New York, NY.
3. KIMMEL, C. A. 1988. Current status of behavioral teratology: Science and regulation. *In* CRC Critical Reviews in Toxicology. Vol. 19: 1-10. CRC Press. Boca Raton, FL.
4. U.S. Environmental Protection Agency. 1986. Guidelines for the health assessment of suspect developmental toxicants. Fed. Regist. **51:** 34028-34040.
5. U.S. Environmental Protection Agency. 1988. Diethylene glycol butyl ether and diethylene glycol butyl ether acetate. Test standards and requirements. Final rule. Fed. Regist. **53:** 5932-5953.

Evolution of American Attitudes Toward Substance Abuse

DAVID F. MUSTO

Child Study Center and History of Medicine
Yale University School of Medicine
333 Cedar Street
New Haven, Connecticut 06510

Anyone who has followed the drug problem for the last ten or fifteen years will have noted an interesting transformation. Cocaine has moved from being perceived as a relatively harmless tonic worthy, according to some drug experts in the 1970s, of decriminalization on those grounds, to being seen as a most dangerous substance with no redeeming qualities. Its earlier merits, euphoria and central nervous system stimulation, are now seen as seductive dangers.[1] This change in attitude toward cocaine may be a paradigm of our pattern of response to a number of powerful chemicals—opium, morphine, cannabis and alcohol. What is even more interesting, this evolution of American attitudes toward substance use and abuse has not happened only once. One might expect that a lesson is learned once and for all, but curiously, in some instances, changes in attitude recur. We may not recall the earlier change in attitude toward cocaine around 1900, but we have been experiencing a close parallel to that cocaine epidemic, at least to 1988. Perhaps the public's almost total lack of knowledge of that earlier time is one powerful reason why we have repeated this "experiment in nature."

Let us think back to that first epidemic. For millenia persons indigenous to the Andean highlands had used the coca leaves growing there as a mild stimulant, mainly by chewing. Spanish conquistadores quickly prohibited use of the leaves, but it was said that coca allowed the workers in mines and elsewhere to work longer, harder, and with fewer complaints; therefore, coca leaf chewing again became acceptable.[2]

Conflicting stories about the properties of the coca leaf and its unknown active principles led to more intensive chemical investigation. Shortly before our Civil War, Albert Nieman in Austria isolated an active ingredient and named it cocaine. One of the popularizers of coca was Angelo Mariani who concocted a wine containing an extract of coca leaves. *Vin Mariani,* as the product was known, had prestigious admirers all over the Western world. Thomas Edison valued it and Pope Leo XIII awarded Mariani a gold medal.[3]

In the mid-1880s a major event changed the pattern of coca use: purified cocaine began to be produced in commercial quantities. The pharmaceutical industry had established efficient international marketing procedures. Merck and Co. produced it in Germany and exported it to the United States, where the Parke, Davis Co. was equally engaged with cocaine production, distribution and promotion.[4] The value of cocaine and its apparent harmlessness greatly encouraged not only pharmaceutical manufacturers but also medical experts who wrote essays of praise with considerable conviction. Writers not uncommonly referred to their own positive experiences with the drug.[5] These were instances of an author going into a topic and the topic going into the author.

In this regard I cannot avoid referring to Dr. William A. Hammond, who enjoyed great credibility as a spokesman for cocaine. A professor at several medical schools and considered one of the founders of the specialty of neurology, he had been Surgeon General of the U.S. Army during the Civil War and even wrote plays and novels.[6] Dr. Hammond, an expert on the effects of cocaine by any objective criterion, could find no fault with the drug. More than that, he recommended it for common human failings—not merely for the serious problem of melancholia, but for when feeling down. He even perfected the ideal "coca wine," two grains of cocaine to a pint of wine, and drank a glass of this with his meals.

"What is true of the wine," Dr. Hammond told the Virginia Medical Society in 1887, "is more emphatically true of the active principle, cocaine." Some physicians questioned his faith in the safety of cocaine, but Dr. Hammond brushed their doubts aside. He said he was "not aware that a fatal dose of cocaine [had] yet been indicated by actual fact." Well, then, was cocaine not addictive? Not at all, replied the great neurologist. He denied "that there is such a thing as a cocaine habit, pure and simple, which the individual cannot, of his own effort, altogether arrest."[7]

Moving from the medical world to the vast public arena, we observe that cocaine use spread amid equal enthusiasm. Cocaine was the first simple remedy for a very annoying ailment, hay fever. At the time, hay fever was considered a problem of the more civilized people of the world, a sign of extreme refinement. American experts in this area proudly claimed we had more hay fever than any other nation.[8] Cocaine was adopted as the official remedy of the Hay Fever Association.[9]

Turning from the needs of those with a physical or emotional complaint to the entire population, we come to one of the most popular beverages in the world's history, Coca-Cola. As first sold at a soda fountain in 1886, Coca-Cola was a *temperance* coca beverage. The formula appears to have been an imitation of the famous French coca wines, such as *Vin Mariani,* but without alcohol. Those who feared the effects of alcohol could still obtain the benefits of the coca plant. The advertising slogans were explicit about exactly what the Coca-Cola drinker could expect. In 1890 the drink was described as "the wonderful nerve and brain tonic and remarkable therapeutic agent." In 1893 customers were urged to buy "the ideal brain tonic" and by 1899 you could learn that "Coca-Cola makes the flow of thought more easy and reasoning power more vigorous."[10] Between 1900 and 1903 the Coca-Cola company removed cocaine from the formula. The fraction of cocaine in the formula by the time it was removed was one four-hundredth per cent.[11]

When we come to the removal of cocaine from Coca-Cola we have reached a crisis in the earlier wave of cocaine use. In the first known advertisement of Coca-Cola in 1886 the proprietors proudly announced a drink "containing the properties of the wonderful Coca plant."[12] Within fifteen years cocaine had shifted from being a reason to drink Coca-Cola to being so negatively perceived that not a milligram could be present in the "pause that refreshes." Clearly a change had taken place in the public's attitude toward cocaine. By 1903 the Atlanta City Council passed an ordinance prohibiting cocaine from being dispensed at a soda fountain. In 1910 the President of the United States sent a Report to Congress that declared, "The misuse of cocaine is undoubtedly an American habit, the most threatening of the drug habits that has ever appeared in this country."[13] In 1912 the United States presided over the Hague Opium Convention which also dealt with the menace of cocaine in the treaty written there and submitted to the nations of the world.[14] In 1914 the Harrison Act was signed by President Wilson. That law, considered by its framers as the domestic implementation of the Hague Opium Treaty, severely restricted the availability of cocaine without a physician's prescription.[15] Reviewing, then, the time-line of cocaine's introduction into America, about fifteen years passed from commercial availability to removal from a popular drink and fifteen more years until the substance was prohibited from almost all nonmedical use. Of course, cocaine continued to be used recreationally, compulsively and illegally, but the consensus among the many institutions of American society that cocaine was without any merit—except in limited medical uses as a block to nerve conduction—appears to have been the bedrock upon which a reduction in demand was built. Cocaine had disappeared in soft drinks, hay fever remedies and as an easily obtainable commodity from mail order houses. The public had grown extremely alarmed by the substance and those who used it.[16]

During the two decades after 1914 cocaine use declined until only occasionally was the drug seized and were users arrested. In 1900 cocaine was everywhere and in everything from Coca-Cola to hay fever remedies, but by 1940 cocaine use had become uncommon. By the time I took the medical school course in pharmacology in 1960, cocaine was a memory for the professors and news to the students.

The campaign against cocaine was successful, although the length of the battle was longer than those alarmed by it would have liked. The change in attitude toward cocaine, however, involved more than just the fear of cocaine's effects—causing agitation, violence and a lack of judgment. An extreme fear of cocaine's liability to create violence appears to have led some Americans to link it with other fears then prominent. These links extended beyond the murky underworld of crime and prostitution. Prior to World War I a linkage between cocaine and Blacks became a commonplace accusation. Although both blacks and whites used cocaine, the link with blacks was emphasized. One can speculate that whites who feared black hostility—and raised lynching to a peak around 1900—were happy to locate a chemical reason why blacks were hostile to civic repression.[17]

Thus the decline in demand for cocaine was not an unalloyed crusade. The fear of drugs spilled over into other areas providing, for example, in the case of Southern Blacks, a simplistic explanation for hostility.

I have dwelt on the first cocaine epidemic for two reasons: I believe the history is of particular interest now when we can see parallels between that change in attitude and the one we have lived through in the last fifteen years or so. The other reason is that I have space only to mention some of the other examples of change in attitude toward seductive chemicals, and the first cocaine epidemic is a convenient model to which these can be compared.

Morphine and other opiates have had a more gradual rise in use and a decline perhaps less precipitous than cocaine. Opiate consumption in the United States peaked in the 1890s after rising throughout the 19th century in an open market.[18] The lack of restrictions on opiates until very late in the century and the total lack of any national controls were both due to our Federal form of government as practiced in the last century, that is, a strict reservation of police power—under which antidrug activities generally operate—to the states. Opiate use, furthermore, did not fade as completely as cocaine and began a gradual rise in the 1950s, earlier than cocaine which came back about 1970.

Alcohol is perhaps the most important substance about which the United States has witnessed recurrent waves of use and alterations of attitude from positive to negative. It is important, I believe, to stress that the changes in attitude from tolerance to intolerance are not just to be found in the decades leading up to national prohibition in 1920 and the backlash to prohibition that began after 1933. This view too easily makes of the antialcohol movement and Prohibition a mere aberration in our social history, a peculiar event that can safely be forgotten. As I have suggested in regard to our first cocaine epidemic, we can easily forget antidrug campaigns, but it is to our loss that we do so.

The first antialcohol movement which led to widespread prohibition in the United States began early in the 19th century. Alcohol had been thought a tonic, a remedy for disease and an aid to physical labor. Record consumption of distilled spirits about 1830 worried many Americans who noticed that alcohol in large amounts did not seem to match the claims for it. Consumption levels declined and about a dozen states enacted prohibitory laws.[19]

Perhaps the Civil War absorbed these reforming energies, but whatever the reason observance of the laws declined in the 1860s and once again consumption climbed. In the 1890s the Anti-Saloon League was formed to combat the most offensive expression of alcohol, the saloon.[20] Gradually the focus of antagonism spread from the saloon to alcohol itself, just as antagonism to distilled spirits in the 1830s gradually grew to encompass all forms of alcohol. By January 1919 the thirty-sixth state had ratified the 18th Amendment to the Constitution and a year later we entered national prohibition. In the 1920s we hit the lowest level of alcohol consumption in our nation's history.[21]

The eventual repeal of Prohibition stemmed from a combination of factors. First, unlike cocaine, there was a cultural acceptance of alcohol among tens of millions of Americans. Although the amount consumed was greatly reduced, the use of alcohol could not be extinguished to the degree that had been accomplished with smoking opium, with other opiates and with cocaine. Then the onset of the Depression made Repeal an attractive stimulation of employment and needed revenue.[22] Repeal, however, came with a backlash, a weariness with talk of controlling alcohol and alcohol-related problems. Fifty years would have to pass before popular movements like Remove Intoxicated Drivers (RID) and Mothers Against Drunk Drivers (MADD) could again raise questions about alcohol without being apologetic or defensive.

Now we are, I believe, entering a new temperance era, a growing awareness of the negative side of alcohol.[23] Several crucial elements of earlier temperance movements can be seen. First, an aspect of alcohol's social impact abhorrent both to drinkers and to abstainers has been identified and broadcast: I refer to the drunk driving problem. Second, the multiple, distinctive forms of alcohol, spirits, wine and beer are collapsing into one significant common denominator: they are all alcohol and the other characteristics are irrelevant. Third, alcohol is moving from a substance helpful, or at least harmless, when taken in moderation toward being a poison, damaging to the extent that it is consumed. Significant factors in this last transformation are studies on the Fetal Alcohol Syndrome and, more recently, warnings against the male partner's consumption of alcohol near conception.[24]

The battle against alcohol and the other chemicals I've mentioned easily become moral contests in which no quarter can be given to the hated enemy. The path toward prohibition is logical and ethical to many combatants against dangerous substances. If we are entering another era of temperance, we can greatly benefit from knowledge of similar past trends. History does not, of course, prescribe our future actions, but it can cause us to reflect on our efforts and their possible outcomes, to expand the factors we employ in analysis and to take into keen consideration the long-term consequences of victory.

One of the saddest aspects of Prohibition was the backlash that inhibited direct and frank consideration of the alcohol problem for half a century afterward. The task of persons deeply concerned about the impact of alcohol and other chemicals on the health of the born and unborn is to consider how to create lasting changes in behavior that will not be subject to the wide swings in attitude that have characterized past antialcohol campaigns. This consideration may be frustrating when the value of abstinence appears obvious, but the most satisfying strategies are those that produce enduring healthful changes.

REFERENCES

1. MUSTO, D. F. 1987. The American Disease: Origins of Narcotic Control. Expand. edit. Oxford University Press. New York, NY. p. 264ff.
2. FREUD, S. 1884. Ueber coca. *In* Cocaine Papers by Sigmund Freud, R. Byck, Ed.: 50. Stonehill Publishing Co. New York, NY.
3. Contemporary Celebrities from the Album Mariani of Paris, France. 1901. Mariani & Co. New York, NY. pp. 4-5.
4. Coca Erythroxylon and its Derivatives. 1885. Parke, Davis & Co. Detroit, MI.
5. Cf. Freud and Hammond articles in Byck, *op. cit.*
6. HAMMOND, W. A. 1932. *In* Dictionary of American Biography. D. Malone, Ed. Vol. **8:** 210-211. Charles Scribner's. New York, NY.
7. HAMMOND, W. A. 1887. Coca: Its Preparations and Their Therapeutical Qualities, with Some Remarks on the So-called "Cocaine Habit." Transactions of the Medical Society of Virginia. pp. 212-226. Richmond, VA.
8. BEARD, G. M. 1881. American Nervousness: Its Causes and Consequences. G. P. Putnam's. New York, NY.
9. HAMMOND, *op. cit.*
10. MUNSEY, C. 1972. The Illustrated Guide to the Collectibles of Coca-Cola. Hawthorn Books. New York, NY.
11. Coca-Cola Bottling Co. of Shreveport, Inc. *et al.* v. The Coca-Cola Co. (Civil Action No. 83-95). April 29, 1983. Opinion of the U.S. District Court for the District of Delaware. p. 15.
12. MUNSEY, *op. cit.*
13. Opium Problem. 1910. U.S. Senate, 61st Congress, 2nd Session, Document No. 377, Government Printing Office. Washington, DC p. 50.
14. MUSTO, *op. cit.,* p. 50ff.
15. Public Law No. 223, 63rd Congress (1914).
16. MUSTO, *op. cit.,* p. 6ff.
17. MUSTO, *loc. cit.* and p. 46.
18. MUSTO, *op. cit.,* p. 5.
19. RORABAUGH, W. J. 1979. The Alcoholic Republic: An American Tradition. Oxford University Press. New York, NY.
20. CLARK, N. H. 1976. Deliver Us from Evil: An Interpretation of American Prohibition. Oxford University Press. New York, NY.
21. GUSFIELD, J. 1986. Symbolic Crusade: Status Politics and the American Temperance Movement. 2nd edit. University of Illinois Press. Urbana, IL.
22. KYVIG, D. E. 1979. Repealing National Prohibition. University of Chicago Press. Chicago, IL. p. 131ff.
23. MUSTO, D. F. 1984. New Temperance vs. Neo-Prohibition. Wall Street Journal. June 25, 1984.
24. LITTLE, R. E. & C. F. SING. 1986. Association of Father's Drinking and Infant's Birth Weight. N. Engl. J. Med. **314:** 1644-1645.

Methodological Issues in the Measurement of Substance Use

NANCY L. DAY AND NADINE ROBLES

Western Psychiatric Institute and Clinic
University of Pittsburgh
School of Medicine
3811 O'Hara Street
Pittsburgh, Pennsylvania 15213

There are two ways to measure drug and alcohol use, questions, and laboratory assessments. Questions allow researchers to differentiate patterns of use, and can ascertain use over longer time periods. Laboratory assessments are more precise, but they measure only current use, and cannot give an estimate of pattern of use. This discussion will focus on the measurement of substance use by questionnaire and some of the problems of measurement of substance use during pregnancy using questionnaires.

The first issue to be considered is conceptual. What is it that we are measuring and what variables best define a behavior such as drinking or taking drugs? Substance use as a behavior can be described by measuring three parameters: (1) quantity, (2) frequency, and (3) duration of use. Quantity is a measure of dose, and is represented by the amount per occasion. Quantity is also a measure of the style of use. For example, whether one drinks moderately, or to intoxication, smokes a joint or smokes three or four, represents not just different exposures but different styles of use.

Quantity as a variable can be described further by three separate components: usual, maximum, and minimum quantity. Usual quantity is a measure of socially acceptable levels of drinking. Maximum quantity represents the largest amount consumed, and minimum quantity represents the smallest amount that is used. It has been the tradition, particularly in drug research, to ask only about usual quantity, thereby eliciting the socially acceptable response. Data will be presented that estimate the amount of error in only ascertaining usual quantity.

An additional feature is the issue of strength, or concentration. This is somewhat easier for alcohol researchers than for drug researchers since the amount of absolute alcohol in liquor is legislated and is clearly defined in the "proof" of the liquor consumed. Although the absolute alcohol content of beer and wine can vary, it varies within a defined range. A recent problem is the development of new ways of marketing wine and beer, including wine and beer coolers and light beer and wine, each of which has a different amount of absolute alcohol.

It has been traditional in survey research on alcohol use to assume that "a drink is a drink is a drink."[1] In other words, all drinks are equivalent in terms of the amount of absolute alcohol. The amount of absolute alcohol contained in the standard 12-oz bottle of beer is roughly equivalent to the amount of absolute alcohol contained in the standard mixed drink and a 4-oz glass of wine. However, not all people actually drink according to these standard drink sizes. Heavy drinkers are more likely to mix larger drinks than are light drinkers, and the dose will therefore be mis-estimated.

8

Translating data that are collected in terms of drinks into equivalents of absolute alcohol does not resolve this problem, since the underlying data are still inaccurate.

The problem with alcohol, however, seems relatively simple when other substances are considered. Illicit drugs are not nicely legislated for the concentration of various constituents. Marijuana, for example is a garbage-can of components, and the relative composition of these components varies from sample to sample. In addition, for street drugs, we must consider the presence of diluents, adulterants and additives, fake, look-alikes and substitutes. Although the subject may not be able to tell the difference, the teratogenic potential is likely to be quite different.

Frequency is a measure of how often a substance is used, and is, therefore, a measure of how much use is part of a life style. For example, marijuana plays a very different role in the lives of subjects who smoke on a daily basis, compared to those who only use marijuana on an infrequent basis. In general, researchers have not allowed frequency to vary, but this flies somewhat in the face of reality, since we know that the frequency of use varies seasonally, at times of stress, and during holidays.

Duration of use is a measure of the level of experience a subject has with the substance. It is, in addition, a way to separate long-term chronic exposure from relatively acute or short-term exposures. There has been little research on the effects of duration of use on teratogenic effects. However, it would seem to be an area worthy of exploration since chronicity of use is likely to be correlated with psychosocial and biological differences between subjects.

Thus, quantity measures tell how much of a substance is used per occasion. Frequency defines how often this happens within a given unit of time and duration of use anchors this behavior on a time continuum.

How are these underlying constructs translated into real data? In the process of creating questions, several factors need to be considered:

1. Understandability of the questions,
2. Correct ascertainment of patterns of use,
3. Memory, and
4. Truthfulness.

When we began our study we tested several sets of questions to assess both marijuana and alcohol use. We experimented with the use of some of the standard alcohol questions including the Cahalan volume-variability[2] and the Khavari KAT scale.[3] It was our experience, however, that our subjects had difficulty answering these questions.

A glance at some of the standard questions makes it clear why they are so difficult to answer. Most scales ask about frequency of use, and then ask subjects to partition frequency into the portion of time spent consuming various quantities. This requires rather sophisticated mathematical thinking to describe behavior that is often poorly remembered. When the complexity of the questions is so great, subjects either resort to guessing, or bias their response, as subjects in their frustration answer with one set of answers consistently. The worst form of response bias from frustrating questions is, of course, "No, I never did that."

We asked our subjects to describe their use in their own terms. What emerged was that most of the women in our sample first described marijuana and alcohol use in terms of quantity, and then, often as a result of some probing, in terms of frequency. Our questions were developed to enable subjects to report quantity first and then frequency. They required no analytical thinking on the part of the respondents, and showed high reliability with blood alcohol measures in a separate study.

There are a number of ways to check whether the subject understands the questions. One is to use two sets of questions and compare the answers. Presumably, if you get different estimates from the two sets, it means that one set is not working properly. Another option is to ask respondents what their understanding of the questions is and what their answers to the questions mean.

The second issue of measurement is correct ascertainment of patterns. Most assessments of substance use measure frequency and usual quantity. In our study, we found that the answers to usual quantity represented only 37% of the total marijuana use reported during the first trimester. Maximum quantity contributed an additional 45% to the overall total marijuana use and minimum quantity of marijuana contributed an additional 17% to our estimates. Therefore, to measure only usual quantity gives a serious underestimate of consumption. And further, this underestimate is a biased underestimate, since maximum quantity and minimum quantity are not reported at the same rate across different levels of marijuana use. Particularly for studies of toxic effects, not only is this underestimate a serious problem, but the absence of information on variability in use means that we may be missing important effects that relate to specific patterns of use.

The third issue is the question of memory. By their very nature, most questionnaires are retrospective in design, and therefore, must ask subjects to remember behaviors over a period of time. We also know from a wealth of research in the substance abuse field, that the longer the time span, the greater the difficulty of recall. In our study we asked one group of women to report on their first trimester alcohol use in the fourth month of pregnancy and again at the seventh month of pregnancy.[4] A second group was asked about first trimester use at the fourth month and at delivery. The correlation between use reported at fourth and seventh month was 0.61. The correlation between first trimester use reported at month four and at delivery was 0.53. Among those women who reported differing rates at the two time periods, the reported amount was more likely to increase than to decrease, a finding reported by other investigators as well.[5] It is difficult to know from these findings whether we are actually dealing with a problem of memory, or a greater feeling of safety that the women may have farther from the event when they are reporting on a labeled behavior.

An additional problem in ascertaining use during pregnancy is that women may not know or remember or think about when pregnancy began. We developed a technique to measure marijuana and alcohol use during each month of the first trimester. This is crucial since one of the major difficulties in assessing the effect of a teratogen is obtaining careful measures of exposure during the first trimester.

At the beginning of the interview, women are asked to indicate on a calendar: (a) when they got pregnant, (b) when they realized they were pregnant, and (c) when pregnancy was diagnosed. After the marijuana questions, the interviewer returns to the calendar and asks, for the time periods between conception and recognition and recognition and confirmation, whether the subject was using marijuana more like her prepregnancy pattern or more like what she reported for her first trimester. Sixty-six percent of the women reported that from conception to recognition of pregnancy, their marijuana use was similar to their prepregnancy pattern rather than what they had reported as their first trimester pattern.[6] Thirty-three percent reported that from recognition to diagnosis, they were still using marijuana at their prepregnancy rate rather than their reported first trimester rate.

The dates of conception, recognition and diagnosis are used to calculate a month-by-month rate of marijuana use and a weighted estimate of the average daily use for the first trimester (TABLE 1). In our cohort, 11.2% of the women reported using marijuana at the rate of 1 or more joints per day whereas, when we calculated what the rate should have been, 19.5% of the women were using marijuana at this rate.

TABLE 1. The Reported and Calculated Prevalence of Marijuana Use during the First Trimester of Pregnancy in the Study Cohort

Average Daily Use	First Trimester Reported Use		First Trimester Calculated Use						Total First Trimester Calculated Use	
			Month 1		Month 2		Month 3			
	N	(%)	N	(%)	N	(%)	N	(%)	N	(%)
Heavy	63	(11.2)	136	(24.1)	102	(18.1)	70	(12.4)	110	(19.5)
Moderate	22	(3.9)	32	(5.7)	23	(4.1)	23	(4.1)	29	(5.1)
Light	109	(19.3)	132	(23.4)	143	(25.4)	119	(21.1)	161	(28.5)
Abstainer	370	(65.6)	261	(46.3)	293	(52.0)	349	(61.9)	261	(46.3)
Total N	564		561[b]		561[b]		561[b]		561[b]	

[a] Definitions: *Heavy* = an average of one or more joints per day; *Moderate* = an average of at least three joints per week but less than one per day; *Light* = >0 to 2.9 joints per week; *Abstainer* = no use.
[b] This average could not be calculated for 3 subjects.

Also, 65.3% reported no use during the trimester when only 46.3% were actually nonusers. Thus, when women are asked to report their first trimester use, the use patterns that they report do not take into consideration their pattern of marijuana use prior to their recognition of pregnancy, even though they had been instructed to think back to the very beginning of pregnancy.

The fourth issue defined is that of truthfulness. This is a particularly thorny problem when we are asking women to report on a behavior such as alcohol use which is proscribed during pregnancy, or drug use, which is illegal. There are multiple ways to approach this problem. Clearly, the context in which the interview takes place is an important component. Women are not likely to answer questions honestly in the presence of another person, and they are less likely to give accurate data to an authority figure, and/or in any situation where they feel that their answers are not confidential or that the answers they give could have repercussions.

Techniques for getting around these problems including choosing a safe and private environment for the interview, preferably one that is removed from the institution. Interviewers must also be carefully chosen. The presentation of the interviewer, the sex of the interviewer and subject, and the abstainer/user status of the interviewer all influence the reporting of substance use.

We have also modified a technique called the 'bogus pipeline' to increase the accuracy of reporting in our sample. The bogus pipeline is a method of convincing our subjects that we do have a measure of their use, even when we really do not.[7] In our experience, this increases the reporting of marijuana by 10% and of other illicit drugs by 50%.

CONCLUSIONS

This discussion began by pointing out that the measurement of substance use is a complicated issue and we have tried to highlight some of the areas of difficulty. It is essential that valid instruments be developed to measure substance use and that, particularly for studies of use during pregnancy, these questions be designed to give information about pattern of use in addition to average use. There is currently little research that focuses specifically on the methodological issues of measurement, and yet an evaluation of the adequacy of these data is an essential factor in determining the effects of substance use on the fetus.

REFERENCES

1. ROOM, R. 1977. The measurement and distribution of drinking patterns and problems in general populations. *In* Alcohol-Related Disabilities. G. Edwards, M. Gross & M. Keller, Eds. Offset Publication No. 32: 2-38. World Health Organization. Geneva.
2. CAHALAN, D., I. CISIN & H. M. CROSSLEY. 1969. American Drinking Practices. College & University Press. New Haven, CT.
3. KHAVARI, K. & P. FARBER. 1978. A profile instrument for the quantification and assessment of alcohol consumption. J. Stud. Alcohol. **39:** 1525-1539.
4. ROBLES, N. & N. DAY. 1989. Recall of alcohol consumption during pregnancy. J. Stud. Alcohol. In press.

5. LITTLE, R. E., W. MANDELL & F. A. SCHULTZ. 1977. Consequences of retrospective measurement of alcohol consumption. J. Stud. Alcohol. **38**(9): 1777-1780.
6. DAY, N., D. WAGENER & P. TAYLOR. 1985. Measurement of substance use during pregnancy: Methodological issues. *In* Current Research on the Consequences of Maternal Drug Abuse. T. Pinkert, Ed. Vol. **59**: 36-48.
7. JONES, E. & H. SIGALL. 1979. The bogus pipeline: A new paradigm for measuring affect and attitude. Psychol. Bull. **76**: 349-364.

Epidemiology of Substance Abuse Including Alcohol and Cigarette Smoking

EDGAR H. ADAMS, JOSEPH C. GFROERER,
AND BEATRICE A. ROUSE

National Institute on Drug Abuse
Division of Epidemiology and Statistical Analysis
5600 Fishers Lane
Room 11A55
Rockville, Maryland 20857

Recent studies of both animals and humans have indicated the adverse effects of perinatal exposure in pregnancy outcomes, fetal characteristics, and infant development from numerous pharmacological substances. Such substances have included amphetamines, barbiturates, PCP, cocaine, heroin, methadone, cannabis, tobacco, caffeine, and alcohol. Chasnoff *et al.,*[1] for example, found cocaine use during pregnancy associated with genitourinary tract malformations in newborns. Golden *et al.*[2] found infants with PCP exposure during pregnancy had significantly poorer attention, hypertonia, and depressed neonatal reflex. In general, infants born to drug-dependent women have a poorer outcome and more abnormalities.[3-6]

The dangers of smoking and drinking during pregnancy have been known for a number of years, as have the problems of babies born to heroin-addicted mothers. However, recent clinical reports about large increases in the number of babies born to cocaine-using mothers have increased public awareness and heightened public concern about the overall problem of drug use in pregnant women.

Because of these concerns, this paper includes data on a group of women at high risk for both pregnancy and substance abuse, that is, women between the ages of 15 and 44. This paper will address three questions: (1) the prevalence of drug use, in particular the use of cigarettes, alcohol, marijuana, and cocaine in women aged 15 to 44; (2) the association between drug use and various sociodemographic characteristics in women aged 22 to 44 and; (3) drug use by marital and parental status in white women aged 22 to 25.

METHODOLOGY

Data for this report were obtained from the 1985 National Household Survey on Drug Abuse (NHSDA). The NHSDA is a general population survey in which individuals selected through a multistage, stratified probability sample are interviewed in the household regarding their alcohol, tobacco, and illicit drug use which includes

14

the nonmedical use of licit psychotherapeutic drugs. The survey covers the household population of the coterminous United States in the ages 12 and older. For this study, women in the primary reproductive years of 15 to 44 were chosen for analysis. Men of the same age group were chosen for comparison. Data were available from 3,144 women and 2,455 men.

Because the analysis of various sociodemographic characteristics contained variables generally associated with the adult population, such as education, employment, marital status, and number of children, analysis of these sociodemographic characteristics was restricted to women aged 22 to 44. There were 2,136 women in this group. Because the relationships of parity and marital status with prevalence of substance abuse are confounded by age and race, the third analysis of prevalence by marital and parental status was restricted to white females aged 22 to 25. Three groups were analyzed: women who were married with children (n = 76), women who were married and had no children (n = 44), and women who had never married and had no children (n = 74).

Comparisons between prevalence rates discussed in the Results section are based on the results of *t* tests, except for the marital and parental status analysis of 22-25-year-old white women. Because of the relatively small sample sizes for the three comparison groups in this portion of the analysis, testing was not done and results are considered as only suggestive.

RESULTS

Prevalence of Drug Use among the Population Aged 15 to 44

Almost 90 percent of the women have tried alcohol and almost three-quarters have tried smoking cigarettes (TABLE 1). Approximately 44 percent have tried marijuana and 14 percent have tried cocaine. Interestingly, the lifetime prevalence rates for these two illicit drugs are basically the same for the 15-21-year-old age group and the 22-44-year-old age group, while rates of cigarette and alcohol use are higher among the 22-44-year-olds. The prevalence of current (use in the past month) alcohol and cigarette use is also greater in the 22-44-year-old age group, but the prevalence of marijuana and cocaine use is greater in the younger, that is the 15-21-year-old age group. This results in an estimate of approximately 6 million women aged 15 to 44 who are current users of marijuana. Two million of these women are aged 15 to 21 and approximately 4 million are aged 22 to 44. This difference is noted because while the rate of use is greater for the 15-21-year-old women, the population denominator in the 22-44-year-old group is much larger. An estimate was also made of the prevalence of current use of any illicit drug (including nonmedical psychotherapeutic use). This resulted in an overall estimate that of the 56 million women in this age group, 15 percent have tried at least one of the 10 illicit drugs or drug classes included in the NHSDA in the past month; that is, there were approximately 8 million current users of an illicit drug.

The prevalence of use of licit as well as illicit drugs is generally higher in males than in females. This is true for both lifetime prevalence and current prevalence or past month use (TABLE 2).

TABLE 1. Prevalence of Drug Use among 15-44-Year-Old Women (n = 3,144)[a]

Age	Cigarettes %	Alcohol %	Marijuana %	Cocaine %
Lifetime use				
15-21	60.1	82.2	42.5	14.8
22-44	78.6	90.8	44.4	14.2
Total	74.5	88.9	43.9	14.3
Past month use				
15-21	25.7	50.4	17.9	5.3
22-44	35.6	63.9	9.2	3.0
Total	33.4	60.9	11.2	3.5

[a] Source: 1985 National Household Survey on Drug Abuse, NIDA.

Sociodemographic Characteristics

The lifetime prevalence of use of cigarettes, alcohol, marijuana, and cocaine is greater among white women than in black or Hispanic women. With the exception of cigarettes, the prevalence of drug use increases somewhat with education. In general, the lifetime prevalence of cigarette smoking is higher among those women who are divorced or separated and those who are living as married when compared to women who have never married or are married. Lifetime prevalence for most drugs is lower among married women. Lifetime prevalence of drug use appears to decrease with the number of children, with the exception of cigarette smoking. Also, women with two or more children have much lower rates of marijuana and cocaine use. It is possible that this result is confounded by the fact that these women may be older. The prevalence of drug use is lower in the older age groups. In general, the lifetime prevalence of drug use is less in homemakers than in the employed or unemployed populations (TABLE 3).

The prevalence of drug use in the past month by the same variables is shown in TABLE 4. Whereas the lifetime prevalence of drug use was greater among whites than blacks or Hispanics, with the exception of current alcohol use, however, the prevalence

TABLE 2. Prevalence of Drug Use among 15-44-Year-Old Men (n = 2,455)[a]

Age	Cigarettes %	Alcohol %	Marijuana %	Cocaine %
Lifetime use				
15-21	68.0	85.1	50.3	18.5
22-44	86.7	95.5	58.6	24.6
Total	82.3	93.0	56.6	23.2
Past month use				
15-21	29.1	62.7	25.0	7.6
22-44	44.3	78.0	17.5	5.5
Total	40.7	74.3	19.3	6.0

[a] Source: 1985 National Household Survey on Drug Abuse, NIDA.

of past month use among black women is equal to or greater than that of either whites or Hispanics. This implies that while white women may experiment more with drugs, the rate of continuation is higher among black women. The rate of current smoking decreases with education, a pattern not noted with other drugs. As with lifetime prevalence, the current prevalence of drug use tends to be lower in married women and highest in those women who are living as married. For alcohol, marijuana, and cocaine the rate of current drug use appears to decrease in women with children. As noted earlier for lifetime use of marijuana and cocaine, this may be confounded by age.

TABLE 3. Prevalence of Lifetime Use of Selected Drugs among Women Aged 22-44 Years (n = 2,136)[a]

	Cigarettes %	Alcohol %	Marijuana %	Cocaine %
Race				
White	83.4	94.2	48.0	15.8
Black	71.7	83.3	42.6	9.8
Hispanic	48.6	70.9	18.3	6.3
Education				
0-11 yrs	75.2	80.9	38.1	9.7
12 yrs	83.6	90.4	42.2	11.1
13+ yrs	75.2	94.8	48.7	18.6
Marital status				
Never married	73.7	90.2	57.4	21.3
Married	77.8	90.2	38.5	10.4
Divorced/separated	87.3	93.7	54.4	19.8
Living as married	81.8	97.6	66.8	36.9
Number of children				
0	75.7	94.6	59.5	25.1
1	79.8	91.6	52.1	16.1
2+	79.6	88.7	34.6	8.3
Employment status				
Employed	79.4	92.8	47.2	15.0
Unemployed	83.9	90.4	50.0	18.2
Homemaker	75.5	86.7	34.8	10.8

[a] Source: 1985 National Household Survey on Drug Abuse, NIDA.

The current prevalence of cigarette smoking is much greater in unemployed women than either employed women or homemakers. In general, the prevalence of use of alcohol and marijuana is less in homemakers.

Prevalence of Drug Use by Marital Status and Parental Status

Married women with children have a higher lifetime prevalence of cigarette smoking and a higher rate of cigarette use in the past month when compared to married

TABLE 4. Prevalence of Past Month Use of Selected Drugs among Women Aged 22-44 Years (n = 2,125)[a]

	Cigarettes %	Alcohol %	Marijuana %	Cocaine %
Race				
White	36.2	68.3	9.6	3.2
Black	42.1	55.6	12.1	3.3
Hispanic	24.2	44.5	3.2	1.2
Education				
0-11 yrs	52.5	49.7	8.5	2.0
12 yrs	41.0	60.8	8.3	3.2
13+ yrs	24.5	72.1	10.3	3.2
Marital status				
Never married	38.6	70.0	15.4	6.1
Married	29.5	59.4	6.3	1.7
Divorced/separated	56.4	76.4	13.5	4.2
Living as married	53.0	84.9	25.2	12.4
Number of children				
0	34.8	75.4	14.9	4.6
1	42.9	66.8	11.1	5.2
2+	33.5	57.6	5.9	1.5
Employment status				
Employed	35.0	69.5	9.9	3.0
Unemployed	60.8	59.7	14.6	1.3
Homemaker	27.5	50.5	5.8	3.7

[a] Source: 1985 National Household Survey on Drug Abuse, NIDA.

women with no children and women who are not married and have no children. It is possible that women who are married with children at this relatively young age have lesser education. As noted earlier, women with less education have higher rates of cigarette smoking. In contrast, the lifetime prevalence of alcohol use is relatively the same across all three groups, while current alcohol use is lowest among those who are married with children (TABLE 5). Current use of marijuana is also lower in women who are married and lowest in women who are married with children.

The rates of any illicit past month use are very similar in the three groups of women. The rate of any illicit past month use in unmarried women and married women without children could be explained almost entirely by their current marijuana use. This does not exclude the possibility that they might be also using other illicit drugs currently. In contrast, current marijuana use could account for only half the rate of illicit drug use in married women with children. It is possible that the pattern of current drug use in married women with children may vary when compared to other women. For example, it may be that married women with children have replaced their use of marijuana with other illicit drugs or the nonmedical use of licit psychotherapeutic drugs.

Among males aged 22 to 25, the prevalence of past month cigarette use as well as lifetime cigarette use was also greater in married men with children. However, unlike the women, there was no diminution of drug use in married men with children when compared to either married men or unmarried men.

DISCUSSION AND CONCLUSIONS

The prevalence of drug use in the population of women at greatest risk of pregnancy is high. Approximately 34 million of the 56 million women in this age group are current drinkers, more than 18 million are current smokers, and more than 6 million are current marijuana users. While there may be a reduction of alcohol, cigarette, and marijuana use during pregnancy, there is some suggestion from other studies that women may not alter their drug use patterns until the pregnancy is actually diagnosed. Since this may occur as long as two months after conception, damage to the fetus may have already occurred. We also noted more than 3 million women with children were current users of illicit drugs. This behavior has serious implications because of the possible effects that current drug use in women may have on parenting and also on an increase in the probability of drug use in their offspring. A study by Gfroerer[7] indicated that in families where older siblings or parents used drugs, the prevalence of drug use was greater in the younger children than in families where there was no drug use by parents or older siblings.

Both the attitudes and behavior of young girls suggest that the risk of drug use during pregnancy remains high. For example, the results of the 1987-1988 National Adolescent Student Health Survey[8] indicated that more than 50 percent of 10th grade girls thought that it was acceptable to have sex with a steady friend. About 13 percent of the girls were currently using marijuana, 50 percent were using alcohol, and 29 percent were using cigarettes.

While these data do not answer the question of the prevalence of drug use among pregnant women, the widespread use of alcohol, cigarettes, and marijuana in this population, coupled with the fact that pregnancy may not actually be diagnosed until well into the first trimester, make it prudent to recommend that physicians include information on the woman's substance use prior to pregnancy as part of the medical

TABLE 5. Prevalence of Drug Use among 22-25-Year-Old White Women by Marital and Parental Status[a]

	Married with Children (n = 76) %	Married No Children (n = 44) %	Not Married No Children (n = 74) %
Cigarettes past month	49.7	27.3	36.0
Cigarettes lifetime	88.6	76.9	75.4
Alcohol past month	61.2	73.5	80.5
Alcohol lifetime	95.9	94.0	95.3
Marijuana past month	9.3	13.4	19.4
Marijuana lifetime	75.4	55.7	65.0
Cocaine past month	7.5	*	5.0
Cocaine lifetime	23.2	19.4	20.2
Any illicit past month	18.2	14.9	20.2
Any illicit lifetime	79.9	58.2	66.0

[a] Source: 1985 National Household Survey on Drug Abuse, NIDA.
* Less than 0.5%.

history and pregnancy care. While many clinicians have encountered substance abuse among their minority patients, these data suggest the need to determine substance use in white, educated women as well in order to appropriately care for the pregnant woman and her developing child. Furthermore, clinicians may want to counsel any one planning a pregnancy to cease all drug use prior to conception.

REFERENCES

1. CHASNOFF, I. J., G. M. CHISUM & W. E. KAPLAN. 1988. Maternal cocaine use and genitourinary tract malformations. Teratology 37(3): 201-204.
2. GOLDEN, N. L., B. R. KUHNERT, R. J. SOKOL, S. MARTIER & T. WILLIAMS. 1987. Neonatal manifestations of maternal phencyclidine exposure. J. Perinat. Med.15(2):185-191.
3. CHASNOFF, I. J., K. A. BURNS, W. J. BURNS & S. H. SCHNOLL. 1986. Prenatal drug exposure: Effects on neonatal and infant growth and development. Neurobehav. Toxicol. Teratol. 8(4): 357-362.
4. CULVER, K. W., A. J. AMMANN, J. C. PARTRIDGE, D. F. WONG, D. W. WARA & M. J. COWAN. 1987. Lymphocyte abnormalities in infants born to drug-abusing mothers. J. Pediatr. 111(2): 230-235.
5. RYAN, L., S. EHRLICH & L. FINNEGAN. 1987. Cocaine abuse in pregnancy: Effects on the fetus and newborn. Neurobehav. Toxicol. Teratol. 9(4): 295-299.
6. DOBERCZAK, T. M., J. C. THORTON, J. BERTSTEIN & S. R. KANDALL. 1987. Impact of maternal drug dependency on birth weight and head circumference of offspring. Am. J. Dis. Child. 141(11): 1163-1167.
7. GFROERER, J. 1987. Correlation between drug use by teenagers and drug use by older family members. Am. J. Drug Alcohol Abuse 13(182): 95-108.
8. 1987-1988 National Adolescent Student Health Survey Final Report. 1989. American Alliance for Health, Physical Education, Recreation and Dance. Reston, VA. In press.

Pharmacological Concepts and Developmental Toxicology

RICHARD G. SKALKO

Department of Anatomy
East Tennessee State University
Quillen-Dishner College of Medicine
P.O. Box 19960A
Johnson City, Tennessee 37614

INTRODUCTION

The embryonic development of multicellular organisms is dependent upon the precisely timed transformation from the zygote to the adult, and it occurs as the consequence of a progressive change in the potential of their constituent cells. The completion of this process of development at the cellular, tissue and organ level is dependent upon two major factors: the differential expression of the components of the genome (genetic factors) and the modulating influence of the environment in which these cells reside at any given moment (epigenetic factors). These two crucial elements, the genome and the environment, are, in fact, interdependent. Consequently, as development proceeds, there is a constant interaction between genetic and epigenetic inputs which lead to the phenotype observed in the mature cell, tissue, organ or organism.

The major thrust of current efforts within developmental biology has been to produce a mechanistic assessment of these two elements that is effective and testable. There are several models which have been proposed to explain those internal mechanisms which control the orderly progress of gene activity (or, as it is alternatively described, differential gene activation).[1] These include suggestions that alterations in the genetic expression of developing cells are mediated within the genome itself.[2-4] In addition, the ability of the environment to modulate gene expression has produced theoretical constructs in which environmental change (in the form of cyclic nucleotides and inorganic ions) or alterations in information flow from the environment into the cell through the inductive action of cell-surface receptors, lead to altered developmental paths.[3,6] Indeed, current thinking tends to look upon developmental events as the manifestation of a sequential signal-response system in which those cellular activities which developing organisms possess in common: cell division, cell movement, cell death, cell adhesion and induction, interact with epigenetic signals to produce the intact organism. To appreciate the results of this precise interplay of genes, cells and environment, it is useful to envision the developing organism as containing a set of signals and a set of specific receptors for those signals. The genome has the responsibility to produce both the signal substances (as inductive molecules) and the receptors (which mediate inductive interaction at the level of the nucleus and the cytoplasm). This constant interaction between signal and receptor allows the cells within the embryo to communicate and, through specific receptors and specific signals, control activation and inhibition of cellular activities and produce the essential transformation from a one-dimensional genetic code to a three-dimensional organism.[7,8] Scientists in developmental biology and developmental toxicology are encouraged by research efforts currently being performed in the discipline of cell biology where there are analogous attempts to explain the ontogeny of immune function in response to an antigenic stimulus[9] and the tissue-specific response to inducers of gene activity.[10]

Abnormal Development

In recent years, there has been a dialogue within the discipline of developmental toxicology to employ the principles and concepts which are used in several companion disciplines (developmental biology, cell biology, pharmacology and toxicology) to develop useful mechanistic hypotheses to explain the ability of exogenous agents to interfere with the normal progression of developmental events and to produce phenotypically abnormal cells, organs and tissues. Indeed, the experimental production of structural (and functional) abnormalities in response to external stimuli, which are collectively described as teratogens, must be understood from the perspective of time, the genome and the environment. The fundamental issue is time, *i.e.*, the time in development during which the embryo is exposed to an external chemical or agent. Experimental data, which have been collected over the past 70 years of research in this discipline, have delineated the concept of "stage specificity" in response to xenobiotics. Of particular significance to modern biology is the appreciation that the type of developmental effect that is seen is a function of the time, in development, when the xenobiotic agent or teratogen is present in the embryo.[11,12] Through the careful manipulation of this parameter of time, it has been repeatedly shown that, under controlled conditions, the (morphological) responses that are observed are highly repeatable and, consequently, assume a specificity of expression which demonstrates that the exogenous agents are effective because they are modulating developmental events which are occurring at the time of exposure.[13]

It has been suggested that quantifiable structural abnormalities produced by exposure to teratogens occur in response to changes at specific sites within the cells of the developing embryo (the intracellular compartment of nucleus and cytoplasm) at the cell surface, within the extracellular matrix, at the level of cell-to-cell interaction and in the fetal environment proper (FIG. 1).[14] Additionally, the concept of "stage-specificity" can be evaluated by an appreciation of the state of development in which susceptible cell types find themselves at the time of exposure. These include: determination, proliferation, organization, migration and morphogenetic cell death (FIG. 2).[14] In this context, it is certainly possible to look at a susceptible cell population and to assess its response to an external influence in a reasonably clear and useful paradigm (FIG. 3)[15] which addresses issues of altered cell structure and function under these conditions.[15] Under normal circumstances as, *e.g.*, the response of cells to a mitogenic stimulus, there is a cascade of events (binding of a molecule such as platelet-derived growth factor to a cell surface receptor, a complex set of alterations within the membrane, cytosol and nucleus) which leads, ultimately, to cell division.[16] Additionally, cyclic AMP, the putative second messenger involved in altered cellular activity, is developmentally regulated during the ontogeny of the rodent secondary palate.[17] This event is mediated by prostaglandins and agents which impair this event (as, *e.g.*, the glucocorticoids), *i.e.*, the arachidonic acid stimulation of cyclic AMP in the palatine shelves, are documented cleft-palate producing agents. In this instance, the signal (dexamethasone), through its actions mediated by the glucocorticoid receptor, interferes with the mobilization of endogenous arachidonic acid and the sub-

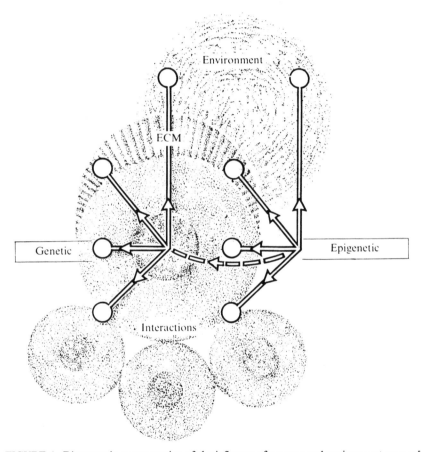

FIGURE 1. Diagramatic representation of the influence of genome and environment on a cell undergoing cytodifferentiation. Epigenetic factors (signals) may interact with the cellular environment, the cell surface or directly with the genome. They may also mediate cell-cell interactions. Gene products, acting through specific mRNA molecules, may influence phenotypic change at the same levels. (From Saxen.[14] Reprinted by permission from the *Journal of Embryology and Experimental Morphology.*)

sequent stimulation of cyclic AMP to eventually contribute to the formation of a cleft of the secondary palate.[17] The central role that receptors play in several critical biological processes, at all levels of cellular activity, has a meaningful impact on our ability to describe embryotoxic events in mechanistic and cellular terms.

Pharmacological Principles in Developmental Toxicology

Research efforts in developmental toxicology have appropriately focused on an assessment of the effects of a broad spectrum of xenobiotics on the developing mammal. It is assumed that the effects that are observed are due to the exposure and response

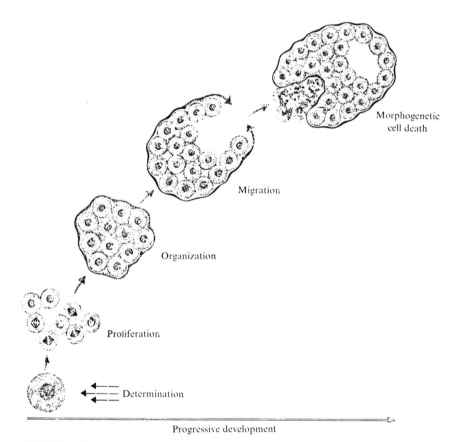

FIGURE 2. Changes in the cellular program that are common to many developing systems. Subsequent to determination of the eventual phenotype (through differential gene expression), cellular clones pass through a time-dependent continuum of organization, migration and morphogenetic cell death to complete morphogenesis. (From Saxen.[14] Reprinted by permission from *The Journal of Embryology and Experimental Morphology.*)

of "sensitive cell populations"[18] within the embryo. However, exposure of the cells contained in the embryo to a known or suspected developmental toxicant does not occur directly but is mediated by the physiological state of the pregnant dam. Several important factors are known which control the delivery of any xenobiotic to the embryo compartment, and all of them have an important role to play in the assessment

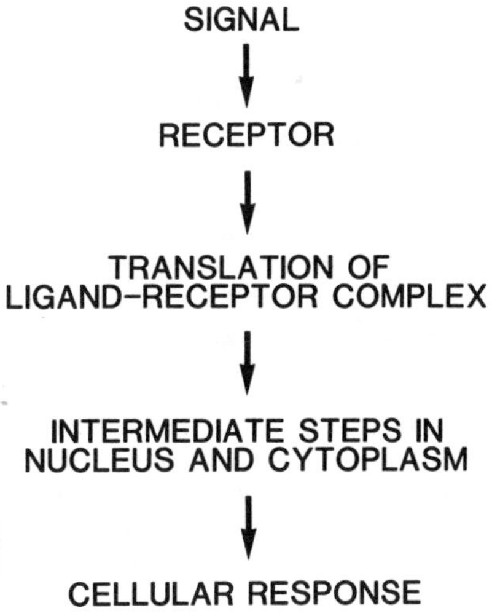

SIGNAL

↓

RECEPTOR

↓

FIGURE 3. A proposed sequence of events for the response of sensitive cell populations in the embryo to epigenetic cues (signals). These may be normal metabolites or developmental toxicants.

TRANSLATION OF
LIGAND–RECEPTOR COMPLEX

↓

INTERMEDIATE STEPS IN
NUCLEUS AND CYTOPLASM

↓

CELLULAR RESPONSE

of an observed embryotoxic response. These are listed in TABLE 1. Under *in vivo* conditions, the critical issue becomes one of being able to interpret an observed response in mechanistic terms. Traditionally, this is done by the utilization of an analytical procedure which defines the dose-response characteristics of the observed effect. For an effect to have a characteristic dose-response, three interdependent factors[15,19,20] are necessary. These are:

1. There is a receptor present;
2. The observed effect is related to the concentration of the agent at the receptor; and
3. The concentration at the receptor is a function of the administered dose.

Critical to the application of these factors is an appreciation of the impact that the important maternal variables play in controlling the concentration of the xenobiotic at its receptor *in situ*. These factors (TABLE 1) are of paramount importance in attempts to delineate the mechanisms which underly the documented strain and species differences which are seen in response to treatment with the same drug or chemical.[21-23]

TABLE 1. Factors Which Influence Drug Delivery to the Fetus[a]

1. Maternal absorption
2. Maternal distribution
3. Plasma and tissue binding
4. Elimination by metabolism or excretion
5. Embryo distribution and tissue binding
6. Embryo metabolism

[a] Based on Nau.[21]

Model Agents and Current Approaches

Of the several chemicals which are known to interfere with embryonic development, there are three which show much promise as model compounds for the delineation of underlying cellular mechanisms of action. These are: the glucocorticoids,[24] ethanol[25] and the retinoids.[21] The morphological consequences of exposure to these teratogenic agents show that the glucocorticoids are properly described as "site-specific" teratogens[26] in that the principal malformation produced by *in vivo* treatment is cleft palate.[24] On the other hand, ethanol[25,27–29] and the retinoids[30–34] are considered "uniform"[26] or "stage-specific" teratogens, since the effects observed are determined by the stage of intrauterine development at which the embryo is exposed.

Each of these chemicals satisfies the specific criteria described above to consider teratogens as agents which produce their toxic effects by serving as epigenetic signals. For the glucocorticoids, their action on the "target" cell type, the palatal mesenchyme, is mediated through the glucocorticoid receptor,[24,35] which produces an inhibition of RNA synthesis[36] and an inhibition of the developmentally regulated rise in cyclic AMP activity.[17] When ethanol is employed as a teratogen, the effects seen are dose- and stage-dependent,[25,28] they are correlated with the tissue levels of ethanol which are measured subsequent to acute exposure,[25] and there is an accumulating body of evidence which suggests that ethanol toxicity may be mediated through the benzo-diazepine receptor.[37,38]

The retinoids, by and large, are the agents of choice in current studies which attempt to delineate cellular mechanisms of toxicity. In recent years, two of these chemicals, all-trans retinoic acid[32] and 13-cis retinoic acid,[34] have been subject to extensive experimental analysis. Their biological activity, in several developing systems, provides strong evidence in support of the concept that phenotypic alterations are a consequence of the response that developing cells have to epigenetic signals in their environment. All-trans retinoic acid is a naturally occurring form of vitamin A and, under specific experimental conditions, acts as a "morphogen",[39] an agent which promotes the expression of specific cellular patterns by acting through the mechanism of differential gene expression. As a consequence, low concentrations of retinoic acid induce pattern duplications in the digits of the developing chick limb.[40,41] Retinoic acid also enhances forelimb regeneration in the axolotl,[42] larval anurans[43] and larval urodeles.[44,45] That these responses are clearly dose-dependent is supported by several studies which have shown that retinoic acid either stimulates[46] or inhibits[46–48] chon-drogenesis in mouse limb primordia or in isolated limb mesenchyme, the effect obtained being directly related to the dosage employed.

Retinoic acid has its own specific intracellular receptor, cellular retinoic acid-binding protein (cRABP).[49] This protein has been localized in several developing tissues with documented responsiveness to retinoic acid including the mouse limb bud,[50] the chick limb bud[51] and the limb of the axolotl.[52] Evidence suggests that, in consort with other proteins which play critical roles in developmental events, the appearance of cRABP may be under stringent developmental control and be associated with incipient morphogenesis and cytodifferentiation.[52] Detailed assessment of the molecular biology of the receptor indicates that it is similar to the glucocorticoid, estrogen and thyroid receptors.[53,54] These observations are of potentially major significance in the study of abnormal developmental mechanisms in view of the central role that the glucocorticoid receptor has been shown to play in glucocorticoid-mediated teratogenesis.[24,35]

When the retinoids have been studied in standard whole animal experiments, it has been shown that, at equivalent dosages and at equivalent stages of development, all-trans retinoic acid is a more potent teratogen than is its isomer, 13-cis retinoic acid.[55,56] Basing their experiments on a literature which showed that the two analogs had different pharmacokinetic profiles in intact mice,[57-59] Kochhar and Nau and their collaborators[56,60,61] have provided substantial evidence which shows that the differential toxicity between the two isomers is a direct consequence of a differential in trans-placental kinetics of the parent compounds and the toxic 4-oxo-metabolites of those compounds. The all-trans isomer is readily transported across the placenta at levels that approach 200 times the transport of an equivalent dosage of the 13-cis isomer. As a consequence, it is reasonable to conclude that the differential toxicity that is observed *in vivo* is due to a difference in concentration of the two compounds and their metabolites at the several target sites within the embryo. Support for this inter-pretation has been provided by a recent observation which has shown that, under *in vitro* conditions, the two isomers suppress chondrogenesis in limb bud mesenchymal cells at comparable dosages (IC_{50} for all-trans retinoic acid $= 5 \times 10^{-8}$ M; for 13-cis retinoic acid $= 6 \times 10^{-8}$ M).[62] These results provide important preliminary evidence that the differential toxicity is not due to either a difference in tissue levels of cRABP (since the cells were isolated under identical conditions) or in the binding of the retinoid to the receptor (because of their equivalence in suppressing chondro-genesis).

The putative intracellular site for the biological activity of the retinoids is the nucleus. In keeping with the model currently being utilized to describe the action of steroids on responsive cells,[63] retinoic acid would enter the cytoplasm, bind to cRABP and be translocated to the nucleus where the complex would bind to, and interact with, the genome to alter gene expression. This would lead to altered gene activity and a subsequent alteration in the synthesis of cell-specific products (FIG. 3). Support for this working hypothesis comes from several sources which have documented the role of the nucleus in retinoid-mediated alterations in phenotype and the critical role that cRABP plays in these changes.[49,64] Additionally, Horton *et al.*[65] have reported that exposure of chondrocytes isolated from chick embryos to retinoic acid produces major alterations in the expression of the chondrocyte phenotype.

SUMMARY

This communication provides evidence to support the concept that developmental toxicants (teratogens) produce their effect by either interfering with or enhancing the time-dependent signal-response mechanisms within the embryo. Essential to this hy-pothesis is the need to show that an observed effect is a function of the administered dose, that there is a positive correlation between the observed effect and pharmacok-inetic parameters and that there is evidence for the existence of a specific receptor for the toxicant. While extensive effort is required for ultimate validation of this concept, it serves to emphasize the value of applying known pharmacological principles in defining a mechanistic framework for the biological activity of developmental toxicants.

REFERENCES

1. DAVIDSON, E. H. 1986. Gene Activity in Early Development. 3rd edit. Academic Press. Orlando, FL.
2. CAPLAN, A. I. & C. P. ORDAHL. 1978. Irreversible gene repression model for control of development. Science **201**: 120-130.

3. SATOH, N. 1982. Timing mechanisms in early embryonic development. Differentiation 22: 156-163.
4. BAILEY, D. W. 1986. Genetic programming of development. Differentiation 33: 89-100.
5. McMAHON, D. 1974. Chemical messengers in development. Science 185: 1012-1021.
6. BRUNNER, G. 1977. Membrane impression and gene expression. Towards a theory of cytodifferentiation. Differentiation 8: 123-132.
7. BONNER, J. T. 1987. The next big problem in developmental biology. Am. Zool. 27: 715-723.
8. EDELMAN, G. M. 1984. Expression of cell adhesion molecules during embryogenesis and regeneration. Exp. Cell Res. 161: 1-16.
9. ALT, F. W., K. BLACKWELL & Y. D. YANCOPOULOS. 1987. Development of the primary antibody repertoire. Science 238: 1079-1087.
10. MANIATIS, T., S. GOODBURN & J. A. FISCHER. 1987. Regulation of inducible and tissue-specific gene expression. Science 236: 1237-1245.
11. STOCKARD, C. R. 1921. Developmental rate and structural expression: An experimental study of twins, "double monsters" and single deformities and the interaction among embryonic organs during their origin and development. Am. J. Anat. 28: 115-277.
12. WILSON, J. G. 1960. General principles in experimental teratology. In First International Conference on Congenital Malformations. M. Fishbein, Ed.: 187-194. J. B. Lippincott. Philadelphia, PA.
13. RUNNER, M. N. 1965. General mechanisms in teratogenesis. In Teratology, Principles and Techniques. J. G. Wilson & J. Warkany, Eds.: 95-111. University of Chicago Press. Chicago, IL.
14. SAXEN, L. 1976. Mechanisms of teratogenesis. J. Embryol. Exp. Morphol. 36: 1-12.
15. SKALKO, R. G. 1985. Cellular mechanisms in teratogenesis. In Basic Concepts in Teratology. T. V. N. Persaud, A. E. Chudley & R. G. Skalko, Eds.: 103-118. Alan R. Liss. New York, NY.
16. ROZENGURT, E. 1986. Early signals in the mitogenic response. Science 234: 161-166.
17. GREENE, R. M. & M. P. GARBARINO. 1984. Role of cyclic AMP, prostaglandins, and catecholamines during normal palate development. Curr. Top. Dev. Biol. 19: 65-78.
18. SKALKO, R. G. 1981. Biochemical mechanisms in developmental toxicology. In Developmental Toxicology. C. A. Kimmel & J. Buelke-Sam, Eds.: 1-11. Raven Press. New York, NY.
19. JUSKO, W. J. 1972. Pharmacodynamic principles in chemical teratology: Dose-effect relationships. J. Pharmacol. Exp. Ther. 183: 469-480.
20. KLAASSEN, C. D. & J. DOULL. 1980. Evaluation of safety: Toxicological evaluation. In Cassarett and Doull's Toxicology. 2nd edit. J. Doull, C. D. Klaassen & M. D. Amora, Eds.: 17-22. MacMillan. New York, NY.
21. NAU, H. 1986. Species differences in pharmacokinetics and drug teratogenesis. Environ. Health Perspect. 70: 113-129.
22. JOHNSON, E. M. 1988. Cross-species extrapolations and the biological basis for safety factor determinations in developmental toxicology. Regul. Toxicol. Pharmacol. 8: 22-36.
23. NEUBERT, D. 1988. Significance of pharmacokinetic variables in reproductive and developmental toxicity. Xenobiotica 18 (Suppl. 1): 45-58.
24. PRATT, R. L. & D. S. SALOMON. 1981. Biochemical basis for the teratogenic effects of glucocorticoids. In The Biochemical Basis of Chemical Teratogenesis. M. R. Juchau, Ed.: 179-199. Elsevier/North Holland. New York, NY.
25. WEBSTER, W. S., D. A. WALSH, A. H. LIPSON & S. E. McEWEN. 1980. Teratogenesis after acute alcohol exposure in inbred and outbred mice. Neurobehav. Toxicol. Teratol. 2: 227-234.
26. NEUBERT, D., I. CHAHOUD, T. PLATZEK & R. MEISTER. 1987. Principles and problems in assessing prenatal toxicity. Arch. Toxicol. 60: 238-245.
27. STREISSGUTH, A. P., J. C. LANDESMAN-DWYER, J. C. MARTIN & D. W. SMITH. 1980. Teratogenic effects of alcohol in humans and laboratory animals. Science 209: 353-361.
28. SULIK, K. K., M. C. JOHNSTON & M. A. WEBB. 1981. Fetal alcohol syndrome: Embryogenesis in a mouse model. Science 214: 936-938.
29. WEST, J. B., A. C. BLACK, JR., P. C. REIMANN & R. L. ALKANA. 1981. Polydactyly and polysyndactyly induced by prenatal exposure to ethanol. Teratology 24: 13-18.
30. KOCHHAR, D. M. & E. M. JOHNSON. 1965. Morphological and autoradiographic studies

of cleft palate induced in rat embryos by maternal hypervitaminosis A. J. Embryol. Exp. Morphol. **14:** 223-238.

31. SHENEFELT, R. E. 1972. Morphogenesis and malformations in hamsters caused by retinoic acid: Relation to dose and stage of treatment. Teratology **5:** 103-118.

32. KWASIGROCH, T. E., R. G. SKALKO & J. K. CHURCH. 1984. Mouse limb bud development in submerged culture: Quantitative assessment of the effects of *in vivo* exposure to retinoic acid. Teratogen. Carcinogen. Mutagen. **4:** 311-326.

33. KISTLER, A. & H. HOMMLER. 1985. Teratogenesis and reproductive safety evaluation of the retinoid etretin (Ro 10-1670). Arch. Toxicol. **58:** 50-56.

34. LAMMER, E. J., D. T. CHEN, R. M. HOAR, N. D. AGNISH, P. J. BENKE, J. T. BRAUN, C. J. CURRY, P. M. FERNHOFF, A. W. GRIX, JR., I. T. LOTT, J. M. RICHARD & S. C. SUN. 1985. Retinoic acid embryopathy. N. Engl. J. Med. **313:** 837-841.

35. SALOMON, D. S. 1983. Hormone receptors and malformations. *In* Teratogenesis and Reproductive Toxicology. E. M. Johnson & D. M. Kochhar, Eds.: 113-134. Springer-Verlag. Berlin.

36. ZIMMERMAN, E. F., F. ANDREW & H. KALTER. 1970. Glucocorticoid inhibition of RNA synthesis responsible for cleft palate in mice: A model. Proc. Natl. Acad. Sci. **67:** 779-785.

37. SUZDAK, P. D., J. R. GLOWA, J. N. CRAWLEY, R. D. SCHWARTZ, P. SKOLNICK & S. M. PAUL. 1986. A selective imidazodiazepine antagonist of ethanol in the rat. Science **234:** 1243-1247.

38. TICKU, M. K. & S. K. KULKARNI. 1988. Molecular interactions of ethanol with GABAergic system and potential of RO15-4513 as an ethanol antagonist. Pharmacol. Biochem. Behav. **30:** 501-510.

39. EICHELE, G. & C. THALLER. 1987. Characterization of concentration gradients of a morphogenetically active retinoid in the chick limb bud. J. Cell Biol. **105:** 1917-1923.

40. TICKLE, C., J. LEE & G. EICHELE. 1985. A quantitative analysis of the effect of all-trans-retinoic acid on the pattern of chick wing development. Dev. Biol. **109:** 82-95.

41. EICHELE, G. 1986. Retinoids induce duplications in developing vertebrate limbs. Bioscience **36:** 534-540.

42. MADEN, M., S. KEEBLE & R. A. COX. 1985. The characteristics of local application of retinoic acid to the regenerating axolotl limb. Roux's Arch. Dev. Biol. **194:** 228-235.

43. MADEN, M. 1983. The effect of vitamin A on limb regeneration in *Rana temporaria.* Dev. Biol. **98:** 409-416.

44. NIAZI, I. A., M. J. PESCITELLI & D. L. STOCUM. 1985. Stage-dependent effects of retinoic acid on regenerating urodele limbs. Roux's Arch. Dev. Biol. **194:** 355-363.

45. LHEREUX, E., S. D. THOMAS & F. CAREY. 1986. The effects of two retinoids on limb regeneration in *Pleurodeles waltl* and *Triturus vulgaris.* J. Embryol. Exp. Morphol. **92:** 165-182.

46. KWASIGROCH, T. E., J. F. VANNOY, J. K. CHURCH & R. G. SKALKO. 1986. Retinoic acid enhances and depresses *in vitro* development of cartilaginous bone anlagen in embryonic mouse limbs. In Vitro **22:** 150-156.

47. KISTLER, A., M. MISLIN & A. GEHRIG. 1985. Chondrogenesis of limb-bud cells: Improved culture method and the effect of the potent teratogen retinoic acid. Xenobiotica **15:** 673-679.

48. ZIMMERMAN, B. & D. TSAMBAOS. 1985. Retinoids inhibit the differentiation of embryonic-mouse mesenchymal cells. Arch. Dermatol. Res. **277:** 98-104.

49. CHYTIL, F. & D. E. ONG. 1984. Cellular retinoid-binding proteins. *In* The Retinoids, vol. 2. M. B. Sporn, A. B. Roberts & D. S. Goodman, Eds.: 89-123. Academic Press. Orlando, FL.

50. KWARTA, R. F., JR., C. A. KIMMEL, G. L. KIMMEL & W. SLIKKER, JR. 1985. Identification of the cellular retinoic acid binding protein (cRABP) within the embryonic mouse (CD-1) limb bud. Teratology **32:** 103-111.

51. MADEN, M. & D. SUMMERBELL. 1986. Retinoic acid-binding protein in the chick limb bud: Identification at developmental stages and binding affinities of various retinoids. J. Embryol. Exp. Morphol. **97:** 239-250.

52. KEEBLE, S. & M. MADEN. 1986. Retinoic acid-binding protein in the axolotl: Distribution in mature tissues and time of appearance during limb regeneration. Dev. Biol. **117:** 435-441.

53. PETKOVICH, M., N. G. BRAND, A. KRUST & P. CHAMBON. 1987. A human retinoic acid receptor which belongs to the family of nuclear receptors. Nature **330:** 444-450.

54. GIGUERE, V., E. S. ONG, P. SEGUI & R. M. EVANS. 1987. Identification of a receptor for the morphogen retinoic acid. Nature **330:** 624-629.

55. KOCHHAR, D. M., J. D. PENNER & C. I. TELLONE. 1984. Comparative teratogenic activities of two retinoids: Effects on palate and limb development. Teratogen. Carcinogen. Mutagen. **4:** 377-387.

56. KOCHHAR, D. M., J. KRAFT & J. NAU. 1987. Teratogenicity and disposition of various retinoids *in vivo* and *in vitro*. *In* Pharmacokinetics and Teratogenesis. Vol. 2. H. Nau & W. J. Scott, Jr., Eds.: 173-186. CRC Press. Boca Raton, FL.

57. WANG, C.-C., S. CAMPBELL, R. L. FURNER & D. L. HILL. 1980. Distribution of all-trans- and 13-cis-retinoic acids and n-hydroxyethylretinamide in mice after intravenous administration. Drug Metab. Dispos. **8:** 8-11.

58. KALIN, J. R., M. E. STARLING & D. L. HILL. 1981. Disposition of all-trans-retinoic acid in mice following oral doses. Drug. Metab. Dispos. **9:** 196-201.

59. KALIN, J. R., M. J. WELLS & D. L. HILL. 1982. Disposition of 13-cis-retinoic acid and N-(2-hydroxyethyl) retinamide after oral doses. Drug Metab. Dispos. **10:** 391-398.

60. NAU, H., D. M. KOCHHAR, J. M. CREECH CRAFT, B. LOEFBERG, J. REINERS & T. SPARENBERG. 1987. Teratogenesis of retinoids: Aspects of species differences and transplacental pharmacokinetics. *In* Approaches to Elucidate Mechanisms in Teratogenesis. F. Welsch, Ed.: 1-15. Hemisphere. Washington, DC.

61. CREECH CRAFT, J., D. M. KOCHHAR, W. J. SCOTT & H. NAU. 1987. Low teratogenicity of 13-cis-retinoic acid (isotretinoin) in the mouse corresponds to low embryo concentrations during organogenesis: Comparison to the all-tran isomer. Toxicol. Appl. Pharmacol. **87:** 474-482.

62. REINERS, J., B. LOFBERG, J. CREECH CRAFT, D. M. KOCHHAR & H. NAU. 1988. Transplacental pharmacokinetics of teratogenic doses of etretinate and other aromatic retinoids in mice. Reproductive Toxicol. **2:** 19-29.

63. HARRISON, R. W. 1983. Cellular factors which modulate hormone responses: Glucocorticoid action in perspective. Int. Rev. Cytol. (Suppl. 15): 1-16.

64. SHERMAN, M. I. 1986. How do retinoids promote differentiation? *In* Retinoids and Cell Differentiation. M. I. Sherman, Ed.: 161-186. CRC Press. Boca Raton, FL.

65. HORTON, W. E., Y. YAMADA & J. R. HASSELL. 1987. Retinoic acid rapidly reduces cartilage matrix synthesis by altering gene transcription in chondrocytes. Dev. Biol. **123:** 508-516.

Concepts in Teratology and Developmental Toxicology Derived from Animal Research

CHARLES V. VORHEES

Institute for Developmental Research
Children's Hospital Research Foundation
and
Departments of Pediatrics, Developmental Biology and
Environmental Health
University of Cincinnati
Cincinnati, Ohio 45229-2899

The purpose of this paper is to review the basic concepts of teratology and developmental toxicology, most of which have arisen from experimental research in laboratory animals. There continues to be some debate over the definition of teratology versus developmental toxicology and related terms. Some prefer to use teratology strictly in the narrow sense of a malformation-inducing agent and further insist that the term apply only to those teratogens which act at substantially nonmaternally toxic exposure levels.[1] There are compelling reasons for rejecting such a narrow interpretation and these have been outlined recently by Nelson.[2] The narrow definition of teratology, while understandable from the traditional perspectives of anatomy and embryology, became unsatisfactory as research expanded far beyond the limited view of abnormal development as the sole province of gross malformations.

Perhaps the clearest and most forward-looking definition of teratology came from the early work of the late James G. Wilson. From the mid-1960s onward he began writing of teratology as encompassing all aspects of abnormal development and by 1973 published a definition that is the one that will be followed herein. Wilson[3] defined teratogenesis as manifesting itself as death, malformation, growth retardation or abnormal function in the offspring as a result of early insult. While today, growth retardation might be best framed as growth abnormality so as to include both reduced and greater than normal growth, as in conditions such as macrosomia, otherwise this definition has stood the test of time.

In recent years the term developmental toxicology has emerged more strongly and is perceived by some as being one that is more generic in terms of all of the end points of abnormal development and also encompassing more stages of development. Even though Wilson[3] stated that teratology theoretically embraces all of development, the field has *de facto* behaved as if it is exclusively the study of congenital anomalies. Because of this practice, the term developmental toxicology breaks free of this connotation, and insofar as it does, is advantageous. On the other hand, the latter incorporates the term 'toxicology' in it which inevitably carries with it some unwanted connotative baggage. The most obvious of these is toxicology's traditional meaning as the study of poisons. This seems to preclude the study of inherited developmental abnormalities or those arising from maternal infectious disease. Because teratology actively embraces investigations of genetic and disease-induced developmental disorders, the term developmental toxicology may not prove to be optimal. Given that neither of the principal terms for this field is ideal, the present discussion will, for the sake of simplicity, treat them synonymously.

BASIC CONCEPTS OF TERATOLOGY AND DEVELOPMENTAL TOXICOLOGY

TABLE 1 presents a reformulated version of the basic principles of teratology/developmental toxicology drawn primarily from the work of Wilson[3,4] and his successors. The basic tenets have been reworded and slightly condensed with an aim towards updating and clarification. Note that Principle 4, related to critical periods of vulnerability, is the one that most sharply distinguishes this discipline from general toxicology or medicine.

Although Wilson stated early that teratology includes the study of developmentally induced dysfunctions, the inclusion of the latter in his writings was conspicuous in part by the lack of research in the field to support it. The absence of such research did not change until the area of behavioral teratology emerged. The term behavioral teratology was introduced in 1963 by Jack Werboff.[5] Werboff's concept was backed by a series of exploratory investigations in rats which empirically established that nonmalforming doses of some psychotherapeutic agents could induce behavioral reactions in the offspring. Studies of this type, however, were not new and may be traced in the experimental animal behavior literature for many years prior to 1963.[6] Nevertheless, Werboff's work and his concepts triggered surprisingly strong resistance among traditional birth defect investigators, so that the new data were treated as if they did not exist. Teratologists' attitudes towards behavioral teratology ranged from neglect to hostility. As a result, the area of behavioral teratology did not really gain credence until the 1970s.

Several important concepts were brought to the field by the explorations undertaken in pursuit of the phenomenon of behavioral teratogenesis in the 1970s. These are given

---

TABLE 1. Basic Concepts of Teratology and Developmental Toxicology[a]

1. Embryo/fetal toxic effects are expressed as death, malformation, growth disorder, or abnormal function.

2. Embryo/fetal toxic effects are a function of the organism's genetic endowment and its environment.

3. Embryo/fetal toxic effects are a function of the dose of the agent reaching the target tissue.

4. Embryo/fetal toxic effects are a function of the developmental stage of the organism at the time of insult. The most sensitive period occurs during organogenesis (embryogenesis).

5. The observed developmental disorder is the final expression of the molecular mechanisms of injury which exceed the compensatory influences of intracellular repair capacities and cell reserves (excess numbers).

---

[a] Adapted from Wilson.[3,4]

TABLE 2. Contributions Arising from Functional/Behavioral Teratology[a]

1. Developmental injuries to the nervous system have a protracted period of susceptibility which extends beyond organogenesis.

   For the central nervous system (CNS) this includes the events of:
   a. Neurogenesis
   b. Neuronal differentiation and migration
   c. Arborization and synaptogenesis
   d. Functional synaptic organization
   e. Myelination
   f. Gliogenesis, glial migration, and glial differentiation

   Corollary: While the most sensitive period is during organogenesis, vulnerability extends to and throughout the fetal and neonatal periods and into infancy.

2. The most frequent injuries to the developing nervous system do not result in CNS malformation, but rather in functional abnormalities. Such effects are often not detectable at birth, *i.e.,* the organism may be said to 'grow into its deficit.'

3. There is a consistent ordinal relationship between the different manifestations of developmental toxicity, but there are noteworthy exceptions, *e.g.,* most substances of abuse.

[a] Adapted from Butcher *et al.,*[7] Hutchings,[8] Vorhees & Butcher,[9] Hutchings,[10] Vorhees.[11]

in TABLE 2.[7-11] Perhaps the most important of these is Principle 1, which arose from early studies which unequivocally demonstrated that for the nervous system the window of vulnerability to insult could not be as conveniently demarcated as it could be for malformations to the period of organogenesis. Simultaneously, the new data revealed a second generality, *viz.,* that the dose-response curve for functional disorder lay to the left of those for malformations and fetal death. The traditional view is illustrated in FIGURE 1. Compare this to the new view introduced by behavioral teratology as illustrated in FIGURE 2.

Rapidly the importance of these two observations, *viz.,* a wider window of vulnerability and greater sensitivity to injury, was appreciated and behavioral teratologists undertook a flurry of research to demonstrate these two themes with every drug and environmental agent that investigators could pursue. More recently, an effort has been made to fit the curve of growth disorders among those for the other end points, and this hypothesized relationship is shown in FIGURE 3.[11] Unfortunately, little research yet exists on the validity of this hypothesis.

Another concept emerged from research in behavioral teratology that has contributed a great deal to the acceptance of the term 'developmental toxicity.' First, behavioral research began to probe for responses to broader periods of exposure than just the period of organogenesis, as mentioned above. This action immediately led to a broader conception of the field so that the term 'developmental' became more appropriate. Second, behavioral research also looked for the consequences of early injury at long intervals after the exposure occurred, not just at birth. This lent another basis to the broader term 'developmental toxicology.' The search for consequences resulting from early exposures then rapidly moved from early postnatal development to assessments during adulthood and even extending into advanced age. Once this process began it was inevitable that new effects would be found, many of which were not related to the central nervous system. As this happened, behavioral teratology became functional teratology and accordingly, greatly broadened in perspective.

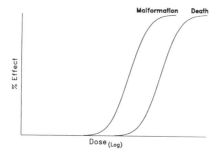

FIGURE 1. Theoretical dose-response curves for congenital malformations and fetal death as traditionally conceived.

THE RELATIONSHIP BETWEEN HUMAN AND ANIMAL FINDINGS

In general, two situations occur with respect to human developmental damage and these are listed in TABLE 3, *i.e.,* either developmental toxicity has been discovered in animals before it is in humans or *vice versa.* Two prime examples of human teratogens predicted by animal data are retinoids and maternal phenylketonuria (PKU) (see TABLE 4[12–40]). The malformation potential of retinoids was established in rodents in the early 1950s using vitamin A. A more dramatic case occurred recently with iso-tretinoin, a retinoid marketed because of its efficacy in treating severe acne. Had reasonable alternatives been available a predictable teratogen such as isotretinoin would undoubtedly never have been introduced, but given the lack of such alternatives the drug was produced and despite warnings, a number of malformed children were born.

Maternal PKU describes the situation where only the mother has the disease and the conceptus is phenotypically normal (*i.e.,* is heterozygous for PKU, which since PKU is recessive, means that such individuals are unaffected). The high incidence of congenital functional and structural teratogenicity in these women's children is striking and all the more remarkable when it is remembered that the damage to the conceptus is entirely due to transplacental hyperphenylalaninemia. Such effects were clearly predicted from animal data as early as 1970.[36]

FIGURE 2. Theoretical dose-response curves for congenital malformations and fetal death in relation to the curve for functional disorders.

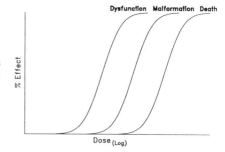

FIGURE 3. Theoretical dose-response curves for malformations, fetal death, and dysfunction, with the curve for ponderal effects inserted between the curves for dysfunction and malformation. The curve for ponderal teratogenesis is in an hypothesized position.

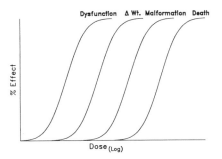

When it comes to the subject of this conference, substances of abuse, the author could not identify any compound that had been adequately tested in animals and was expected to be functionally or structurally teratogenic in humans before it became a widespread abuse problem. Passively affected infants turning up in neonatal intensive care units and pediatric clinics have been the first harbinger of things to come in almost every case.

This situation, where developmental abnormalities have been discovered in humans and only later confirmed in animals, has unfortunately represented the predominant sequence of events for all agents, not only drugs of abuse. Commonly recognized reasons for this are listed in TABLE 5 and less well-recognized reasons are listed in TABLE 6. This unfortunate state of affairs can only change through better regulatory science, which is based on the new developments occurring today in developmental toxicology. The role of animal research which occurs after identification of a hazard in humans is summarized in TABLE 7. Such research is the best avenue currently known for preventing recurrence of similar situations in the future.

A partial list of the functional and structural teratogens first identified in humans is provided in TABLE 8. A number of these are subjects of this conference and will be described in some detail elsewhere in these proceedings.

Abuse agents represent a special group of developmental toxins and some of this group's characteristics are listed in TABLE 9. One of the most important of these centers around dosage. Whereas dose and duration of exposure to prescription and over-the-counter drugs, food additives, and occupational chemicals follow guidelines which are designed to maintain a safety margin consistent with accumulated toxicity and efficacy data, abuse agents are taken at doses near or sometimes even above those which are toxic. For these drugs, dosage is user determined and is a consideration only in so far as it induces an acceptable level of stimulation. In such a context, drugs are often consumed at doses that, while usually not acutely toxic, are frequently chronically toxic. Moreover, the doses that come to be tolerated by the mother may

TABLE 3. Relationship between Animal and Human Teratogenicity/Developmental Toxicity

1. Animal findings presage discovery of human teratogenicity/developmental disability.

2. Human findings uncover disorder, which triggers subsequent animal research.

TABLE 4. Examples of the Predictive Power of Animal Studies for Human Teratogenicity

---

1. Retinoids

a. For malformations:

1. In animals:

a. Hypervitaminosis A: Produces malformations in multiple species.[12–16]
b. *trans*-retinoic acid: Produces malformations in multiple species.[12–19]
c. Isotretinoin (13-*cis*-retinoic acid, Accutane®): Produces malformations in multiple species[16] (also Hoffmann-LaRoche preclinical studies).

Retinoids predicted to be human structural teratogen

2. In humans:

a. Hypervitaminosis A: Suspected teratogen, but there is a paucity of cases.[20]
b. *trans*-retinoic acid: Not taken by humans.
c. Isotretinoin: Established human teratogen.[21]

b. For dysfunctions:

1. In animals:

a. Hypervitaminosis A: Behavioral teratogen in rats.[22–32]
b. *trans*-retinoic acid: Behavioral teratogen in rats.[33–34]
c. Isotretinoin: Under investigation in rats.

Retinoids predicted to be human behavioral teratogen[7,35]

2. In humans:

a. Hypervitaminosis A: Few cases & not examined for functional effects.
b. *trans*-retinoic acid: Not taken by humans.
c. Under investigation (J. Adams, personal communication, 1988).

2. Maternal Phenylketonuria (PKU)

a. For malformations:

1. In animals

Maternal hyperphenylalaninemia: Produces increased fetal loss and intrauterine growth retardation, slight increase in structural defects in rat offspring[36] (also Vorhees & Berry, unpublished observations).

2. In humans:

Maternal PKU: Produces high incidence of intrauterine growth retardation, microcephaly, & increased incidence of cardiac defects.[37–39]

b. For dysfunctions

1. In animals:

Maternal hyperphenylalaninemia: Produces learning impairments and altered locomotor activity in rat offspring.[36,40]

2. In humans:

Maternal PKU (untreated): > 90% of such women have delivered at least one mentally retarded child.[37–39]

Maternal PKU (treated): Produces mental retardation in most cases, but number of cases is small.[37]

Abuse Compounds: No known examples.

TABLE 5. Why Has Developmental Hazard Prediction Not Been Better from Animal Data?

Conventional reasons:

1. Assessment methodology is relatively new and even today is only partially standardized.

    Assessment guidelines for developmental **structural defects** have been standardized at FDA since 1965, but at EPA only since 1985 for toxic substances and are still not standardized for pesticides. Few data have accrued from the EPA's efforts and much of what does exist is proprietary and therefore unavailable.

    Assessment guidelines for developmental **functional defects** is nonexistent at FDA and is only in the draft stage at EPA.

2. Problems exist concerning cross-species extrapolation. False positive and miss rates are largely unknown. Problem of how to interpret different defects in different species is unresolved.

3. Dosage differences. Experimental teratologists often work at doses above those used in humans.

4. Ascertainment differences. It is often difficult to confirm or refute that an agent is a human teratogen, especially when:

    a. frequency of occurrence of the effects is low,

    b. it is a defect not easily detected at birth,

    c. the defects are not easily categorized, and

    d. the type of defect is common or does not co-occur with other defects to form a distinctive syndrome.

TABLE 6. Why Has Developmental Hazard Prediction Not Been Better from Animal Data?

Less well-known reasons:

1. Problems of selective elimination of cases: If an animal screen has a hit, *i.e.,* detects a new chemical as a teratogen, it is generally not marketed. Since such agents never reach humans, the correct positive rate of the screening method is never known.

    If the animal test scores a false positive, the agent is not marketed, and hence the false positive rate of the test is never known.

    Only correct negatives and misses (false negatives) in animal testing routinely reach the market. Misses are often incorrectly construed as indicative that animal screening tests are invalid.

2. Use of many potential human teratogens in humans predates the introduction of standardized structural and functional animal assessment regulations.

3. Use of many potential human teratogens were approved based on inadequate animal data, *e.g.,* most chemicals in commerce, many medical devices, numerous toxic substances, and some drugs (those that are exempted from testing for various reasons or are marketed in countries where only partial testing is required, *e.g.,* the United States).

4. Some agents are untested because they are not legally marketed, *e.g.,* abuse compounds.

TABLE 7. Role of Animal Research When Discovery of Developmental Toxicity First Occurs in Humans

1. To establish cause and effect with strict control of confounding variables
2. To define dose-effect relationships
3. To determine critical periods of vulnerability
4. To assess interacting variables
5. To investigate pathophysiology
6. To test mechanistic hypotheses
7. To uncover general principles which may aid in preventing recurrent incidences

TABLE 8. Human Findings Uncover Disorder, Which Triggers Subsequent Animal Research.

Examples:

a. Thalidomide
b. High dose X-irradiation
c. Infections: Toxoplasmosis, rubella, CMV, herpes, syphilis, etc.
d. Androgenic hormones
e. Aminopterin and other folic acid antagonists
f. Ethanol
g. Methylmercury
h. Warfarin and other oral anticoagulants
i. Some alkylating agents, *e.g.,* cyclophosphamide
j. Anticonvulsants
    1. Valproic acid
    2. Phenytoin
    3. Phenobarbital
    4. Trimethadione
    5. Carbamazepine (newly implicated[41])
k. Lead
l. PCB's
m. cigarettes
n. heroin and methadone (functional effects only)
o. cocaine (probable)

TABLE 9. Special Considerations for Substances of Abuse

1. Unlike most other agents, abuse compounds may be intentionally taken at maternally toxic doses.

2. Abuse compounds may be more likely to be inadvertently taken at toxic doses due to lack of control of quality of material and because of taking combinations of agents.

3. Substance abuse may lead to secondary changes in self-care habits and nutritional practices which may compound effects of the agent of abuse.

4. Most abuse substances do not produce birth defects and thus, "easy" to detect newborn markers of injury are not present. Effects are either predominantly or exclusively functional.

5. Length of interval between period of exposure and detection of functional problems in the child (at school age) is long which makes linkage to the mother's prenatal drug history problematic.

6. The known beneficial effects of routine prenatal care are often not utilized by those abusing substances.

7. Ascertainment of actual exposure period and dosage are rarely possible.

be substantially above the tolerances of the embryo and fetus. Therefore, the abuse population represents one of the highest drug exposure groups encountered in humans.

It is also evident that many abuse agents do not possess the classic developmental toxicity pattern presented in FIGURE 3. Often the pattern more closely resembles that depicted in FIGURE 4, where dysfunction and ponderal changes may be seen at doses far removed from those inducing malformations or early death. The weight change and dysfunction curves may even be superimposed, or the weight change curve may lie to the left of the dysfunction curve. Ethanol and cocaine are candidates for these patterns. FIGURE 5 shows a case where an agent may have no or no practical dose-response curve at all for malformations or early death. Opiates may represent this pattern. Finally, the dysfunction and ponderal change curves may occur close together for some abuse agents (as in FIG. 4) while there may be no establishable malformation curve. Cigarette smoking may represent a case fitting this pattern.

It is not possible to determine at this juncture how many different patterns there may be, but it is clear that abuse agents will continue to provide new information that can be beneficial to future research designed to uncover, treat, and prevent developmental disorders.

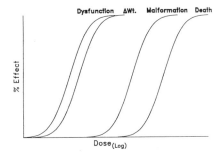

FIGURE 4. Theoretical dose-response curves for dysfunction, ponderal abnormalities, malformation, and death, with the former two depicted as being in close proximity.

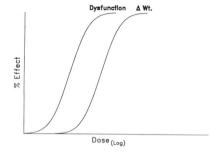

FIGURE 5. Theoretical dose-response curves for dysfunction and ponderal abnormalities alone, with no curves for malformation or death. This pattern may hold for some abuse substances.

REFERENCES

1. JOHNSON, E. M. 1986. False positives/false negatives in developmental toxicology and teratology. Teratology **34**: 361-362.
2. NELSON, B. K. 1987. "Teratogen": A case against redefinition. Response to Johnson's editorial comment re: "Teratogen." Teratology **36**: 399-400.
3. WILSON, J. G. 1973. Environment and Birth Defects. Academic Press. New York, NY.
4. WILSON, J. G. 1977. Current status of teratology—General principles and mechanisms derived from animal studies. *In* Handbook of Teratology. J. G. Wilson & F. C. Fraser, Eds., Vol. **1**: 47-74. Plenum Press. New York, NY.
5. WERBOFF, J. & J. S. GOTTLIEB. 1963. Drugs in pregnancy: Behavioral teratology. Obstet. Gynecol. Surv. **18**: 420-423.
6. VORHEES, C. V. 1986. Origins of behavioral teratology. *In* Handbook of Behavioral Teratology. E. P. Riley & C. V. Vorhees, Eds.: 3-22. Plenum Press. New York, NY.
7. BUTCHER, R. E., K. HAWVER, T. BURBACHER & W. SCOTT. 1975. Behavioral effects from antenatal exposure to teratogens. *In* Aberrant Development in Infancy: Human and Animal Studies. N. R. Ellis, Ed.: 161-167. Erlbaum & Associates. Hillsdale, NJ.
8. HUTCHINGS, D. E. 1978. Behavioral teratology: Embryopathic and behavioral effects of drugs during pregnancy. *In* Early Influences. G. Gottlieb, Ed.: 7-35. Academic Press. New York, NY.
9. VORHEES, C. V. & R. E. BUTCHER. 1982. Behavioral teratogenicity. *In* Developmental Toxicology. K. Snell, Ed.: 249-298. Praeger Press, New York, NY.
10. HUTCHINGS, D. E. 1985. Prenatal opioid exposure and the problem of causal inference. *In* National Institute on Drug Abuse Research Monograph Series, No. 59: Current Research on the Consequences of Maternal Drug Abuse. T. M. Pinkert, Ed.: 6-19. Alcohol, Drug Abuse and Mental Health Administration, Public Health Service, U.S. Department of Health and Human Services. Washington, DC.
11. VORHEES, C. V. 1986. Principles of behavioral teratology. *In* Handbook of Behavioral Teratology. E. P. Riley & C. V. Vorhees, Eds.: 23-48. Plenum Press. New York, NY.
12. COHLAN, S. Q. 1953. Excessive intake of vitamin A as a cause of congenital anomalies in the rat. Science **117**: 535-536.
13. COHLAN, S. Q. 1953. Excessive intake of vitamin A during pregnancy as a cause of congenital anomalies in the rat. Am. J. Dis. Child. **86**: 348-349.
14. KALTER, H. 1968. Teratology of the Central Nervous System. University of Chicago Press, Chicago, IL pp. 47-56.
15. GEELAN, J. A. G. 1979. Hypervitaminosis A induced teratogenesis. CRC Crit. Rev. Toxicol. **6**: 351-376.
16. Teratology Society Position Paper. 1987. Recommendations for vitamin A use during pregnancy. Teratology **35**: 269-275.
17. KOCHHAR, D. M. 1967. Teratogenic activity of retinoic acid. Acta Pathol. Microbiol. Scand. **70**: 398-404.

18. KOCHHAR, D. M. 1973. Limb development in mouse embryos. I. Analysis of teratogenic effects of retinoic acid. Teratology 7: 289-298.
19. NOLEN, G. A. 1972. The effects of various levels of dietary protein on retinoic acid-induced teratogenicity in rats. Teratology 5: 143-152.
20. ROSA, F. W., A. L. WILK & F. O. KELSEY. 1986. Teratogen update: Vitamin A congeners. Teratology 33: 355-364.
21. LAMMER, E. J., D. T. CHEN, R. M. HOAR, N. D. AGNISH, P. J. ENDKE, J. T. BRAUN, C. J. CURRY, P. M. FERNHOFF, A. W. GRIX, I. T. LOTT, J. M. RICHARD & S. C. SUN. 1985. Retinoic acid embryopathy. N. Engl. J. Med. 313: 837-841.
22. BUTCHER, R. E., R. L. BRUNNER, T. ROTH & C. A. KIMMEL. 1972. A learning impairment associated with maternal hypervitaminosis-A in rats. Life Sci. 11: 141-145.
23. HUTCHINGS, D. E., J. GIBSON & M. A. KAUFMAN. 1973. Maternal vitamin A excess during the early fetal period: Effects on learning and development in the offspring. Dev. Psychobiol. 6: 445-457.
24. HUTCHINGS, D. E. & J. GASTON. 1974. The effect of vitamin A excess administered during the mid-fetal period on learning and development in rat offspring. Dev. Psychobiol. 7: 225-233.
25. VORHEES, C. V. 1974. Some behavioral effects of maternal hypervitaminosis A in rats. Teratology 10: 269-274.
26. HUTCHINGS, D. E., J. GIBBON, J. GASTON & L. VACCA. 1975. Critical periods in fetal development: Differential effects on learning and development produced by maternal vitamin A excess. In Aberrant Development in Infancy: Human and Animal Studies. N. R. Ellis, Ed.: 177-185. Erlbaum & Associates. Hillsdale, NJ.
27. COYLE, I. R. & G. SINGER. 1975. The interaction of post-weaning housing conditions and prenatal drug effects on behaviour. Psychopharmacologia 41: 237-244.
28. VORHEES, C. V., R. L. BRUNNER, C. R. MCDANIEL & R. E. BUTCHER. 1978. The relationship of gestational age to vitamin A induced postnatal dysfunction. Teratology 17: 271-276.
29. VORHEES, C. V., R. L. BRUNNER & R. E. BUTCHER. 1979. Psychotropic drugs as behavioral teratogens. Science 205: 1220-1225.
30. MOONEY, M. P., K. T. HOYENGA, K. B. HOYENGA & J. R. C. MORTON. 1981. Prenatal hypervitaminosis A and postnatal behavioral development in the rat. Neurobehav. Toxicol. Teratol. 3: 1-4.
31. ADAMS, J. 1982. Ultrasonic vocalizations as diagnostic tools in studies of developmental toxicity: An investigation of the effects of hypervitaminosis A. Neurobehav. Toxicol. Teratol. 4: 299-304.
32. SAILLENFAIT, A. M. & B. VANNIER. 1988. Methodological proposal in behavioural teratogenicity testing: Assessment of propoxyphene, chlorpromazine, and vitamin A as positive controls. Teratology 37: 185-199.
33. NOLEN, G. A. 1985. An industrial developmental toxicologist's view of behavioral teratology and possible guidelines. Neurobehav. Toxicol. Teratol. 7: 653-657.
34. NOLEN, G. A. 1986. The effects of prenatal retinoic acid on the viability and behavior of offspring. Neurobehav. Toxicol. Teratol. 8: 643-654.
35. VORHEES, C. V. 1986. Retinoic acid embryopathy. N. Engl. J. Med. 315: 262-263.
36. BUTCHER, R. E. 1970. Learning impairment associated with maternal phenylketonuria in rats. Nature 226: 555-556.
37. LENKE, R. R. & H. L. LEVY. 1980. Maternal phenylketonuria and hyperphenylalaninemia: An international survey of the outcome of untreated and treated pregnancies. N. Engl. J. Med. 303: 1202-1208.
38. LEVY, H. L. & S. E. WAISBREN. 1983. Effects of untreated maternal phenylketonuria and hyperphenylalaninemia on the fetus. N. Engl. J. Med. 309: 1269-1274.
39. LEVY, H. L., R. R. LENKE & A. C. CROCKER. 1981. Maternal PKU: Proceedings of a Conference. U.S. Department of Health and Human Services, Health Services Administration, Washington, DC.
40. VORHEES, C. V., R. E. BUTCHER & H. K. BERRY. 1981. Progress in experimental phenylketonuria: A critical review. Neurosci. Biobehav. Rev. 5: 177-190.
41. JONES, K. L., R. V. LACRO, K. A. JOHNSON & J. ADAMS. 1988. Pregnancy outcome in women treated with Tegretol. Teratology 37: 468-469.

Maternal-Fetal Pharmacokinetics and Fetal Dose-Response Relationships

HAZEL H. SZETO

Department of Pharmacology
Cornell University Medical College
1300 York Avenue
New York, New York 10021

INTRODUCTION

Our primary concern in the use of both licit and illicit drugs during pregnancy is the adverse effects that these drugs may produce on the developing fetus. It is now evident that the placenta does not act as a barrier to protect the fetus against exposure to most drugs consumed by the mother. There is little doubt that drugs that have ready access into the central nervous system will also distribute readily across the placenta and exert direct actions on the fetus. The intensity of adverse effects on the fetus would therefore depend on the extent of drug distribution to the fetus. A thorough understanding of the effects of maternal drug use on the developing fetus would thus require knowledge of both the maternal-fetal pharmacokinetics of the drug and its pharmacodynamic actions on the fetus.

Information on maternal-fetal pharmacokinetics of the drugs of abuse in humans has been restricted for both technical and ethical reasons. Available data are generally limited to single time point determinations of maternal and cord blood levels at the time of delivery. There are great difficulties in interpreting a series of fetal/maternal concentration ratios obtained at different times after drug consumption from pregnant women with varying histories of drug use. Much of our understanding of maternal-fetal pharmacokinetics has necessarily resulted from systematic investigations carried out with the use of animal models. We and others have found the chronically instrumented pregnant sheep model to be particularly well suited for such studies.[1-3] The sheep has a relatively long gestational period (approximately 5 months) and usually carries only one or two fetuses. Most important, the fetus is large enough to permit the implantation of chronic indwelling vascular catheters, which permits repeated collection of fetal blood throughout the third trimester in an unanesthetized, unrestrained animal. The discussion of this paper will be confined to results that have been obtained with this animal model.

Maternal-Fetal Pharmacokinetics

Maternal-Fetal Drug Distribution after Single Dose Exposure

The distribution of several drugs of abuse between the mother and fetus has been studied using the pregnant sheep model. The results of these studies indicated that while all drugs studied to date were distributed to the fetus, there were some differences in their rate and extent of placental transfer.

The placental transfer of most opioid drugs was found to be extremely rapid after intravenous (iv) administration to the mother, with peak fetal blood levels occurring in less than 2 min for alfentanil and meperidine, and in 5-10 min for methadone and morphine.[4-6] Fetal blood levels were similar to maternal blood levels for meperidine, but lower than corresponding maternal levels for alfentanil, methadone and morphine at all times after drug administration. The elimination half-lifes of all four opioid drugs in the fetus were found to be similar to maternal half-lifes, suggesting that elimination of these drugs in the maternal-fetal unit is largely dictated by maternal elimination characteristics.

Rapid bidirectional transfer of drug between the mother and fetus was also reported for ethanol.[3,7,8] The maternal and fetal blood concentration curves were virtually superimposable up to 14 hr after 1 hr infusion of ethanol to the mother. The apparent zero-order elimination rates for maternal blood and fetal blood were similar,[3] suggesting that the elimination of ethanol from the fetus is regulated primarily by maternal hepatic biotransformation, since alcohol dehydrogenase activity in fetal lamb liver has been shown to be less than 10% of that in maternal liver.[9]

On the other hand, the placental transfer of tetrahydrocannabinol (THC) following marijuana smoking was found to be slower than either the opioids or ethanol. THC was barely detectable in fetal plasma even at 30 min after maternal smoke inhalation, and peak blood levels did not occur until 2-4 hr even though peak maternal levels occurred before the marijuana cigarette was completed.[10] Fetal THC levels also remained significantly lower than maternal levels at all times after the cigarette administration. The reason for the apparent slow distribution to the fetus of such an extremely lipid-soluble compound is not known. A possible contributing factor may be the very extensive binding of THC to maternal plasma proteins.

Maternal-Fetal Drug Distribution under Steady State Conditions

Despite the rapid distribution of these drugs to the fetus, it was rather surprising that fetal levels of certain drugs remained consistently lower than maternal levels following single dose exposure. This apparent lack of equilibration between the mother and fetus was initially thought to be due to the rapid elimination of these drugs from the mother. However, even when the opioids were infused to the mother at constant rate until steady state concentrations were reached in both mother and fetus, the ratio of fetal concentration to maternal concentration was still found to be only 0.15 for methadone, 0.13 for morphine, and 0.3 for meperidine.[4,5,11] Studies with many other drugs have revealed that this is a rather universal phenomenon, perhaps with the exception of ethanol (see TABLE 1).

TABLE 1.

Drug	C_F/C_M (Total)	C_F/C_M (Unbound)
Methadone[5]	0.15	0.40
Morphine[11]	0.13	0.13
Meperidine[4]	0.30	0.40
Cimetidine[12]	0.04	0.04
Triamterene[13]	0.17	—
Acetylsalicylic acid[14]	0.22	0.22
Indomethacin[15]	0.28	0.28
Omeprazole[16]	0.47	0.22
Dilantin[17]	0.51	—
Dexamethasone[18]	0.67	0.67
Lidocaine[19]	0.76	—
Acetaminophen[2]	0.77	0.77
Ethanol[20]	1.00	1.00

It has been suggested that this observed maternal-fetal concentration gradient may be due to differences in the extent of drug binding in maternal and fetal plasma, since total drug concentrations were used in the calculation of these ratios. However, as indicated in TABLE 1, fetal levels of unbound drug were still lower than maternal levels for all drugs in which this was examined.

Proposed Pharmacokinetic Models for the Maternal-Fetal Unit

Pharmacokinetic modelling has been used to explain this persistent maternal-fetal gradient and the large variation seen in the distribution of various drugs between the mother and the fetus.[1,2,11,21] As with any mathematical modelling, the purpose was to reduce the complex biological system into simpler systems which we could fully describe mathematically, and for which we were able to obtain experimental data and compare with the theoretical estimates. It is this last requirement that has generally prevented us from proposing more complicated models which would perhaps be a closer approximation to the real biological system.

The simplest model that could be proposed for the maternal-fetal unit would be a two-compartment model wherein the mother and fetus are each represented as a single compartment. As illustrated in FIGURE 1, there are three possible types of two-compartment models. They differ only in that the drug may be eliminated from the maternal compartment only (Model 1a), from the fetal compartment only (Model 1b), or from both maternal and fetal compartments (Model 1c).

Model 1a had been proposed by some investigators in the past based on the assumption that the fetus does not have significant ability to eliminate drugs. Since the fetal compartment is closed in this model, the intercompartmental clearances must be equal ($CL_{MF} = CL_{FM}$), and fetal concentration would be the same as maternal concentration under steady state conditions.[21] This model would therefore be adequate for ethanol where fetal concentrations were found to be always equal to maternal concentrations,[3,7,8,20] and suggests that elimination of ethanol by the fetus is insignificant, and that elimination of ethanol from the maternal-fetal unit is entirely driven by maternal drug elimination.

In view of the finding that fetal concentrations do not approach maternal concentrations for practically all other drugs studied in the sheep model, a slightly more complicated model, Model 1c, has been proposed.[21] In this model, the clearance of drug from the fetal compartment results in a persistent net flux of drug from the maternal compartment to the fetal compartment, thus resulting in lower drug concentrations in the fetus. The extent of fetal exposure, expressed mathematically as the ratio of fetal concentration to maternal concentration, is therefore determined by:

$$(C_F/C_M = CL_{MF}/(CL_{FM} + CL_{FO})$$

In the past, it was often thought that if fetal drug concentration was lower than maternal drug concentration at steady state, it would imply that there was a "placental barrier" limiting diffusion of the drug from the mother to the fetus. However, this mathematical model suggests that a fetal-maternal steady state concentration ratio of less than one could only result from elimination of the drug by the fetus.

This model has been used for the determination of transplacental clearances and fetal clearance of several drugs, including morphine,[11] methadone,[11] and acetaminophen.[2] These clearance values are shown in TABLE 2. The validity of this compartmental model has been verified by comparing the calculated transplacental clearances with direct measurements using an extraction ratio method.[2] These clearance values suggest that the relatively lower extent of fetal exposure to morphine as compared to methadone is due to a lower transplacental clearance; and that the fetus plays a larger role in the clearance of morphine and methadone as compared with acetaminophen.

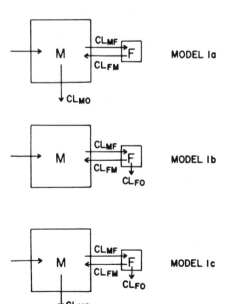

FIGURE 1. Three possible types of two-compartment open models describing the disposition of a drug in the mother and fetus at steady state, where M represents the maternal compartment, and F represents the fetal compartment; CL_{MF} and CL_{FM} are the respective clearances from the maternal compartment to the fetal compartment, and from the fetal compartment to the maternal compartment; CL_{MO} and CL_{FO} are the respective nonplacental clearances from the maternal and fetal compartments. (From Szeto.[1] Reprinted by permission from the *Annual Review of Pharmacology*.)

TABLE 2.

Drug	CL_{MF} (ml/min)	CL_{FM} (ml/min)	CL_{MO} (ml/min)	CL_{FO} (ml/min)	$CL_{FO}/(CL_{FO} + CL_{FM})$
Morphine[11]	25	58	2797	126	67.4
Methadone[5]	390	504	7571	3810	42.8
Acetaminophen[2]	61	58	913	23	27.2

These results illustrate how pharmacokinetic modelling can provide a better understanding of the factors that govern drug distribution to the fetus.

Evidence for Fetal Elimination of Drugs

Several attempts have been made to obtain direct evidence for fetal drug elimination in support of Model 1c. Drug elimination in the fetus may occur via renal excretion and/or biotransformation. Direct evidence for renal clearance has been reported for a number of drugs, including meperidine,[22,23] cimetidine,[12] omeprazole[16] and acetaminophen.[2] When normalized for differences in weight, renal clearance of cimetidine in the fetus was comparable to that in the mother.[12] In addition, fetal renal clearance of meperidine[23] and cimetidine[12] were both greater than creatinine clearance, suggesting renal tubular secretion. For meperidine, there is evidence that tubular secretion is due to ion trapping.[23] However, as in the adult, the contribution of renal clearance to the overall fetal clearance of these drugs has been small.

Prenatal drug metabolism has been extensively studied using in vitro liver enzyme preparations.[24] Direct in vivo evidence for fetal biotransformation has been more difficult to obtain. The presence of metabolites in fetal plasma alone does not imply that the fetus has biotransformation ability, since some metabolites of maternal origin may be readily distributed to the fetus, as has been demonstrated for normeperidine[4] and acetaldehyde.[3,20] Recently, however, there have been some very elegant studies demonstrating biotransformation ability in the fetal lamb. Wang et al.[2] reported on the presence of both acetaminophen glucuronide and acetaminophen sulfate in fetal plasma following acetaminophen administration to the mother. In a subsequent study, they demonstrated that neither conjugate distributes across the placenta to any significant extent, thus providing evidence that these metabolites must be of fetal origin.[25] These conjugates are highly polar and are eventually excreted into fetal urine via glomerular filtration.[25] Using a similar argument, the presence of morphine glucuronide in the fetus following morphine administration to the mother indicates the ability of the fetus to biotransform morphine.[6] However, there is as yet no quantitative determination of in vivo hepatic drug clearance in the fetus. Thus it is not yet possible to assess the contribution of biotransformation to overall fetal drug clearance.

Distribution of Drugs into Amniotic Fluid

There is experimental evidence that many drugs can be detected in amniotic fluid following maternal administration. These include meperidine,[22] lidocaine[26] and ethanol.[3] The appearance of drug in amniotic fluid is usually delayed following a single iv dose to the mother, but the concentration in amniotic fluid gradually increases, and peak concentration usually far exceeds the concurrent concentrations in maternal and fetal plasma. Metabolites, such as normeperidine[4] and acetaldehyde[20] have also been detected in amniotic fluid. The delay in appearance of drug in amniotic fluid suggests that a major source of drug comes from fetal urine. Since many of the drugs of abuse and their metabolites are weak bases, accumulation in amniotic fluid can result due to the lower pH of amniotic fluid, thus resulting in a reservoir of drug *in utero.* Elimination of drugs from the amniotic fluid may occur via diffusion across membranes into the fetal and/or maternal circulation and by fetal swallowing of amniotic fluid. For lipid-soluble drugs such as meperidine, diffusion across the membranes into maternal circulation has been shown to be the predominant pathway.[4]

Correlation between Maternal-Fetal Pharmacokinetics and Pharmacodynamics

The fundamental premise in pharmacology states that there is a relationship between the dose of a drug and the magnitude of response it elicits (*i.e.,* the dose-response relationship). Applying the Law of Mass Action, the intensity of effect is directly related to the log dose (or concentration) in a sigmoidal manner.[27] If this dose-response relationship can also be presumed in the fetus, then the magnitude of pharmacologic response in the fetus should be directly proportional to the extent of fetal exposure.

Pharmacokinetic studies have demonstrated that there can be significant differences in the extent of fetal exposure to different drugs, even within the same class of pharmacologic agents such as the opiates. For instance, our data showed that the extent of fetal exposure to methadone is three times greater than to morphine.[11] We would then expect the fetal response to maternally-administered methadone to be three times greater than that to morphine. To illustrate this relationship between pharmacokinetics and pharmacodynamic response, we have compared the effects of maternal administration of morphine and methadone on fetal behavioral activity using the pregnant sheep model.

Behavioral activity in the fetal lamb can be assessed using intrauterine polygraphic recordings of electrocortical activity (EEG), eye movements and muscle tone.[28] Under normal physiological conditions, less than 10% of the time can be classified as the state of arousal in the fetus, and the remainder of time is evenly divided between quiet sleep and rapid eye movement sleep.[28] Direct administration of either methadone or morphine to the fetus resulted in an increase in arousal and a suppression of quiet sleep in the fetal lamb,[29,30] as shown in FIGURE 2. There was no significant difference

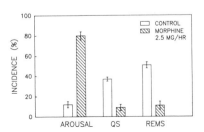

FIGURE 2. Effects of morphine administration to the fetus (2.5 mg/hr) on the incidence of arousal, quiet sleep (QS) and rapid eye movement sleep (REMS).

between the response to equal doses of morphine and methadone, suggesting that morphine and methadone were equi-effective in stimulating arousal and suppressing quiet sleep in the fetal lamb[30] (FIG. 3). However, when equivalent doses of morphine and methadone were administered to the mother, the response was threefold less for morphine compared to methadone[30] (FIG. 3). This is in complete agreement with the threefold difference in the extent of fetal exposure to the two opioid drugs.[11]

These studies represent the first attempt to correlate pharmacodynamic effects in the fetus with maternal-fetal pharmacokinetics, and support the notion that the intensity of drug effects in the fetus consequent to maternal drug use is determined by the extent of fetal drug exposure. More investigations in this area would provide greater support for the need of pharmacokinetic studies in the maternal-fetal unit.

Fetal Dose-Response Relationships

It was mentioned earlier that a full understanding of the effects of maternal drug use on the fetus would require a knowledge of the pharmacokinetics of the drug in the maternal-fetal unit and a knowledge of the pharmacodynamic actions of the drug in the fetus. While there has been much interest in quantitative analysis of drug disposition in the maternal-fetal unit, there have been fewer attempts to analyze dose-response relationships in the fetus quantitatively. We recently carried out some studies on the pharmacodynamic actions of morphine in the fetus and the findings not only revealed some unconventional dose-response relationships in the fetus but also suggested that fetal response to maternal drug consumption can be both *qualitatively* and *quantitatively* affected by the extent of fetal drug exposure.

There has been much confusion in the literature regarding the effects of morphine on fetal breathing movements (FBM). Morphine has been reported to both stimulate and suppress FBM in the fetal lamb.[30-35] The data in these conflicting reports were very difficult to compare, since different doses and routes of administration were employed in these studies. Some used constant rate iv infusions of morphine to the mother,[30] while others used iv bolus,[33,34] constant rate iv infusions,[30-32] or intracerebroventricular injections[35] to the fetus. This confusion prompted us to explore the full dose-response characteristics of morphine's effect on FBM. Interpretation of the data was facilitated by examining effects of morphine at steady state fetal plasma morphine levels achieved with constant rate iv infusions to the fetus.

When a large range of doses was examined in the fetal lamb, morphine was found to result in stimulation of FBM in some fetuses and suppression of FBM in others[36]

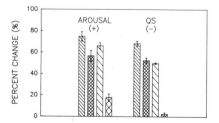

FIGURE 3. Percent changes in the incidence of arousal and quiet sleep (QS) during opiate infusion to either mother or fetus. □—morphine infusion to fetus, 2.5 mg/hr; □—methadone infusion to fetus, 2.5 mg/hr; □—morphine infusion to mother, 0.3 mg/kg/hr; □—methadone infusion to mother, 0.3 mg/kg/hr.

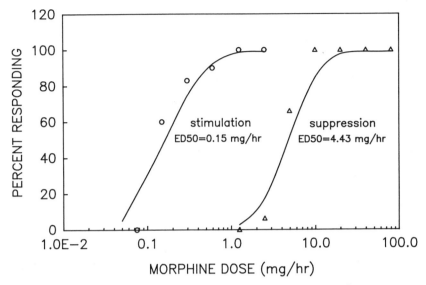

FIGURE 4. Quantal dose-response curve for stimulation ○ and suppression △ of FBM due to morphine administration. The ordinate corresponds to the percentage of fetuses responding. (From Szeto *et al.*[36] Reprinted by permission from the *Journal of Pharmacology and Experimental Therapeutics.*)

(FIG. 4). At doses ranging from 0.15 to 2.5 mg/hr, increasing morphine doses resulted in an increase in the percentage of animals responding by stimulation of FBM. At doses greater than 2.5 mg/hr, an increasing number of animals responded by a decrease in FBM. Probit analysis revealed that there was a 30-fold difference between the ED_{50} for stimulation and for suppression[36] (FIG. 4). These data illustrate that the quantal dose-response relationship is upheld in the fetus, and that morphine can exert opposing actions on FBM depending on the extent of fetal drug exposure.

The graded dose-response curve for the effects of morphine on the incidence of FBM was found to be biphasic (FIG. 5, top panel), with a dose-dependent increase at lower doses and a dose-dependent decrease at higher doses with total apnea observed in all animals at 80 mg/hr.[36] This transition from stimulation to suppression of FBM occurred over a very narrow dose range, and there is a certain dose along this curve that morphine would appear to have no effect. This dose-response relationship appears to be unique to the fetus as such dramatic respiratory stimulation is not seen in the adult, and stresses the importance of systematic pharmacodynamic investigation in the fetus.

Due to the biphasic nature of the graded dose-response curve, it could not be analyzed using conventional analytical procedures. We therefore sought to gain further understanding of these data by utilizing mathematical models to describe the interaction of morphine with its receptor-effector systems. It is important to emphasize that, as in pharmacokinetic modelling, such mathematical models are not meant to be exact representations of the enormously complicated chain of events leading from the contact between the molecules of drug and a biological entity to the ensuing effect.[37] Such biphasic curves have been predicted in the functional antagonism model

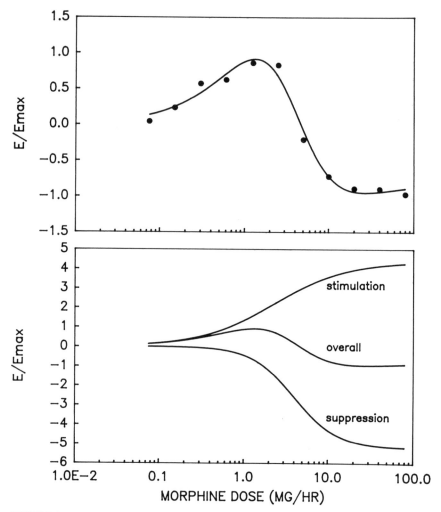

FIGURE 5. *Top panel* illustrates the best-fit curve obtained using the functional antagonism model (see APPENDIX 1) to describe the biphasic effects of morphine on FBM as a sum of two individual dose-response curves. *Bottom panel* is a computer simulation showing the contribution of the separate stimulation and suppression curves toward the overall response. (From Szeto *et al.*[36] Reprinted by permission from the *Journal of Pharmacology and Experimental Therapeutics.*)

proposed by Ariens *et al.*[38] It is proposed that the drug interacts with two independent receptor-effector systems, R1 and R2, causing effects that counteract each other. The overall effect would therefore be governed by the sum of the two independent dose-response curves (APPENDIX 1). When our data were fitted to the mathematical function describing such a model, an excellent fit was obtained as demonstrated by the curve in the top panel of FIGURE 5. With the parameter estimates obtained, we were able to simulate the two individual dose-response curves which are illustrated in the bottom panel of FIGURE 5. The parameter estimates revealed that there was a four-fold difference between the ED_{50} for stimulation and that for suppression of FBM.

The excellent fit of our data to the functional antagonism model suggests that the observed effect of morphine on FBM may be mediated via two different receptor-effector systems. Bennett et al.[35] have demonstrated that the suppression of FBM by morphine can be reversed by naloxone. We have evidence that the stimulation of FBM can also be abolished by naloxone pretreatment,[36] thus indicating that both effects are mediated by opioid receptors. However, due to the lack of specificity of naloxone,[39] it is possible that the dual action of morphine may involve two different opioid receptor

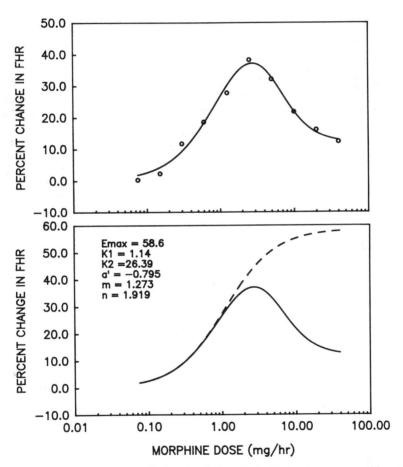

FIGURE 6. *Top panel* illustrates the best-fit solution obtained using the noncompetitive auto-inhibition model (see APPENDIX 2) to describe the bell-shaped dose-response curve of morphine on FHR. *Bottom panel* shows the best-fit curve (*solid line*) and the theoretical curve (*dashed line*) of morphine-induced tachycardia in the absence of autoinhibition. (From Zhu and Szeto.[43] Reprinted by permission from the *Journal of Pharmacology and Experimental Therapeutics.*)

subtypes. This proposal is supported by the relative lack of specificity of morphine for the different receptor subtypes,[39,40] and the qualitative differences between the actions of mu and delta agonists on adult respiratory function.[41,42] We are currently investigating the mechanisms of action of morphine on FBM.

Another unconventional dose-response relationship was seen when we examined the effect of morphine on fetal heart rate (FHR).[43] Doses of morphine ranging from 0.15 mg/hr to 2.5 mg/hr produced an increase in FHR. Further increase in dose, however, was associated with a decrease in the magnitude of response. This resulted in a bell-shaped dose-response curve as illustrated in the top panel of FIGURE 6. This dose-response relationship also appears to be unique to the fetus since bradycardia was not observed even at doses which completely abolished FBM and resulted in a slowing of the EEG.

Mathematical modelling was also attempted for the effects of morphine on FHR. Since bradycardia was never observed, it was felt that the noncompetitive autoinhibition model[44] would be more appropriate for these data. In this model, it is proposed that the drug interacts with two receptor-effector systems, R1 and R2. As a result of the interaction of the drug with R2, the affinity or intrinsic activity of the drug-receptor complex formed with R1 may be reduced. At high enough doses, the effect may become zero (APPENDIX 2). An excellent fit was also obtained for our data using this autoinhibition model[43] (FIG. 6, top panel). The dashed line in the bottom panel of FIGURE 6 illustrates the predicted dose-response curve in the absence of autoinhibition.

The excellent fit to the autoinhibition model suggested to us that the bell-shaped dose-response curve may again be due to morphine's interaction with multiple opioid receptor subtypes. We recently completed a series of studies exploring the effects of specific mu and delta agonists on FHR. Our results clearly indicate that mu agonists (DAGO) caused a dose-dependent tachycardia in the fetal lamb, while delta agonists (DPDPE) did not significantly affect FHR.[45] Thus interaction of morphine with the delta receptor would reduce the maximal effect that would be produced by its interaction with the mu receptor. The difference in affinity of morphine to R1 and R2 was estimated to be approximately 20-fold from the model, which is quite reasonable compared to the relative selectivity of morphine for the mu and delta receptor which has been shown to be approximately 10-fold in *in vitro* assays.[39,40]

CONCLUSIONS

It is hoped that this review has served to illustrate the complexities of drug action in the maternal-fetal unit. Mathematical modelling has been shown to be useful in enhancing our understanding of both maternal-fetal pharmacokinetics and pharmacodynamics. The magnitude of adverse effects in the fetus consequent to maternal drug use is clearly determined by the extent of fetal drug exposure. But in addition to maternal-fetal pharmacokinetics, drug effects may be further complicated by unconventional dose-response relationships in the fetus. Investigations to date indicate that fetal response to maternal drug consumption can be both qualitatively and quantitatively affected by the extent of fetal drug exposure. There continues to be a great need for systematic investigations of both pharmacokinetics and pharmacodynamics in the maternal-fetal unit.

REFERENCES

1. SZETO, H. H. 1982. Pharmacokinetics in the ovine maternal-fetal unit. Annu. Rev. Pharmacol. Toxicol. **22:** 221-243.
2. WANG, L. H., A. M. RUDOLPH & L. Z. BENET. 1986. Pharmacokinetic studies of the disposition of acetaminophen in the sheep maternal-placental-fetal unit. J. Pharmacol. Exp. Ther. **238:** 198-205.
3. BRIEN, J. F., D. W. CLARKE, B. RICHARDSON & J. PATRICK. 1985. Disposition of ethanol in maternal blood, fetal blood, and amniotic fluid of third trimester pregnant ewes. Am. J. Obstet. Gynecol. **152:** 583-590.
4. SZETO, H. H., L. I. MANN, A. BHAKTHAVATHSALAN, M. LIU & C. E. INTURRISI. 1978. Meperidine pharmacokinetics in the maternal-fetal unit. J. Pharmacol. Exp. Ther. **206:** 448-459.
5. SZETO, H. H., J. F. CLAPP, R. LARROW, J. HEWITT, C. E. INTURRISI & L. I. MANN. 1981. Disposition of methadone in the ovine maternal-fetal unit. Life Sci. **28:** 2111-2117.
6. GOLUB, M. S., J. H. EISELE & J. H. ANDERSON. 1986. Maternal-fetal distribution of morphine and alfentanil in near-term sheep and rhesus monkeys. Dev. Pharmacol. Ther. **9:** 12-22.
7. COOK, P. S., R. M. ABRAMS, M. NOTELOVITZ & J. E. FRISINGER. 1981. Effect of ethyl alcohol on maternal and fetal acid-base balance and cardiovascular status in chronic sheep preparations. Br. J. Obstet. Gynecol. **88:** 188-194.
8. CUMMING, M. E., B. Y. ONG, J. G. WADE & D. S. SITAR. 1984. Maternal and fetal ethanol pharmacokinetics and cardiovascular responses in near-term pregnant sheep. Can. J. Physiol. Pharmacol. **62:** 1435-1439.
9. CUMMING, M. E., B. Y. ONG, J. G. WADE & D. S. SITAR. 1985. Ethanol disposition in newborn lambs and comparisons of alcohol dehydrogenase activity in placenta and maternal sheep, fetal and neonatal lamb liver. Dev. Pharmacol. Ther. **8:** 338-345.
10. ABRAMS, R. M., C. E. COOK, K. H. DAVIS, K. NEIDERREITHER, M. J. JAEGER & H. H. SZETO. 1985. Plasma delta-9 tetrahydrocannabinol in pregnant sheep and fetus after inhalation of smoke from a marijuana cigarette. Alcohol Drug Res. **6:** 361-369.
11. SZETO, H. H., J. G. UMANS & J. MCFARLAND. 1982. A comparison of morphine and methadone disposition in the maternal-fetal unit. Am. J. Obstet. Gynecol. **143:** 700-706.
12. MIHALY, G. W., D. B. JONES, D. J. MORGAN, M. S. CHING, L. K. WEBSTER, R. A. SMALLWOOD & K. J. HARDY. 1983. Placental transfer and renal elimination of cimetidine in maternal and fetal sheep. J. Pharmacol. Exp. Ther. **227:** 441-445.
13. PRIUTT, A. W., J. L. MCNAY & P. G. DAYTON. 1975. Transfer characteristics of triamterene and its analogs. Central nervous system, placenta and kidney. Drug Metab. Dispos. **3:** 30-41.
14. ANDERSON, D. F., T. M. PHERNETTON & J. G. H. RANKIN. 1980. The placental transfer of acetylsalicylic acid in near-term ewes. Am. J. Obstet. Gynecol. **136:** 814-818.
15. ANDERSON, D. F., T. M. PHERNETTON & J. G. H. RANKIN. 1980. The measurement of placental drug clearance in near-term sheep: Indomethacin. J. Pharmacol. Exp. Ther. **213:** 100-104.
16. CHING, M. S., D. J. MORGAN, G. W. MIHALY, K. J. HARDY & R. A. SMALLWOOD. 1986. Placental transfer of omeprazole in maternal and fetal sheep. Dev. Pharmacol. Ther. **9:** 323-331.
17. SHOEMAN, D. W., R. E. KAUFFMAN, D. L. AZARNOFF & B. M. BOULOS. 1972. Placental transfer of diphenylhydantoin in the goat. Biochem. Pharmacol. **21:** 1237-1243.
18. ANDERSON, D. F., M. K. STOCK & J. H. G. RANKIN. 1979. Placental transfer of dexamethasone in near-term sheep. J. Dev. Physiol. **1:** 431-436.
19. BIEHL, D., S. M. SHNIDER, G. LEVINSON & K. CALLENDER. 1978. Placental transfer of lidocaine: Effects of fetal acidosis. Anesthesiology **48:** 409-412.
20. BRIEN, J. F., D. W. CLARKE, G. N. SMITH, B. RICHARDSON & J. PATRICK. 1987. Disposition of acute, multiple-dose ethanol in the near-term pregnant ewe. Am. J. Obstet. Gynecol. **157:** 204-211.
21. SZETO, H. H., J. G. UMANS & S. I. RUBINOW. 1982. The contribution of transplacental

clearances and fetal clearance to drug disposition in the ovine maternal-fetal unit. Drug Metab. Dispos. **10:** 382-386.

22. SZETO, H. H., R. F. KAIKO, J. F. CLAPP, R. W. LARROW, L. I. MANN & C. E. INTURRISI. 1979. Urinary excretion of meperidine by the fetal lamb. J. Pharmacol. Exp. Ther. **209:** 244-248.

23. SZETO, H. H., J. F. CLAPP, R. W. LARROW, C. E. INTURRISI & L. I. MANN. 1980. Renal tubular secretion of meperidine by the fetal lamb. J. Pharmacol. Exp. Ther. **213:** 346-349.

24. DUTTON, G. J. & J. E. A. LEAKEY. 1982. The perinatal development of drug metabolizing enzymes. Prog. Drug. Res. **25:** 189-273.

25. WANG, L. H., A. M. RUDOLPH & L. Z. BENET. 1986. Distribution and fate of acetaminophen conjugates in fetal lambs *in utero*. J. Pharmacol. Exp. Ther. **235:** 302-307.

26. MORISHIMA, H. O., M. FINSTER, H. PEDERSON, A. FUKUNAGA, R. RONFELD, H. G. VASSALLO & B. G. COVINO. 1979. Pharmacokinetics of lidocaine in fetal and neonatal lambs and adult sheep. Anesthesiology **50:** 431-436.

27. CLARK, A. J. 1937. General Pharmacology. *In* Heffter's Handbuch der Exp. Pharmakol., Vol. IV. Springer. Berlin.

28. SZETO, H. H. & D. J. HINMAN. 1985. Prenatal development of sleep-wake patterns in sheep. Sleep **8:** 347-355.

29. SZETO, H. H. 1983. Effects of narcotic drugs on fetal behavioral activity: Acute methadone exposure. Am. J. Obstet. Gynecol. **146:** 211-217.

30. UMANS, J. G. & H. H. SZETO. 1983. Effects of opiates on fetal behavioral activity. Life Sci. **33:** 639-642.

31. OLSEN, G. D., A. R. HOHIMER & M. D. MATHIS. 1983. Cerebral blood flow and metabolism during morphine-induced stimulation of breathing movements in fetal lambs. Life Sci. **33:** 751-754.

32. OLSEN, G. D. & G. S. DAWES. 1983. Morphine effects on fetal lambs. Fed. Proc. **42:** 1251.

33. SHELDON, R. E. & P. L. TOUBAS. 1984. Morphine stimulates rapid, regular, deep and sustained breathing efforts in fetal lambs. J. Appl. Physiol. **57:** 40-43.

34. TOUBAS, P. L., A. L. PRYOR & R. E. SHELDON. 1985. Effect of morphine on fetal electrocortical activity and breathing movements in fetal sheep. Dev. Pharmacol. Ther. **8:** 115-128.

35. BENNET, L., B. M. JOHNSTON & P. D. GLUCKMAN. 1986. The central effects of morphine on fetal breathing movements in the fetal sheep. J. Dev. Physiol. **8:** 297-305.

36. SZETO, H. H., Y. S. ZHU, J. G. UMANS, G. DWYER, S. CLARE & J. AMIONE. 1988. Dual action of morphine on fetal breathing movements. J. Pharmacol. Exp. Ther. **245:** 537-542.

37. VAN DER BRINK, F. G. 1977. General theory of drug-receptor interactions: Drug receptor interaction models and calculations of drug parameters. *In* Kinetics of Drug Action. J. M. van Rossum, Ed.: 169-254. Springer-Verlag. Berlin.

38. ARIENS, E. J., J. M. VAN ROSSUM & A. M. SIMONIS. 1956. A theoretical basis of molecular pharmacology. Part III. Interactions of one or two compounds with two independent receptor systems. Arch. Forsch. **6:** 737-746.

39. KOSTERLITZ, H. W., J. A. H. LORD, S. J. PATERSON & A. A. WATERFIELD. 1980. Effects of changes in the structure of enkephalins and of narcotic analgesic drugs on their interactions with mu and delta receptors. Br. J. Pharmacol. **68:** 333-342.

40. MOSBERG, H. I., R. HURST, V. J. HRUBY, K. GEE, H. I. YAMAMURA, J. J. GALLIGAN & T. F. BURKS. 1983. Bis-penicillamine enkephalins possess highly improved specificity toward opioid receptors. Proc. Natl. Acad. Sci. USA **80:** 5871-5874.

41. HADDAD, G. G., J. I. SCHAEFFER & K. J. CHANG. 1984. Opposite effects of the delta and mu receptor agonists on ventilation in conscious adult dogs. Brain Res. **323:** 73-82.

42. MORIN-SURUN, M. P., E. BOUDINOT, G. GACEL, J. CHAMPAGNAT, B. ROQUES & M. DENAVIT-SAUBIE. 1984. Different effects of μ and δ opiate agonists on respiration. Eur. J. Pharmacol. **98:** 235-240.

43. ZHU, Y. S. & H. H. SZETO. 1988. Morphine-induced tachycardia in fetal lambs: A bell-shaped dose-response curve. J. Pharmacol. Exp. Ther. In press.

44. ARIENS, E. J., J. M. VAN ROSSUM & A. M. SIMONIS. 1957. Affinity, intrinsic activity and drug interactions. Pharmacol. Rev. **9:** 208-269.

45. ZHU, Y. S., L. Q. CAI & H. H. SZETO. 1988. Differential effects of mu and delta opioid peptides on fetal heart rate. Submitted.

APPENDIX 1

The Functional Antagonism Model[38]

It is supposed that drug A acts on two different receptors, R1 and R2, to produce two opposite effects, stimulation of FBM (E1) and suppression of FBM (E2). In this case, the overall effect of drug A is described by the sum of the two opposite effects:

$$E = E1 + E2 = \frac{Emax1}{1 + k1/[A]^m} + \frac{Emax2}{1 + k2/[A]^n}$$

where Emax1 and Emax2 are the maximal response produced by system (1) and (2), respectively; k1 is the dissociation constant for system (1) and k2 for system (2); m and n are the respective Hill coefficients for the two systems; and [A] is the concentration of drug A.

APPENDIX 2

The Noncompetitive Autoinhibition Model[43]

It is supposed that the drug A has an affinity to both receptor 1 (R1) and receptor 2 (R2). It produces an effect on R1, but the effect originally produced on R2 may be negligible. As a result of the interaction of A with R2, the dissociation constant or the intrinsic activity of the complex formed by A and R1 may be changed. This interaction is represented by:

$$E = \frac{Emax}{1 + k1/[A]^m} \left(1 + \frac{a'}{1 + k2/[A]^n} \right)$$

where Emax is the maximal response produced by drug A on R1; a' is the intrinsic activity of A on R2 to induce the change in the effect produced by A with R1; k1 is the dissociation constant for [R1A]; k2 is the dissociation constant for [R2A]; m and n are the Hill coefficients for R1 and R2, respectively; and [A] is the concentration of drug A.

Pharmacogenetics of Drugs of Abuse

LOUIS SHUSTER

Department of Pharmacology
Tufts University School of Medicine
136 Harrison Avenue
Boston, Massachusetts 02111

A recurring theme in any consideration of drugs of abuse is the variability of individual responses. For example, half of a group of volunteers who were injected with morphine or heroin found that the experience was pleasurable. The others described it as unpleasant.[1] Obviously, prior experience and expectations are important influences when dealing with agents that are taken for the express purpose of producing euphoria or relaxation. However, variability is also encountered in carefully controlled animal experiments. According to Kreuger *et al.*[2] the lethal doses of morphine sulfate reported in the older literature range from 200 to 1200 mg per kg for "white mice," from 200 to 500 mg per kg for rats, 250 to 2000 mg per kg for guinea pigs, and 190 to 500 mg per kg for rabbits. There is growing evidence that an important component of this variability is genetic makeup. Any study of perinatal effects of drugs of abuse should also take into account genetic predisposition.

Sensitization to Perinatal Morphine

We had observed that the addition of morphine to cultured embryonic chick brain cells increased the activity of the enzymes choline acetyltransferase and acetylcholinesterase. *In vivo* increases were also produced by the injection of levorphanol into the yolk sacs of embryonated chick eggs.[3] When adult mice bearing a neuroblastoma were injected with morphine, enzyme activity was increased in the tumor but not in the mouse's brain.[4] These observations suggested that morphine could affect developing neuronal cells, and led to experiments with newborn mice.

Baby mice were injected subcutaneously twice daily with morphine sulfate or saline for 5 days. Beginning one to two months later, the running response to morphine, 25 mg per kg, was measured repeatedly at intervals of approximately 10 days. Mice that had been pretreated with morphine from days 13 through 17 showed a higher running response than controls that had been injected with saline. Mice that were pretreated with morphine on days 10-14 did not. For all mice the running response to morphine increased 2- to 3-fold during the course of repeated testing (FIG. 1). Perinatal treatment with morphine did not alter the analgesic response to morphine, as measured by the tail-flick assay.[5]

In subsequent experiments it was found that adult mice also displayed a long-lasting sensitization or reverse tolerance in their running response to morphine.[5] Thus the perinatal effects that we observed were actually characteristic of the mature rather than the developing brain. In attempting to explain why these unusual observations had not been reported by other workers we considered the possibility of genetic influences, because the mice we used were hybrids of 2 inbred strains, C57BL/6 and A. We therefore tested the parental strains.

Responses of Inbred Strains

As shown in FIGURE 2, we found that the response of the C57BL/6 strain was similar to that of the B_6AF_1 hybrid. However, mice of the A strain showed little running response to morphine, whether or not they had been pretreated. This finding is one example of the striking differences that one can encounter between inbred strains when studying drugs of abuse.

As indicated by genetic similarity matrix analysis, C57BL/6 mice differ from many other strains, including A, BALB/c and DBA/2, in a large number of genetic loci[6,7] (FIG. 3). Considerable work on genetics of responses to narcotic drugs has been carried out with strains DBA/2 and C57BL/6 (TABLE 1). Diallel analysis of crosses and backcrosses shows that with respect to the running response to morphine the C57BL/6 trait is dominant over DBA/2.[8]

There is considerable genetic correlation between neurochemical and pharmacologic responses to morphine. For example, morphine causes the release of dopamine from the striatum and limbic forebrain in C57BL/6 mice but not in DBA/2 mice.[9] C57BL/6 mice have more enkephalin receptors in the striatum[10] and more beta-endorphin in the pituitary[11] than DBA/2 mice.

In planning experiments on perinatal effects of drugs of abuse, one can select candidate inbred strains of mice or rats on the basis of known differences in their drug responses or in neurochemical parameters such as the activity of neurohormone-synthesizing enzymes.[12–18]

Selective Breeding

Inbred strains are extensively characterized and readily available, but they differ in thousands of genetic determinants. Their choice for perinatal or other experiments would be based on indirect correlations with other genetically controlled responses. A more direct approach to examining the genetic determinants involved would be to carry out selective breeding from an outbred foundation stock for the trait in question, such as perinatal effects. Some examples of selective breeding for responses to drugs of abuse, including ethanol, are listed in TABLE 2.

This procedure has several drawbacks, however.[19] Selective breeding is tedious and expensive, requiring from 20 to 40 generations of inbreeding, preferably from duplicate lines, in order to achieve homozygosity. During this time the genotype is changing continuously, so that replication of experiments, even in the same laboratory, is extremely difficult or impossible. Furthermore, in many cases the specificity of selection is not as clear-cut as one might expect. For example, selective breeding has been used to obtain 2 strains of mice, long-sleep and short-sleep, that differ markedly in their sensitivity to the hypnotic action of ethanol.[20] The genes controlling this difference appear to be pleiotropic, because they also affect the response to barbiturates, adenosine derivatives, and other central nervous system (CNS) depressants.[21,22] Similar results

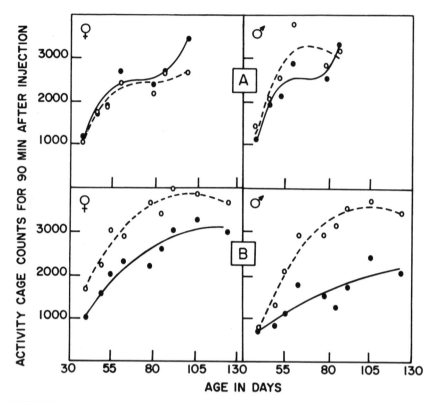

FIGURE 1. Running response to morphine of adult mice that had been pretreated with morphine as babies. Group (**A**) was injected from 10 through 14 days of age; group (**B**), from 13 through 17 days. Treated mice (*open circles*) were injected subcutaneously twice daily with morphine sulfate, 10 mg per kg on the first day, and 25 mg per kg on each of the following 4 days. Control mice (*closed circles*) were injected with 0.15 M sodium chloride. Each point represents the number of light beam interruptions by a group of 3 mice during the first 90 minutes after an intraperitoneal injection of morphine sulfate, 25 mg per kg. (From Shuster *et al.*[5] Reprinted by permission from the *Journal of Pharmacology and Experimental Therapeutics.*)

have been obtained with rats that were selectively bred for alcohol tolerance.[23,24] A genetic difference in responses to barbiturates was also encountered when mice were selectively bred for sensitivity to anesthesia by nitrous oxide.[25] There are cases where selective breeding for an apparently unrelated trait, such as open-field defecation[26] or voluntary saccharine consumption[27] in rats, also appears to select for differences in the consumption of or sensitivity to morphine.

In spite of these difficulties, the homozygous high-responding and low-responding lines obtained by selective breeding are generally better models for neurochemical analysis than widely separated inbred strains. A good example is the selection of alcohol-preferring and -nonpreferring lines of rats that also differ in the serotonin content of various brain regions.[28]

Recombinant-Inbred Strains

One difficulty in the genetic analysis of drug-related traits in inbred lines is the need to perform extensive crosses and back-crosses in attempts to establish linkage. Bailey has developed a series of recombinant-inbred (RI) strains in which the genes of two inbred parental strains are scrambled and then fixed in defined replicable combinations. The RI strains are derived by 40 generations of brother-sister matings from F_2 generation. Comparison of the drug responses of a battery of RI strains with those of the progenitor strains can be used to establish linkage with histocompatibility loci as determined by skin grafting.[29] The probability of detecting linkage depends upon the numbers of markers that have been typed, and on the number of RI strains that are available. For the seven RI strains derived from C57BL/6 and BALB/c, the definition of 80 known loci yields a probability of defining linkage of 0.37. For the 24 strains derived from C57BL/6 and DBA/2, the same number of loci would increase the probability to 0.7.[30] One recently described set, derived from C57BL/6 and the A strain, contains 48 RI lines.[31] A listing of other RI sets is provided by Bailey.[32]

RI analysis is most effective when a large difference between progenitor strains is controlled by a single gene. The results to date with various drugs of abuse have not yielded a clear-cut definition of genetic determinants, although several may fit a 2-locus model.[33,34]

One of the RI strains derived from C57BL/6 and BALB/c differs in its analgesic response to morphine from both progenitors. The low analgesic response seems to

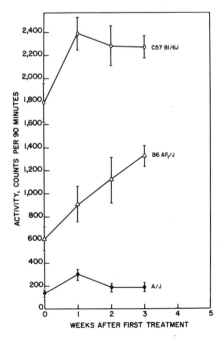

FIGURE 2. Changes in the running response of C57BL/6J, A/J and B_6AF_1/J hybrid mice to repeated injections of morphine sulfate. Each point is the mean ± SEM for 10 male mice tested individually after the i.p. injection of 25 mg per kg morphine sulfate (From Shuster *et al.*[5] Reprinted by permission from the *Journal of Pharmacology and Experimental Therapeutics.*)

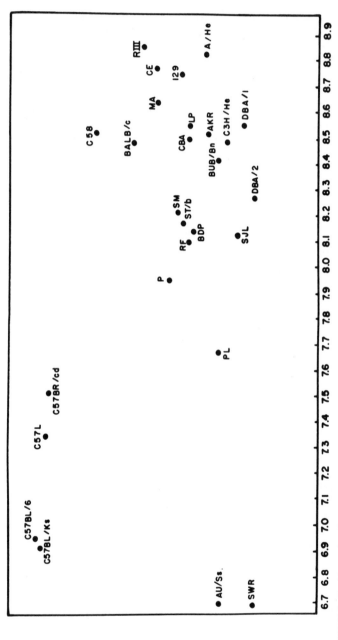

FIGURE 3. Positions of 27 inbred mouse strains in a 2-dimensional genetic similarity matrix (From Taylor.[6] Reprinted by permission from the *Journal of Heredity*.)

TABLE 1. Some Neuropharmacological Differences between C57BL/6 and DBA/2 Mice[a]

Drug or Treatment	Parameter	C57BL/6	DBA/2	Reference
Morphine	analgesia	+	+ +	8
	motor activity	+	0	8
	striatal adenylate cyclose	+	0	9
	striatal GMP	0	+	9
	drinking preference	+	0	53
	plasma CAMP and			
	cGMP	+	0	70
	caudate choline acetylase	−	0	71
	hypothermia	+	+ +	72
	respiratory rate	−	− −	72
Ethyl ketocyclazocine	analgesia	+	+ +	73
Butorphanol	analgesia	0	+	74
Naloxone	motor activity	+	−	75
	discrimination learning	−	+	76
	withdrawal jumping after morphine	+ +	+	77
FK 33-824	motor activity	+	−	78
Pentobarbital	sleep time	+	+ +	79
Ethanol	motor activity	−	+	14
	drinking preference	+	0	80
	sleep time after 3.3 g/kg	28 min	83 min	81
	release of dopamine from straitum	+	+ +	14
	withdrawal seizures	+	+ +	59
	β-endorphin in hypothalamus	−	0	82
Muscimol	motor activity	−	+	83
Apomorphine	motor activity	+ +	−	89
	climbing	+ +	0	
Nicotine	rate of respiration	0	−	84
Tobacco smoke	motor activity	−	+	85
Caffeine	motor activity	+	+ +	86
BDZ antagonist (FG7142)	seizures	+	+ +	87
Loud noise	audiogenic seizures	0	+	88
Electric shock	seizures	+ +	+	88
Stress (defeat)	analgesia	+	+ +	67

[a] Adapted from Shuster.[62] An increase is indicated by +, a decrease by −, and no change by 0.

result from a decreased number of mu receptors in the brain, as defined by the administration of specific agonists[33,35-38] and the binding of various ligands[39,35,40] (FIG. 4). Moskowitz *et al.* have demonstrated regional differences in narcotic receptors.[41] There is apparently no difference in the number of mu receptors in the spinal cord.[38] CXBK mice are also much less sensitive than the progenitors to endogenous opioid peptides released by acupuncture,[42] the stress of defeat[43] or foot-shock.[44]

Bailey[32] has re-analyzed the naloxone-binding data of Baran *et al.*[39] As shown in TABLE 3 and FIGURE 5, the results fit a 2-locus model in which one of the genes has an epistatic effect. With the isolation of mu receptors[45] it may eventually become possible to define these genes in terms of polypeptide chains that make up the receptor.

TABLE 2. Selective Breeding for Responses to Drugs of Abuse

Species	Drug or Treatment	Response	Reference
Mouse	ethanol	sleeptime	20
		withdrawal severity	60, 90
	nitrous oxide	anesthesia and barbiturate hypnosis	24
	morphine	analgesia	91
		running activity	92
	diazepam	ataxia	93
	cold water stress	analgesia after stress or morphine	63
Rat	ethanol	voluntary consumption	23, 27, 55

Congenic Lines and Defined Mutants

Congenic lines have been produced by repeated back-crossing from the F_1 generation to one of the parental strains. The resulting genotypes are very similar to that strain except for the presence of a small portion of one chromosome from the other strain.[46] If they exhibit drug responses attributed to the minor progenitor strain, congenic lines can be used to localize the genetic determinants involved.

More exact definition can sometimes be achieved by screening defined mutants. Examples of mutants of C57BL/6 mice that differ from the parental strain in their responses to morphine are shown in FIGURE 6 and TABLE 4. The genes detected in this way are pleiotropic, because the mutant strains were originally defined on the basis of coat color or physical defects. It is intriguing that the locus of each of the mutants described here is on a different chromosome.

The case of the Beige-J mutant is unusual because this mouse is also immunologically defective. Splenectomy of Beige mice restores their analgesic response to centrally administered morphine. The transfer of B lymphocytes from Beige mice to normal heterozygotic littermates leads to a 75% decrease in the analgesic response to morphine after 8 days. Binding assays have not revealed any difference between mutant and progenitor mice in the number of narcotic receptors in the brain. These findings suggest that B lymphocytes, or some substance produced by them, can influence the response of narcotic receptors in the brain.[47,48]

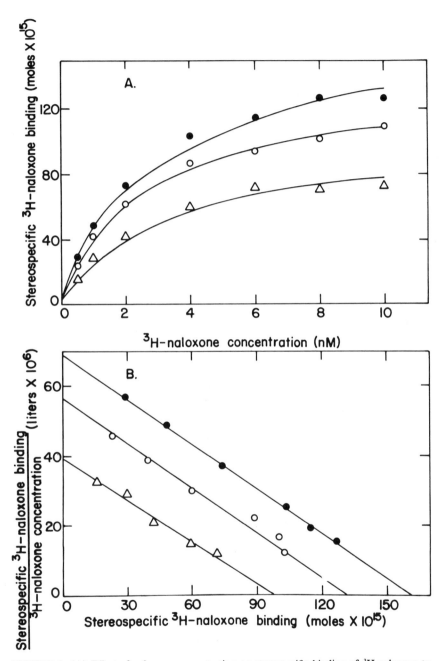

FIGURE 4. (A) Effect of naloxone concentration on sterospecific binding of ^{3}H-naloxone to brain homogenates from different strains. (B) Scatchard plot of ^{3}H-naloxone binding to brain homogenates from different mouse strains. *Closed circles*: CXBH; *triangles*: CXBK; *open circles*: all other strains (From Baran *et al.*[39] Reprinted by permission from *Life Sciences.*)

TABLE 3. A 2-locus Model to Describe the Genetics of Naloxone Binding in RI mice[a]

Strain	Naloxone Bound, cpm per mg protein[b] $+$ SEM	Designated Genotype
CXBH	1044 $\pm$ 33	$A_2A_2B_1B_1$
C57BL6/By	968 $\pm$ 25	$A_2A_2B_2B_2$
BALB/c	948 $\pm$ 26	$A_1A_1B_1B_1$
CXBJ	952 $\pm$ 27	
CXBI	940 $\pm$ 27	
CXBE	934 $\pm$ 25	
CXBD	983 $\pm$ 24	
CXBG	884 $\pm$ 21	
CXBK	609 $\pm$ 30	$A_1A_1B_2B_2$

[a] Adapted from Bailey.[32]
[b] Data from Baran et al.[39]

Much more remains to be done to examine the drug responses of the hundreds of defined mouse mutants that are available.

Subline Comparisons

A small number of genetic differences, attributable to new mutations and residual heterozygosity, serves to distinguish colonies of the same strain that have been maintained in separate laboratories. For example, the Bailey (By) and Jackson (J) sublines of strain C57BL/6 differ by approximately 50 gene pairs.[49] It is extremely unlikely that a difference between these sublines in their response to a particular drug such as morphine could be the result of more than one gene difference. TABLE 5 and FIGURES 7 and 8 illustrate some of the responses of these two sublines to endogenous and

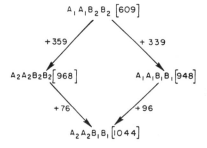

FIGURE 5. Effects of gene substitutions on the binding of naloxone. Phenotypic group means, *in brackets,* and designated genotypes are the same as in TABLE 3 (From Bailey.[32] Reprinted by permission from Academic Press.)

FIGURE 6. Analgesic response to morphine sulfate of C57BL/6J and homozygous and heterozygous single gene mutant mice. Each bar represents the mean ± SEM change in tailflick latency 30 minutes after the injection of morphine. The number of mice in each group is shown in parenthesis. A *star* indicates a significant difference from C57BL/6J, $p < 0.05$. (From Shuster.[67] Reprinted by permission from the National Institute on Drug Abuse.)

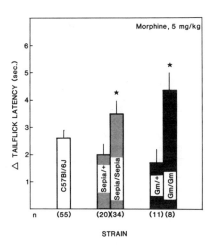

exogenous opioids and to other drugs that act on the CNS. Preliminary measurements suggest that the brains of By mice have a greater number of mu receptors than the brains of J mice.[50]

In the case of the BALB/c strain, mice of the By subline sleep twice as long after the injection of 4 g per kg of ethanol as mice of the J subline.[51] Unrelated adult males of the J subline will attack each other when caged together. Such aggression is not displayed by the NIH or Bailey sublines. Ciaranello *et al.*[52] have reported that mice of the Jackson subline have higher levels of enzymes for synthesizing epinephrine than those of the NIH subline. This difference appears to be controlled by a single dominant gene.

TABLE 4. Responses of Some Defined Mutants of Strain C57BL/6J Mice to Morphine[a]

Mutant	Chromosome Locus	Response	Difference from C57BL/6J	Reference
Pallid	2	motor activity	+	94
		hypothermia	+	94
Sepia	1	analgesia	+	67
		motor activity	+	67
Gunmetal	14	analgesia	+	67
		motor activity	+	67
Albino	7	motor activity	−	95
		hypothermia	−	95
Jimpy	x	analgesia	−	96
Beige-J	13	analgesia	−	47

[a] Adapted from Shuster.[69] + indicates greater than; − indicates less than.

Genetic Differences in Self-Administration

One of the questions that continues to exercise students of drug abuse is why certain individuals exhibit strong craving and drug-seeking behavior while others do not. Strain comparisons and selective breeding have indicated that there is a definite genetic component in these differences. For example, C57BL/6 mice will voluntarily drink enough morphine in a saccharine solution to kill them, whereas DBA/2 mice will not.[53] Lewis rats drink solutions of ethanol or the synthetic narcotic etonitazone more readily than Fisher rats.[54] Alcohol-preferring and -nonpreferring strains of rats have been obtained by selective breeding.[27,55]

In strain comparisons of voluntary oral consumption of drugs of abuse, it is important to take into account the possible role of genetic differences in taste-aversion. Dole et al.[56] have recently suggested, based on measurement of the nongenetic variance in the consumption of ethanol, that the apparent preference for ethanol solutions

TABLE 5. Some Differences in Drug and Stress Responses between the Bailey and Jackson Sublines of C57BL/6 Mice[a]

Drug or Treatment	Parameter	Response[b] By	J	Reference
Morphine	analgesia	++	+	97
	motor activity	+	+	97
d-amphetamine	motor activity	+	++	51
Stress (defeat)	analgesia	++	+	67
Dihydromorphine	binding sites in brain	++	+	50
Apomorphine	climbing	++	+	69
Cocaine	seizures	0	++	98

[a] Adapted from Shuster.[69]
[b] By and J refer to the Bailey and Jackson sublines respectively.

exhibited by C57BL/6 mice is really a reflection of their relative insensitivity to the aversive effects. This complication can be circumvented in animals that are trained to inject drugs through an intragastric catheter. Alcohol-preferring rats consistently consume more ethanol via this route than the nonpreferring strain.[57]

In some cases animals will self-administer ethanol only if they have previously been made physically dependent.[58] This observation raises the possibility that prevention of withdrawal may be a driving force for self-administration by an addicted individual. The availability of inbred[59] and selectively bred[60] strains of mice that differ in severity of withdrawal from ethanol provides useful tools for testing this hypothesis.

Nonspecific Responses

It is theoretically possible to have genetic differences in nonspecific responses to perinatal exposure to drugs of abuse. For example, Kinsley et al. found that heat and

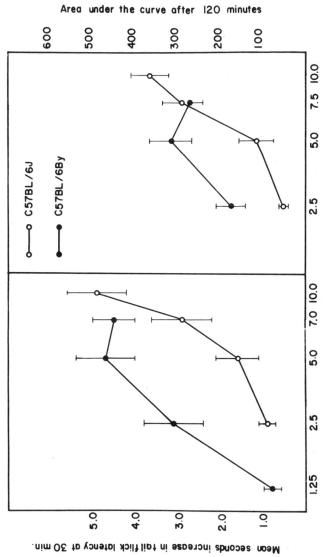

FIGURE 7. Analgesic response to morphine sulfate of the By and J sublines of C57BL/6 mice. Each point represents the mean value for 10 male mice (From Shuster.[68] Reprinted by permission from Academic Press.)

restraint applied to pregnant rats between days 15 and 22 produced a long-lasting alteration in both morphine-induced and stress-induced analgesia in the offspring.[61] Genetic differences in stress-induced analgesia have been described for inbred mouse strains,[62] and high- and low-responding lines have been produced by selective breeding.[63,64] The stress produced by administering and withdrawing drugs such as morphine or cocaine is not readily controlled for by injecting saline, and could easily have confounding effects. It might be helpful, in such experiments, to work with strains that do not exhibit perinatal effects of stress.

Genetic differences in metabolism need to be separated rom genetic differences in drug receptors. For example, the Afghan pika, a rabbitlike animal, does not respond to subcutaneous injections of morphine in doses as high as 500 mg per kg. In this species morphine actually antagonizes the analgesic effects of synthetic narcotics such as etorphine.[65] Forges et al.[66] found the same numbers and types of narcotic receptors in the brain of the pika as in the rabbit brain. They suggest that in the pika morphine may be metabolized to a substance that behaves as a narcotic antagonist.

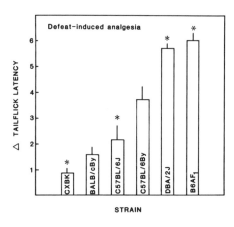

FIGURE 8. Defeat-induced analgesia in mice of 6 different strains. Each bar represents the mean ± SEM increase in tailflick latency after 70 attack bites. An *asterisk* indicates a significant difference from C57BL/6J, $p < 0.05$. (From Shuster.[67] Reprinted by permission from the National Institute on Drug Abuse.)

CONCLUDING REMARKS

Awareness of marked strain differences in responses to drugs of abuse is most helpful in selecting appropriate animal models and in the design of experiments on perinatal effects of drugs. Identification of the genetic determinants of a particular response may lead to new information about mechanisms of action. Many potentially useful strains and mutants have not yet been screened for their responses to drugs of abuse. A great deal remains to be done in terms of receptor mapping, analysis of restriction fragment polymorphisms and sequencing of genes for receptors. In addition, it is important to define genetic differences in pharmacokinetics and drug metabolism. Meanwhile every investigator who is examining perinatal effects of drugs of abuse should be aware that pharmacogenetic variables can confound experimental results, as well as provide new opportunities to ask meaningful questions.

REFERENCES

1. LASAGNA, L., J. M. VON FELSINGER & H. K. BEECHER. 1955. Drug-induced mood changes in man. I. Observations on healthy subjects, chronically ill patients and post-addicts. J. Am. Med. Assoc. **157:** 1006-1020.
2. KREUGER, H., N. B. EDDY & M. SUMWALT. 1941. The pharmacology of the opium alkaloids. Supplement No. 165 to the Public Health Reports: 636. U.S. Public Health Service. Washington, DC.
3. PETERSON, G. R., G. W. WEBSTER & L. SHUSTER. 1974. Effect of narcotics on enzymes of acetylcholine metabolism in cultured cells from embryonic chick brains. Neuropharmacology **13:** 365-376.
4. PETERSON, G. R. & L. SHUSTER. 1973. Effects of morphine on choline acetyltransferase and acetylcholinesterase in cultured mouse neuroblastoma. Proc. West. Pharmacol. Soc. **16:** 129-133.
5. SHUSTER, L., G. W. WEBSTER & G. YU. 1975. Increased running response to morphine in morphine-pretreated mice. J. Pharmacol. Exp. Ther. **192:** 64-72.
6. TAYLOR, B. A. 1972. Genetic relationships between inbred strains of mice. J. Hered. **63:** 83-86.
7. GUTTMAN, R. & L. GUTTMAN. 1974. Nonmetric analysis of genetic relationships among inbred strains of mice. Syst. Zool. **23:** 355-362.
8. CASTELLANO, C. & A. OLIVERIO. 1975. A genetic analysis of morphine-induced running and analgesia in the mouse. Psychopharmacology **41:** 197-200.
9. RACAGNO, G., F. BRUNO, E. JULIANO & R. PAOLETTI. 1979. Differential sensitivity to morphine-induced analgesia and motor activity in two inbred strains of mice: Behavioral and biochemical correlations. J. Pharmacol. Exp. Ther. **209:** 111-116.
10. REGGIANI, A., F. BATTAINI, H. KOBAYASHI, P. SPANO & M. TRABUCCHO. 1980. Genotype-dependent sensitivity to morphine: Role of different opiate receptor populations. Brain Res. **189:** 289-294.
11. CRABBE, J. C., JR., R. G. ALLEN, N. D. GAUDETTE, E. YOUNG, A. KOSOBUD & J. STACK. 1981. Strain differences in pituitary-endorphin and ACTH content in inbred mice. Brain Res. **219:** 219-223.
12. INGRAM, D. K. & T. P. CORFMAN. 1980. An overview of neurobiological comparisons in mouse strains. Neurosci. Biobehav. Rev. **4:** 421-435.
13. KERR, L. M., A. S. UNIS & J. K. WAMSLEY. 1988. Comparison of the density and distribution of brain D-1 and D-2 dopamine receptors in Buffalo vs. Fischer 344 rats. Pharmacol. Biochem. Behav. **30:** 325-330.
14. KIIANMAA, K. & B. TABAKOFF. 1983. Neurochemical correlates of tolerance and strain differences in the neurochemical effects of ethanol. Pharmacol. Biochem. Behav. **18** (Suppl. 1): 383-388.
15. SANGHERA, M. K., I. FUCHS, E. WEIDMER-MIKHAIL & S. G. SPECIALE. 1987. Met-enkephalin levels in midbrain dopamine regions of inbred mouse strains which differ in the number of dopamine neurons. Brain Res. **412:** 200-203.
16. YOSHIMOTO, K. & S. KOMURA. 1987. Reexamination of the relationship between alcohol preferences and brain monoamines in inbred strains of mice including senescence-accelerated mice. Pharmacol. Biochem. Behav. **27:** 317-322.
17. CLEMENT, J., S. SIMLER, L. CIESIELSKI, P. MANDEL, S. CABIBE & S. PUBLISI-ALLEGRA. 1987. Age-dependent changes of GABA levels, turnover rates and shock-induced aggressive behavior in inbred strains of mice. Pharmacol. Biochem. Behav. **26:** 83-88.
18. BOEHME, R. R. & R. D. CIARANELLO. 1981. Dopamine receptor binding in inbred mice: Strain differences in mesolimbic and nigrostriatal dopamine binding sites. Proc. Natl. Acad. Sci. USA **78:** 3255-3259.
19. BROADHURST, P. L. 1978. Drugs and the Inheritance of Behavior. A Study of Comparative Psychopharmacogenetics. Plenum, New York, NY. p. 11.
20. MCLEARN, G. E. & S. M. ANDERSON. 1979. Genetics and ethanol tolerance. Drug Alcohol Depend. **4:** 61-76.
21. MORLEY, R. J., L. L. MINER, J. M. WEHNER & A. C. COLLINS. 1986. Differential effects of central nervous system depressants in long-sleep and short-sleep mice. J. Pharmacol. Exp. Ther. **238:** 1028-1033.

22. McINTYRE, T. D. & H. P. ALPERN. 1985. Reinterpretation of the literature indicates differential sensitivities of long-sleep and short-sleep mice are not specific to alcohol. Psychopharmacology **87**: 379-389.

23. HELLEVUO, K., K. KIIANMAA, A. JUHAKOSKI & C. KIM. 1987. Intoxicating effects of lorazepam and barbital in rat lines selected for differential sensitivity to ethanol. Psychopharmacology **91**: 263-267.

24. MAYER, J. M., M. M. KHANNA, C. KIM & H. KALANT. 1983. Differential pharmacological responses to ethanol, pentobarbital and morphine in rats selectively bred for ethanol sensitivity. Psychopharmacology **81**: 6-9.

25. KOBLIN, D. D., F. W. LURZ, B. O'CONNOR, N. T. NELSON, E. I. EGER II & C. R. BAINTON. 1984. Potencies of barbiturates in mice selectively bred for resistance or susceptibility to nitrous oxide anesthesia. Anesth. Analg. **63**: 35-39.

26. SATINDER, K. P. 1982. Alcohol-morphine interaction: Oral intake in genetically selected Maudsley rats. Pharmacol. Biochem. Behav. **16**: 707-711.

27. LIEBLICH, I., E. COHEN, J. R. GONCHROW, E. M. BLASS & F. BERGMANN. 1983. Morphine tolerance in genetically selected rats induced by chronically elevated saccharine intake. Science **221**: 871-873.

28. LI, T.-K., L. LUMENG, W. J. McBRIDE, M. B. WALLER & J. M. MURPHY. 1986. Studies on an animal model of alcoholism. *In* Genetic and Biological Markers in Drug Abuse and Alcoholism. M. C. Braude & H. M. Chao, Eds.: 41-49. NIDA Research Monograph 66. National Institute on Drug Abuse. Rockville, MD.

29. BAILEY, D. W. 1971. Recombinant inbred strains. Transplantation **11**: 325-327.

30. TAYLOR, B. A. 1978. Recombinant-inbred strains: Use in gene mapping. *In* Origins of Inbred Mice. H. C. Morse III, Ed.: 423-438.

31. NESBITT, M. N. & E. SKAMENE. 1984. Recombinant inbred mouse strains derived from A/J and C57BL/6J: A tool for the study of genetic mechanisms in host resistance to infection and malignancy. J. Leuk. Biol. **36**: 357-364.

32. BAILEY, D. W. 1981. Recombinant inbred strains and bilineal congenic strains. *In* The Mouse in Biomedical Research. H. L. Foster, J. D. Small & J. G. Fox, Eds. Vol. 1: 223-239. Academic Press. New York, NY.

33. SHUSTER, L., G. W. WEBSTER, G. YU & B. E. ELEFTHERIOU. 1975. A genetic analysis of the response to morphine in mice: Analgesia and running. Psychopharmacology **42**: 249-254.

34. OLIVERIO, A., C. CASTELLANO & B. E. ELEFTHERIOU. 1975. Morphine sensitivity and tolerance. A genetic investigation in the mouse. Psychopharmacologia **42**: 219-224.

35. JACOB, J., G. MICHAUD, M. A. NICOLA & N. PRUDHOMME. 1983. Genetic differences in opioid binding sites and in antinociceptive activities of morphine and ethylketo-cyclazocine. Life Sci. **33**(Suppl. I): 645-648.

36. RAFFA, R. B., J. R. MATHIASEN & H. I. JACOBY. 1987. Colonic bead expulsion time in normal and μ-opioid receptor deficient (CXBK) mice following central (ICV) administration of μ- and delta-opioid agonists. Life Sci. **41**: 2229-2234.

37. MOSKOWITZ, A. S., G. W. TERMAN, K. R. CARTER, M. J. MORGAN & J. C. LIEBESKIND. 1985. Analgesic, locomotor and lethal effects of morphine in the mouse: Strain comparisons. Brain Res. **361**: 46-51.

38. VAUGHT, J. L., J. R. MATHIASEN & R. B. RAFFA. 1988. Examination of the involvement of supraspinal and spinal MU and Delta opioid receptors in analgesia using the MU receptor deficient CXBK mouse. J. Pharmacol. Exp. Ther. *245:* 13-16.

39. BARAN, A., L. SHUSTER, B. E. ELEFTHERIOU & D. W. BAILEY. 1975. Opiate receptors in mice: Genetic differences. Life Sci. **17**: 633-640.

40. REITH, M. E. A., H. SERSHEN, C. VADASZ & A. LAJTHA. 1981. Strain differences in opiate receptors in mouse brain. Eur. J. Pharmacol. **74**: 377-380.

41. MOSKOWITZ, A. S. & R. R. GOODMAN. 1985. Autoradiographic analysis of MU_1, MU_2, and delta opioid binding in the central nervous system of C57BL/6By and CXBK (opioid receptor-deficient) mice. Brain Res. **360**: 108-116.

42. PEETS, J. M. & B. POMERANZ. 1978. CXBK mice deficient in opiate receptors show poor electroacupuncture analgesia. Nature **273**: 675-676.

43. MICZEK, K. A., M. L. THOMPSON & L. SHUSTER. 1982. Opioid-like analgesia in defeated mice. Science **215**: 1520-1522.

44. MOSKOWITZ, A. S., G. W. TERMAN & J. C. LIEBESKIND. 1985. Stress-induced analgesia in the mouse: Strain comparisons. Pain 23: 67-72.
45. CHO, T. M., J. I. HASEGAWA, B. L. GE & H. H. LOH. 1986. Purification to apparent homogeneity of a μ-type opioid receptor from rat brain. Proc. Natl. Acad. Sci. (USA) 83: 4138-4142.
46. BAILEY, D. W. 1975. Genetics of histocompatibility in mice: New loci and congenic lines. Immunogenetics 2: 249-256.
47. MATHIASEN, J. R., R. B. RAFFA & J. L. VAUGHT. 1987. C57BL/6J-bg^J (beige) mice: Differential sensitivity in the tail flick test to centrally administered μ- and delta-opioid receptor agonists. Life Sci. 40: 1989-1994.
48. RAFFA, R. B., J. MATHIASEN & E. S. KIMBALL. 1988. Transfer of defective analgesic response to morphine by adoptive transfer of spleen cells. FASEB J. 2: A1261.
49. BAILEY, D. W. 1978. Sources of subline divergence and their relative importance for sublines of six major inbred strains of mice. In Origins of Inbred Mice. H. C. Morse III, Ed.: 197-215.
50. CREMINS, J. & L. SHUSTER. 1982. A genetically controlled difference in morphine analgesia and narcotic receptors in mice. Fed. Proc. 41: 1314.
51. MOISSET, B. 1978. Subline differences in behavioral responses to pharmacological agents. In Origins of Inbred Mice. H. C. Morse III, Ed.: 483-484.
52. CIARANELLO, R. D., H. J. HOFFMAN, J. G. M. SHIRE & J. AXELROD. 1974. Genetic regulation of catecholamine biosynthetic enzymes. II. Inheritance of tyrosine hydroxylase, dopamine hydroxylase and phenylethanolamine methyl transferase. J. Biol. Chem. 249: 4520-4536.
53. HOROWITZ, G. P., G. WHITNEY, J. C. SMITH & F. K. STEPHAN. 1977. Morphine ingestion: Genetic control in mice. Psychopharmacology 52: 119-122.
54. GEORGE, F. R. 1987. Genetic and environmental factors in ethanol self-administration. Pharmacol. Biochem. Behav. 27: 379-384.
55. ERIKSSON, K. & M. RUSI. 1981. Finnish selection studies on alcohol-related behaviors: General outline. In Development of Animal Models as Pharmacogenetic Tools. NIAA Research Monograph 6: 87-117. National Institute on Alcohol Abuse. Rockville, MD.
56. DOLE, V. P., A. HO, R. T. GENTRY & A. CHIN. 1988. Toward an analogue of alcoholism in mice: Analysis of nongenetic variance in consumption of alcohol. Proc. Natl. Acad. Sci. USA 85: 827-830.
57. WALLER, M. B., W. J. MCBRIDE, G. J. GATTO, L. LUMENG & T. K. LI. 1984. Intragastric ethanol self-administration by ethanol-preferring and -nonpreferring lines of rats. Science 225: 78-80.
58. DEUTSCH, J. A. & A. EISNER. 1977. Ethanol self-administration in the rat induced by forced drinking of ethanol. Behav. Biol. 20: 81-90.
59. CRABBE, J. C., JR., E. R. YOUNG & A. KOSOBUD. 1983. Genetic correlations with ethanol withdrawal severity. Pharmacol. Biochem. Behav. 18: 541-547.
60. CRABBE, J. C., JR., A. KOSOBUD & E. R. YOUNG. 1983. Genetic selection for ethanol withdrawal severity: Differences in replicate mouse lines. Life Sci. 33: 955-962.
61. KINSLEY, C. H., P. E. MANN & R. S. BRIDGES. 1988. Prenatal stress alters morphine- and stress-induced analgesia in male and female rats. Pharmacol. Biochem. Behav. 30: 123-128.
62. JACOB, J. J., M.-A. NICOLA, G. MICHAUD, C. VIDAL & N. PRUDHOMME. 1986. Genetic modulations of stress-induced analgesia in mice. Ann. N.Y. Acad. Sci. 467: 104-115.
63. PANOCKA, I., P. MAREK & B. SADOWSKI. 1986. Inheritance of stress-induced analgesia in mice, selective breeding study. Brain Res. 397: 152-155.
64. PANOCKA, I., P. MAREK & B. SADOWSKI. 1986. Differentiation of Neurochemical basis of stress-induced analgesia in mice by selective breeding. Brain Res. 397: 156-160.
65. PUGET, A., J. CROSS & J. C. MEUNIER. 1979. The natural tolerance of the Afghan pika (Ochotona rufescens) to morphine. Eur. J. Pharmacol. 53: 343-349.
66. FARGES, R. C., A. PUGET, C. MOISAND & J. C. MEUNIER. 1988. Opioid receptor types in the brain of the Afghan pika (ochotona rufescens), a species which is naturally tolerant to morphine. Life Sci. 43: 659-664.
67. SHUSTER, L. 1984. Genetic determinants of responses to drugs of abuse: An evaluation of research strategies. In Mechanisms of Tolerance and Dependence. NIDA Research

Monograph 54. C. W. Sharp, Ed.: 50-69. National Institute on Drug Abuse. Rockville, MD.

68. SHUSTER, L. 1987. Pharmacogenetics of drugs of abuse. *In* Genetic and Perinatal Effects of Abused Substances. M. C. Braude & A. M. Zimmerman, Eds.: 27-42. Academic Press. Orlando, FL.

69. SHUSTER, L. 1986. Genetic markers of drug abuse in mouse models. *In* Genetic and Biological Markers in Drug Abuse and Alcoholism. NIDA Research Monograph 66. M. D. Braude & H. M. Chao, Eds.: 71-85. National Institute on Drug Abuse. Rockville, MD.

70. MURAKI, T., H. UZUMAKI & R. KATO. 1982. Strain difference in morphine-induced increase in plasma cyclic AMP and cyclic GMP levels in relation to locomotor activity in male mice. Psychopharmacology 76: 316-319.

71. EBEL, A., T. DURKIN, G. AYAD, G. MACK & P. MANDEL. 1980. Genetically determined cholinergic involvement in morphine-induced behavioral responses in mice. Neuropharmacology 19: 423-427.

72. MURAKI, T. & R. KATO. 1986. Strain difference in the effects of morphine on the rectal temperature and respiratory rate in male mice. Psychopharmacology 89: 60-64.

73. GWYNNE, G. J. & E. F. DOMINO. 1984. Genotype-dependent behavioral sensitivity to mice vs. kappa opiate agonists. II. Antinociceptive tolerance and physical dependence. J. Pharmacol. Exp. Ther. 231: 312-316.

74. FILIBECK, V., C. CASTELLANO & A. OLIVERIO. 1981. Differential effects of opiate agonists—antagonists on morphine-induced hyperexcitability and analgesia in mice. Psychopharmacology 73: 134-136.

75. CASTELLANO, C. & S. PUGLISI-ALLEGRA. 1982. Effects of naloxone and naltrexone on locomotor activity in C57BL/6 and DBA/2 mice. Pharmacol. Biochem. Behav. 16: 561-563.

76. CASTELLANO, C. 1981. Strain-dependent effects of naloxone on discrimination learning in mice. Psychopharmacology 73: 152-156.

77. BRASE, D., H. H. LOH & E. L. WAY. 1977. Comparison of the effects of morphine on locomotor activity, analgesia and primary and protracted physical dependence in six mouse strains. J. Pharmacol. Exp. Ther. 201: 368-374.

78. CASTELLANO, C. 1981. Strain-dependent effects of the enkephalin analogue FK33-824 on locomotor activity in mice. Pharmacol. Biochem. Behav. 15: 729-734.

79. NABESHIMA, T. & I. K. HO. 1980. Pharmacological responses to pentobarbital in different strains of mice. J. Pharmacol. Exp. Ther. 216: 198-204.

80. RODGERS, D. A. 1966. Factors underlying differences in alcohol preference among inbred strains of mice. Psychosom. Med. 28: 498-513.

81. SPUHLER, K., B. HOFFER, N. WEINER & M. PALMER. 1982. Evidence for genetic correlation of hypnotic effects and cerebellar Purkinje neuron depression in response to ethanol in mice. Pharmacol. Biochem. Behav. 17: 569-578.

82. GIANOULAKIS, C. & A. GUPTA. 1986. Inbred strains of mice with variable sensitivity to ethanol exhibit differences in the content and processing of B-endorphin. Life Sci. 39: 2315-2325.

83. VAN ABEELEN, J. H. F. & H. J. L. M. BOERSMA. 1984. A genetically controlled hippocampal transmitter system regulating exploratory behavior in mice. J. Neurogenet. 1: 153-158.

84. MARKS, M. J., J. B. BURCH & A. C. COLLINS. 1983. Genetics of nicotine response in four inbred strains of mice. J. Pharmacol. Exp. Ther. 226: 291-301.

85. BAER, D. S., G. E. MCLEARN & J. R. WILSON. 1980. Effects of chronic administration of tobacco smoke to mice: Behavioral and metabolic measures. Psychopharmacology 67: 131-137.

86. BUCKHOLTZ, N. S. & L. D. MIDDAUGH. 1987. Effects of caffeine and L-Phenylisopropyladenosine on locomotor activity of mice. Pharmacol. Biochem. Behav. 28: 179-185.

87. NUTT, D. J. & R. G. LISTER. 1988. Strain differences in response to a benzodiazepine receptor inverse agonist (FG 7142) in mice. Psychopharmacology 94: 435-436.

88. SCHLESINGER, K. & S. K. SHARPLESS. 1975. Audiogenic seizures and acoustic priming. *In* Psychopharmacogenetics. B. E. Eleftheriou, Ed. Plenum Press. New York, NY.

89. CABIB, S. & S. PUGLISI-ALLEGRA. 1988. A classical genetic analysis of two apomorphine-induced behaviors in the mouse. Pharmacol. Biochem. Behav. **30:** 143-147.

90. GOLDSTEIN, D. B. 1973. Inherited differences in intensity of alcohol withdrawal reactions in mice. Nature **245:** 154-156.

91. BELKNAP, J. K., P. W. DANIELSON, S. E. LAURSEN & B. NOORDEWIER. 1987. Selective breeding for levorphanol-induced antinociception on the hotplate assay: Commonalities in mechanism of action with morphine, pentazocine, ethylketo-cyclazocine, U-50488H and clonidine in mice. J. Pharmacol. Exp. Ther. **241:** 477-481.

92. JUDSON, B. A. & A. GOLDSTEIN. 1978. Genetic control of opiate-induced locomotor activity in mice. J. Pharmacol. Exp. Ther. **206:** 56-60.

93. GALLAHER, E. J., L. E. HOLLISTER, S. E. GIONET & J. C. CRABBE. 1987. Mouse lines selected for genetic differences in diazepam sensitivity. Psychopharmacology **93:** 25-30.

94. KATZ, R. J. & R. L. DOYLE. 1980. Enhanced responses to opiates produced by a single gene substitution in the mouse. Eur. J. Pharmacol. **67:** 301-303.

95. KATZ, R. J. 1980. The albino locus produces abnormal responses to opiates in the mouse. Eur. J. Pharmacol. **68:** 229-232.

96. LAW, P. Y., R. A. HARRIS, H. H. LOH & E. L. WAY. 1978. Evidence for the involvement of cerebroside sulfate in opiate receptor binding: Studies with Azure A and Jimpy mutant mice. J. Pharmacol. Exp. Ther. **207:** 458-468.

97. SHUSTER, L. 1982. A pharmacogenetic approach to the brain. *In* Genetics of the Brain. I. Lieblich, Ed.: 157-176.

98. GEORGE, F. R. & S. R. GOLDBERG. 1988. Genetic differences in responses to cocaine. *In* Mechanisms of Cocaine Abuse and Toxicity. Research Monograph No. 88. D. Clouet, K. Asgar & R. Brown, Eds. 239-249. National Institute on Drug Abuse. Rockville, MD.

Exposure to Passive Cigarette Smoking and Child Development

A Critical Review

D. RUSH [b] AND K. R. CALLAHAN [c]

[b] Human Nutrition Research Center on Aging
Tufts University
711 Washington Street
Boston, Massachusetts 02111
and
[c] Division of Western Hemisphere Research
Beecham Products
1500 Littleton Road
Parsippany, New Jersey 07054

INTRODUCTION

While maternal cigarette smoking during pregnancy is profoundly related to the growth and survival of the fetus,[1] the nature and extent of effects on later development of the child are not at all clearly understood. In an attempt to clarify current knowledge, we will describe the design and some of the strengths and weaknesses of each of the studies known to us, and then summarize, across studies, relationships with somatic, cognitive, and behavioral development. The results of all studies are presented in detail in the tables.

Possible Confounding by Undercontrol

The major problem of drawing inference from observational studies comparing developmental outcomes of offspring of smokers and nonsmokers is undercontrol for social differences, since both the independent and dependent variables are strongly related to social status.

It is imperative to be cautious in assuming that we can efficiently match or statistically control for differences in all factors from the social environment that may be associated both with imputed causes and effects, such as the ones under consideration here. Smokers are known to be different in behavior, personality, and social status

[a] Supported by National Institute of Child Health and Human Development Grant RO1-HD13347.

from nonsmokers,[2-6] and such factors are strongly related to child development. Thus, while it is necessary to control for such differences in analysis it is almost surely illusory to assume that we can do so fully, since, within any stratum comparable on some index, such as occupational status, the smokers, are, on average, very likely to still be at a disadvantage.

Precisely this effect was observed by Rantakallio[7] in her study in northern Finland of development at age fourteen of children whose mothers had smoked during pregnancy, compared to a group of children matched on mother's marital status, age, parity, and place of residence. She found that within "each social class of the husband, the smoking mother was in a less favorable position in terms of (unemployment, sick leave or sick pension, not living with the family, or having died) than her nonsmoking counterpart (with minor exceptions)." Thus, within social class strata, smoking was associated with consistently adverse conditions for child development.

However, many of the differences in cognitive and neurological development in childhood reported in many studies to be associated with parental smoking were only minimally controlled for social factors, and while they may have been highly significant statistically, they cannot be straightforwardly interpreted as having been caused by smoking.

REVIEW OF SPECIFIC STUDIES

The National Child Development Study (NCDS) (TABLE 1)

All 16,000 children born in one week in March 1958 in Great Britain were studied at birth and at ages seven, 11 and 16.[8-12] Measures of physical, behavioral, and cognitive development have been reported from each postnatal follow-up, and those that were related to maternal smoking in pregnancy are presented in TABLE 1.

Definitions of smoking, and analytic procedures varied somewhat at different ages. Raw differences were adjusted for social class and several other pertinent factors for all four outcomes reported at age 11, and for parental height at age seven. For reading and social adjustment at age seven, and for all measures at age 16, the reported results were adjusted for birthweight. Unfortunately, adjusting for birthweight would tend to systematically underestimate the relationship of smoking during pregnancy with later child development, since cigarette smoking in pregnancy causes lowered birthweight. The reported decrements in reading achievement at age seven that were controlled for birthweight (1.0 month in children of light smokers, and 3.9 months in children of heavy smokers) thus were likely to be underestimates of real relationships.

At age seven, much of the relationship between maternal smoking during pregnancy with depressed stature was associated with lowered birthweight: among seven year old children of lighter smokers, the height difference was reduced from 0.60 cm to 0.40 cm by controlling for birthweight, and among children of heavy smokers, from 0.99 cm to 0.65 cm.

At age 11, with adjustment for social class, children of lighter smokers (< 10 cigarettes/day) were shorter by 0.57 cm, and retarded by 4.5 months in general ability, 3.1 months in reading achievement, and 4.7 months in mathematics achievement, compared to children of nonsmokers; for children of heavier smokers, the respective differences were 1.0 cm, 3.6 months, 3.7 months, and 4.9 months, compared to children of nonsmokers. These differences were all highly significant. Controlling for paternal occupational status (as well as the child's sex, maternal age and parity, and the number of younger sibs) caused an average reduction in the association of prenatal smoking to the four outcomes (height, general ability, reading and mathematics) of 48%. At age sixteen, only results adjusted for birthweight were presented. Effects on height were greater among boys, but, overall, differences appeared to be relatively stable over time.

Even though the relationships of maternal smoking to indices of child development at all ages remained highly significant after social class adjustment, it is clear that the profound social and demographic differences between smokers and nonsmokers in characteristics that were strongly associated with the developmental indices under study were unlikely to have been taken fully into account by statistical adjustment procedures, given both incompleteness of, and inherent measurement error in, the set of control variables.

National Collaborative Perinatal Project (NCPP) (TABLE 2)

The NCPP followed 58,000 pregnancies at 12 United States teaching centers, starting in the late 1950's, and most of the surviving children were then periodically examined to age seven. We are aware of six publications that related maternal smoking to later child development.

TABLE 1. Studies for the National Child Development Study (Great Britain). All Children Born 3-9 March 1958, Followed Longitudinally (N = Approx. 16,000)

Authors:
Davie et al.,[10] at seven years of age.
Butler and Goldstein,[11] at eleven years of age.
Fogelman,[12] at sixteen years of age.

Results:
Cognitive/Neurological Development at Age Seven, Percent Abnormal (Not Adjusted for Covariates)

	Maternal Smoking at the Fourth Month of Gestation Cigarettes/Day			
	0	< 10	10+	Significance
Copy designs score < 5	10.5	12.3	12.3	**
Clumsy: certainly	2.0	2.4	2.6	***
: somewhat	10.3	12.1	13.9	
Known handicap	1.2	1.8	2.4	**
Would benefit from special school	1.6	2.3	2.4	***

Differences in Ability and Achievement (in Months, Except as Noted) and in Height (cm), vs. Nonsmokers

| | Cigarettes/Day from Fourth Month of Gestation | | | | | |
| | < 10 | | | 10+ | | |
Age (Years)	Unadjusted	(1)	(2)	Unadjusted	(1)	(2)
General ability						
11	−8.0***	−4.5***		−8.0***	−3.6***	
Reading						
7			−1.0***			−3.9***
11	−7.4***	−3.1***	−.087***[1]	−9.0***	−3.1***	−0.117***[1]
Mathematics						
11	−7.1***	−4.7***		−8.5***	−4.9***	
16			−0.14***[1]			−0.18***[1]
Height						
7	−0.9[2]	−0.60[2]	−0.40[2]	−1.3[2]	−0.99[2]	−0.65[2]
11	−0.95***	−0.57***		−1.6***	−1.0***	

	10 Cigarettes/Day	> 10 Cigarettes/Day
16		
Boys	−0.57*	−0.89*
Girls	0.19	−0.39

(1) Adjusted for age (except at 16), sex, maternal height and parity, paternal occupational status, and n younger sibs.
(2) As (1), plus gestation and birthweight.
[1] SD units (age not included in regression: cannot be translated into months).
[2] Statistical tests not presented.
  * p < 0.05.
 ** p < 0.01.
*** p < 0.001.

Comments:
At age seven, after controlling for all covariates, social adjustment was significantly worse with increased smoking (p < 0.001).

Smoking assessed at fourth month of gestation.

Women who smoked variable amounts from the fourth month of pregnancy were omitted (generally) from analyses.

Garn et al.[13,14] found increased rates both of low neonatal Apgar scores and Bayley motor and mental scores at one year of age among children whose mothers had been heavy smokers during pregnancy, both whites and blacks. The only impressive adverse impact was among infants of the few women who smoked 40 or more cigarettes a day (96 whites and 24 blacks, and somewhat fewer children at one year of age). Other, smaller studies have not been able to replicate these findings (see below). Social and other differences between smokers and nonsmokers were not controlled, and no statistical tests were presented.

TABLE 2. Studies from the National Collaborative Perinatal Project (NCPP)

The National Collaborative Perinatal Project studied 58,000 pregnancies at 12 US teaching centers, starting in the late 1950's. Children were followed to age seven. All studies refer only to maternal smoking during pregnancy, except Broman (1975).

Authors:
Garn et al.[13,14]

Population studied:
43,492 live born singletons

Results:

% Apgar Score < 5

		Cigarettes/Day in Pregnancy		
	0	< 20	21-40	41+
One Minute				
Whites	12.8	14.0	13.7	20.8
Blacks	12.0	13.7	14.2	31.8
Five minute				
Whites	2.2	2.9	3.1	3.3
Blacks	3.5	4.0	7.2	12.5

% Bayley Scores < 26 (Motor) and < 74 (Mental) at Eight Months

		Cigarettes/Day in Pregnancy		
	0	< 20	21-40	41+
Whites				
Motor	10.1	10.2	13.8	15.8
Mental	10.2	10.5	12.5	15.8
Blacks				
Motor	9.7	10.2	11.8	11.8
Mental	15.2	15.2	17.9	23.5

Authors:
Hardy and Mellits[15]

Population studied:
Subjects were 88 infants of women who smoked 10+ cigarettes/day, registered in Baltimore subsample of NCPP.

Controls: (1) 88 infants of nonsmokers matched for race, sex, date of delivery and maternal age and schooling, and (2) 55 infants also matched for birthweight.

Results:
Case-Control Differences

	Weight (g)		Length (cm)		Head Circ. (cm)	
Age	(1)	(2)	(1)	(2)	(1)	(2)
Birth	−250***	−20	−1.34***	−0.26	−0.32	0.01
1 year	−250	170	−0.13*	0.32	−0.36	−0.19
4 years	−110	0	−0.70	0.15	−0.39*	−0.14
7 years	−650	−400	−1.00	0.62	−0.17	−0.07

	(1)	(2)
Mean Apgar score		
Lowest	0.47	0.70
5 min	−0.11	−0.11
% Neurological abnormal	6% (10% vs 4%)	4% (10% vs 6%)
IQ, 4 yoa	−1.20	−0.10
IQ, 7 yoa	−1.35	−1.49
At 7:		
WRAT Spelling	−2.62*	−2.16
Reading	−1.86	−2.36
Math	0.89	−0.37
Bender Gestalt	−0.24	−0.67
Draw a person	−2.91	2.47
ITPA	−0.09	0.69

(1) = vs control subjects not matched for birthweight.
(2) = vs control subjects matched for birthweight.
   * p < 0.05.
 *** p < 0.001.

Comments:
Statistical tests used were not specified.
Only 96 whites and 24 blacks smoked > 40 cigarettes/day for Apgar score analysis, and fewer for Bayley analysis.

No adjustment for any social or other differences between smokers and nonsmokers.

Authors:
Broman et al.[16]

Population studied:
26,789 four year old children classified by whether mothers had *ever* smoked, to time of birth.

Results:

Mean IQ

	Mothers Never Smoked	Mothers Ever Smoked
White	105.3	104.3**
Black	90.8	91.9***

  ** p < 0.01.
 *** p < 0.001.

Comments:
No adjustment for social, demographic, or other differences between smokers and nonsmokers.

No data on outcome related to smoking limited to pregnancy.

Authors:
Nichols and Chen[17]

Population studied:
29,889 seven year old children

Results:
Relative Risk of Children Whose Mothers Smoked 20+ Cigarettes/Day during Pregnancy, vs Children of Nonsmokers

Cigarettes/Day	LD[1]		HI[1]		NS[1]
	All	Severe	All	Severe	
20+	1.25***	1.44***	1.28***	1.32***	1.15**
40+	1.46**	1.66*	1.54**	1.63*	1.34*

   * $p < 0.05$.
  ** $p < 0.01$.
 *** $p < 0.001$.

On discriminant analysis, among pregnancy and delivery factors, number of cigarettes/day was significantly related to LD (3rd strongest discriminator) severe LD (second strongest), HI (strongest), severe HI (strongest), NS (strongest), severe NS (rank order not given).

[1] See *Comments,* below, for definitions.

Comments:
In a study of minimal brain damage at age seven, three factors were extracted from extensive neurological, behavioral and developmental examination, which were called Learning Difficulties (LD) (reading, spelling, arithmetic, audio-vocal association, Bender Gestalt), Hyperkinetic-Impulsive behavior (HI) (hyperactivity, impulsivity, emotional ability, short attention span) and Neurological Soft Signs (NS) (coordination, gait, mirror movements, other abnormal movements, position sense, asteriognosis, nystagmas, reflexes, strabismus).

Relative risks for children of smokers of 1-19 cigarettes/day not presented.

Extent of covariance of smoking and social differences impossible to judge from report; multivariate analysis obscured by simultaneous inclusion of antecedents (*e.g.,* smoking, SES) and outcomes other than MED (*e.g.,* IQ).

Authors:
Naeye and Peters[19]

Population studied:
NCPP population at Boston Lying-In Hospital (482); subset of 2,903 white infants in middle of SES rank, and 578 same sex sibling pairs (presumably from all NCPP sites) among whom mother smoked only in one pregnancy, balanced for bith order.

Results:
Standardized Regression Coefficients at Age Seven with No. of Cigarettes/Day during Pregnancy, Adjusted for Several Factors

Spelling[1]	−0.046***
Reading[1]	−0.042*
Arithmetic[1]	−0.020
Attention span[2]	−0.049***
Activity level[2]	0.043*
(N = 6,482)	

Achievement Scores among Seven Year Old Children of 2903 White Middle SES Women, Unadjusted Results

	Smoking during Pregnancy (Cigarettes/Day)		
	0	1-19	20+
Spelling[1]	27.4	27.0	26.6***
Reading[1]	41.0	39.8	39.2***
Arithmetic[1]	21.6	21.5	21.1***

Sibling Comparisons, Test Scores at Age Seven (578 Pairs)

	Mother Smoked during Pregnancy	
	No	Yes
Spelling[1]	24.8	24.0*
Reading[1]	36.0	34.2**
Arithmetic[1]	20.5	20.1
Attention span[2]	2.95	2.90*
Motor activity[2]	2.91	2.98*

[1] Wide Range Achievement Test scores
[2] Five point scale
* $p < 0.05$.
** $p < 0.01$.
*** $p < 0.001$.

Comments:
Although no formal analysis was presented, depressed achievement among children appeared to be accounted for by shortened attention span.

In sibling study, no information on whether other situational differences existed between pregnancies (*e.g.,* stress) in additional to smoking behavior.

Hardy and Mellits[15] performed a well controlled small study among the Baltimore subsample of the NCPP. They matched 88 infants of women who smoked 10 or more cigarettes a day during pregnancy for race, sex, date of delivery and maternal age and years of schooling, with 88 control subjects; for 55 subjects, they also selected a second control subject matched for birthweight. Since numbers were small, power was low, and few differences could be expected to be significant. At age seven children of smokers were one cm shorter than the children of mothers who had not smoked, but not shorter than the birthweight matched controls: later somatic differences in stature thus appeared to be mediated by prenatal growth retardation. Among cognitive measures, only the spelling scale of the Wide Range Achievement Test (WRAT) was significantly depressed. However, performance by subjects was worse than controls on all subtests.

Broman *et al.*[16] found a small (1.0 point) but significant advantage in IQ at age four among white children whose mothers had never smoked, compared to those whose mothers had ever smoked, and a small but highly significant *advantage* for infants of black smokers compared to infants of black nonsmokers (1.1 points). Social differences were not controlled.

Nichols and Chen[17] performed an elaborate investigation of minimal brain damage (MBD) among 30,000 NCPP children examined at age seven. Maternal smoking during pregnancy was strongly and significantly related to all three components of MBD, learning difficulties (LD), hyperactivity-impulsivity (HI), and neurological soft signs (NS). For instance, children of women smoking more than 20 cigarettes a day during pregnancy were 25% more likely to have LD, 44% severe LD, 28% HI, 32% severe HI, and 15% NS. These results were not controlled for social differences between smokers and nonsmokers.

Naeye[18] presented some results on height at age seven [see TABLE 7]. Among 140 full term white sibling pairs in which the mother smoked in only one pregnancy, the children exposed to cigarette smoke were 1.7 cm shorter at age seven ($p < 0.001$). Among white term children, those of 1634 light smokers during pregnancy (<20 cigarettes/day) were 1.1 cm shorter at age seven, and of 1231 heavy smokers ($20+$ cigarettes/day) 2.1 cm shorter, than children of 1632 nonsmokers (calculated from the author's data). All differences were highly significant. Neither sex nor birth order were controlled in the sibling study; social differences were not controlled, nor was there any explanation why blacks (who comprised nearly half the study population) were not included in analysis.

Naeye and Peters[19] reported on some aspects of the mental development of seven year olds from the Boston Lying-In Hospital population of the NCPP, and also among 578 same sex sibling pairs, balanced for birth order, in which the mother smoked in only one pregnancy, presumably from all NCPP sites.

Among the Boston Lying-In Hospital population there were significant decrements in spelling and reading (but not arithmetic) scales on the WRAT in a regression analysis adjusted for several possible confounding factors. Children of smokers were rated as significantly less attentive and more active on a five point scale (who did the rating was not reported). The five point scales were pathological at both extremes, and the authors' interpretation that the results implied hyperactivity and short attention are thus problematical. The sibling comparisons generated similar results.

In a parallel analysis (personal communication) the same authors related cognition and behavior to smoking among 1578 term sib pairs without major handicap and surviving to age eight, whose mothers smoked only during one pregnancy. There were equal numbers of pairs with mother smoking in the first and second pregnancy; no mention was made of whether women smoked throughout their index pregnancies, or of the amounts smoked. In both sib-pair analyses, it is possible that mothers may have avoided smoking in the second pregnancy *because* their first child had manifested problems. In addition, other kinds of stress may vary between pregnancies which might have led both to the mother's smoking in either pregnancy and to circumstances that were detrimental to the child's development. In spite of these limitations, the results for cognition were impressive, since static environmental, maternal, and familial circumstances (mother's height, intelligence, etc.) would be similar for both sibs. The results for abnormal behavior (activity and attention) were less convincing; the five point scales were pathologic at both extremes, and mean differences on the scales cannot be interpreted as demonstrating pathology.

Seattle Longitudinal Study (TABLE 3)

Martin et al.[20] reported on the first of a series of papers following a cohort of children born to predominantly white middle class pregnant women recruited at two

TABLE 3. Seattle Longitudinal Study

Authors:
Martin *et al.*[20]

Population studied:
Two day old infants in the Seattle studies of the effects of maternal tobacco and alcohol intake on infant and child development, who "evidenced a performance change" on an operant head turning (n = ?63) and two sucking (n = 80) learning tasks. (No definition of performance change given.)

Results:
Head turnings:
"The test of no nicotine main effect adjusted for the alcohol and the interaction terms (between alcohol and tobacco) was rejected with $p = 0.003$. The alcohol by nicotine interaction term adjusted for both main effects was significant at $p = 0.00012$."

Sucking:
"Babies born to mothers who smoked but did not drink during pregnancy had higher performance scores on both tasks than the control babies."
"Maternal alcohol and nicotine consumption in combination resulted in poorer neonatal performance."

Comments:
Fragmentary and qualitative presentation of results.

Authors:
Streissguth *et al.*[21]

Population studied:
Sample of 462 eight month old infants from a cohort of 1,529 predominantly white, middle class mothers interviewed in the fifth month of pregnancy, stratified to maximize the number of heavy smokers and drinkers.

Results:
Partial F test with nicotine exposure during pregnancy adjusting for alcohol and caffeine use, and gestational age.
Bayley Mental development index, $F_{(1,453)} = 0.55$, $p = 0.46$.
Bayley Psychomotor development index, $F_{(1,454)} = 0.10$, $p = 0.76$.

No effect of adjustment for maternal age or parity

Comments:
Associations with alcohol were significant.

Authors:
Landesman-Dwyer *et al.*[22]

Population:
Subsample of 128 four year olds born in the Seattle longitudinal study (see above two references).

Results:
Maternal cigarette smoking unrelated to any subscale of Caldwell's Home Observation for Measurement of the Environment (HOME) scale, nor any of eight behavior patterns assessed at both meal and story time.

From maternal rating of 98 items describing child temperament, offspring of smokers showed:

1) Greater willingness to approach strangers in novel situations
2) Greater persistence, interpreted both as stubbornness and sustained involvement in single activities; and
3) Greater intensity, interpreted as more negative reaction when upset, annoyed, or disciplined.

Comments:
Results adjusted for HOME score, birth order.
No evidence of overactivity.

Authors:
Streissguth *et al.*[23]

Population studied:
452 singleton $4\frac{3}{12}$ year old children from the Seattle longitudinal study (see above). Sample stratified to overrepresent alcohol and cigarette users during pregnancy (14.4% moderate and 18.4% heavy smokers).

Results:
Nicotine score during pregnancy (number of cigarettes/day times amount of nicotine/cigarette) significantly related, on a vigilance task, to errors of omission ($p = 0.016$) commission ($p = 0.035$), ratio of correct/total responses ($p = 0.001$) and to total trails oriented ($p = 0.037$). No significant relationship to reaction time, or to time moving during testing.

Comments:
Results adjusted for birth order, and maternal alcohol and caffeine use, education, and nutrition (method unspecified). Authors state that adjustment for age and sex did not affect results. Adjustment for race not mentioned. (All independent variables log transformed).

Authors:
Streissguth *et al.*[24]

Population studied:
475 $6\frac{1}{2}$ to $8\frac{1}{2}$ year old children in the Seattle study who were presented a laboratory vigilance task.

Results:
Results for relationship to maternal cigarette smoking were not presented directly. However, it was implied that there was no significant relationship to nicotine, since it was stated that cigarette use was retained in the final regression model because it was related to alcohol use, and not because it was related to the outcome measure.

Comments:
No direct presentation of relationship of maternal tobacco use and outcome.

Seattle hospitals. The sample was weighted to overrepresent mothers who were heavy smokers and users of alcohol. Two learning tasks were presented to two day old infants. Sixty three were tested on a head turning task and 80 on two sucking learning tasks. There was a significant relationship between maternal cigarette smoking and less efficient performance on the head turning task and there was also a significant interaction term between alcohol and tobacco use. The magnitude of differences was not reported. On the sucking task, babies born to mothers who smoked and did not drink did better than controls, while combined maternal alcohol and nicotine consumption was associated with poor neonatal performance. The results were presented qualitatively.

Streissguth *et al.*[21] studied 462 eight month old infants in the Seattle study. There was no suggestion of relationship between maternal smoking on either the Bayley mental development index or the Bayley psychomotor development index.

Landesman-Dwyer *et al.*[22] studied 128 four year olds from the same longitudinal study in Seattle. Maternal cigarette smoking during pregnancy was unrelated to any subscale of the Caldwell HOME scale, or to any of eight specific behavior patterns assessed at meal and story time. Mothers ranked their children on 98 items describing the child's temperament, and the offspring of smokers showed significant differences in three groups of items: greater willingness to approach strangers in novel situations;

greater persistence, interpreted both as stubbornness and sustained involvement in single activities; and greater intensity, interpreted as more negative reaction when upset, annoyed or disciplined. (Children of smokers were not inattentive.)

Streissguth et al.[23] studied a vigilance task among 452 singleton four year old children who were part of the same Seattle longitudinal study. Children of smokers during pregnancy made significantly more errors of omission, had a significantly lower ratio of correct to total responses, and had fewer trials in which they were oriented. There was no significant relationship of maternal smoking to reaction time nor to time moving during the testing session. The results were adjusted for birth order, maternal alcohol and caffeine use, and education and nutrition. Adjustment for age and sex did not affect results. It is unclear from the presentation what the magnitude of the deficits associated with tobacco use were, nor the impact of adjustment procedures. While it was stated that Caldwell's HOME score at age one was not associated with alcohol and nicotine use, it is not clear whether any attempts have been made to include assessment of the home environment at age four in the analysis of development at age four.

The same group presented a laboratory vigilance task to 475 of these children between ages of 6 ½ and 8 ½.[24] Results were only presented for alcohol use during pregnancy, but it was implied that there was no relationship with cigarette use, since cigarette use was listed as a variable included in the final regression model only because it was related to alcohol use, and not because it was related to outcome.

Ottawa Prenatal Prospective Study (TABLE 4)

Gusella and Fried,[25] in the first of a series of reports from the Ottawa Prenatal Prospective Study, assessed 84 thirteen month olds. Detailed data on cigarettes smoked, other substances used, and a variety of background factors were gathered three times during pregnancy. The only significant relationship of maternal smoking during pregnancy with any aspect of the Bayley exam, after adjustment for father's education, was with a set of items that the investigators grouped under the rubric of verbal comprehension. Two other sets of indices were related to cigarette consumption *prior* to pregnancy, the psychomotor development index, and an item cluster called fine motor skills.

Three further reports were published by this cohort in 1987.[26–28] These authors found no relationship between cigarette smoking in pregnancy and somatic growth at 12 or 24 months. No quantitative results were presented, and only 67 children of smokers were followed up. In the neonatal period smoking was related to reduced habituation to sound (a direction opposite to that reported in other studies), and increased tremulousness.

Mother's education was reported to be strongly correlated to cigarette smoking during pregnancy ($r = 0.336$, $p < 0.001$) but mother's education was not adjusted in any of the reported results. Further, mother's weight gain, often reported to be depressed with cigarette smoking, and birthweight were used as control variables, maternal weight gain in analyses of somatic growth and neurologic status, and birthweight in the analysis of neurologic status. Since both birthweight (almost surely) and maternal weight gain (in all likelihood) are affected by cigarette smoking, the results were probably overcontrolled and possible effects of smoking would have been understated.

TABLE 4. Ottawa Prenatal Prospective Study

Authors:
Gusella and Fried[25]

Population studied:
Thirteen month old children who were products of 84 consecutive pregnancies, 11/78 to 12/79. Data on cigarette use (and other factors) gathered at three times during pregnancy.

Results:
Maternal Nicotine Consumption before and during Pregnancy Correlated with Bayley Examinations at 13 Months

	Mental Development Index	Psychomotor Development Index	Item Clusters[1]		
			Verbal Comprehension	Spoken Language	Fine Motor
Pre-pregnancy consumption	−0.20*	−0.37***	−0.27**	−0.05	−0.27**
+ adj. for father's education	−0.13	−0.35***	−0.16	—	−0.21*
Pregnancy consumption	−0.06	−0.19*	−0.31**	−0.05	−0.18
+ adj. for father's education	−0.03	−0.15	−0.22*	—	−0.11

— = not presented.
* $p < 0.05$.
** $p < 0.01$.
*** $p < 0.001$.
[1] A priori regrouping of items from Bayley exam.

Authors:
Fried and O'Connell[26]
Fried and Makin[27]
Fried et al.[28]

Population studied:
Volunteers entered the study "after becoming aware of the study either by notices in the media or by signs placed in the offices of their obstetricians." 210 cannabis, alcohol, and/or cigarette users, and 50 control women randomly chosen who used no tobacco, marijuana and little or no alcohol. There were 22 heavy smokers, 61 less heavy smokers and 167 nonusers of cigarettes.

Results:
Postnatal somatic growth:
"Nicotine was not significantly related to any of the outcomes at 12 or 24 months of age." No quantitative results presented, and only 123 children (67 of whose mothers smoked) were followed.

Neonatal behavior:
Smoking significantly related to reduced habituation to sound and increased tremulousness.

Comments:
Recruitment procedure (volunteers) open to selection bias. Mothers education correlated r = 0.336, $p < 0.001$, with nicotine consumption, suggesting very likely confounding of results. (Mother's education not adjusted in any of the reported results.)

Mother's weight gain adjusted in analysis of somatic growth and neurological status, and birthweight controlled in analyses of neurologic status: since birthweight and maternal weight gain are affected by cigarette smoking, results are probably overcontrolled.

Other Studies (TABLE 5)

Wingerd and Schoen[29] demonstrated highly significant depression of height among five year olds whose mothers smoked during pregnancy. Results were controlled for sex, birth order, length of gestation, parental age, education, income and stature, mother's age at menarche, and father's occupational status. The height of the children whose mothers smoked less than 15 cigarettes/day was depressed 0.40 cm, and of those who smoked more than that, 0.90 cm.

Denson et al.[30] matched 20 methylphenidate sensitive hyperkinetic five to fifteen year old children for social class, age and sex with one dyslexic and one normal control. The average number of cigarettes smoked was significantly higher among mothers of subjects than either control group (the number currently smoked was related more strongly to outcome than the amount reported to have been smoked during pregnancy). Sixteen of 20 mothers of subjects had smoked during pregnancy; the rate for controls was not reported. There was no significant association with paternal smoking.

Dunn et al.[31,32] studied all trackable and surviving six and one half year old children born at the Vancouver General Hospital between September, 1958 and March, 1965 with birthweights under four and one half pounds (plus several referred low birthweight children), and normal birthweight control subjects recruited at the end of the study period. Results were presented within birthweight and gestational strata; we combined results by assuming that four percent of births weighed under four and one half pounds. The normal birthweight children were chosen from nonpaying patients in an attempt to control for social disparity, since low birthweight occurs more often among those of lower status. It is not possible to judge, from the reported results, whether this control strategy was successful.

Children of smokers were significantly shorter (2.02 cm, $p < 0.001$) and had significantly lower full scale Wechsler Intelligence Scale for Children (WISC) performance IQ: Bender Gestalt, Knox cubes, sentence repetition and draw a person were not significantly different. Although the overall verbal IQ was not significantly different, children of smokers did significantly worse on three subscales, block completion, coding, and vocabulary.

Teachers reported misbehavior to be more common among boys whose mothers had smoked during pregnancy (n.s., according to the tabulated data) on the Haggerty-Olson-Wickman Behavior Rating Schedule. There were significant relationships of maternal smoking to lower cognition, poorer physical traits, retarded social development, and less stable temperament.

Saxon[33] found four of twenty items on the Brazelton Assessment Scale to be significantly different in 15 four to six day old infants whose mothers had smoked 15 or more cigarettes/day, compared to 17 controls "matched" for maternal age, social class and parity. There was no explanation how there could be more "matched" controls than cases, nor was it stated whether the observer was blind to the child's study status. The author interpreted the direction of all four differences to be adverse, but the tabulated data indicated that infants of smokers habituated more rapidly to an auditory stimulus, a response usually assumed to be positively correlated with later intelligence.

Hingson et al.[34] related one and five minutes Apgar scores to amount of cigarette smoking during pregnancy, assessed by postpartum interview. They found no significant relationships between Apgar scores and cigarette smoking. No numerical results were presented.

TABLE 5. Other Studies of Smoking during Pregnancy and Later Child Development

Authors:
Wingerd and Schoen[29]

Population studied:
Kaiser Permanente Medical Center, Oakland, California

Results:
Case-Control (N = 2,404) Differences in Length (cm)

| | Cigarettes/Day | |
	< 15	15+
Length (cm)		
Birth	−0.49	−0.99***
5 years	−0.40	−0.90***
N	562	741

*** p < 0.001.

Comments:
Results controlled for sex, birth order, length of gestation, parental age, education, income and stature, mother's age at menarche, and father's occupational status.

Authors:
Denson et al.[30]

Population studied:
20 Methylphenidate-sensitive hyperkinetic children, 5-15 years old (18 M, 2 F), in Saskatchewan, Canada.

Matched for SES, age and sex with: a) dyslexic, and b) normal, controls.

Results:
Average Number of Cigarettes/Day Smoked by Mother

	Hyperkinetics	Dyslexic Controls	Normal Controls
In pregnancy	14.3*	6.0	6.3
Currently	23.3***	6.1	8.2

* p < 0.05.
*** p < 0.001.

Comments:
Parents of hyperkinetic children. Significantly more first born hyperkinetic children; 16/20 mothers of cases smoked during pregnancy (no data given for controls). No significant difference in paternal smoking.

Authors:
Dunn *et al.* [31,32]

Population studied:
All infants born at Vancouver General Hospital <2,041 g birthweight from 9/58-3/65 (n = 480) + 17 born elsewhere. 205 controls >2,500 g birthweight, "non-pay" patients, recruited in 1965–66; 234 lbw, 146 fbw followed to 6.5 years.

Results:
Length/Height (cm) [1]

Age	Nonsmokers	Smokers	Difference
Birth	50.90	50.39	0.51
1 year	75.36	74.44	0.92*
4 years	103.19	101.51	1.68**
6.5 years	119.09	117.07	2.02***

Psychological Status, Age 6.5 [1,2]

WISC IQ	Nonsmokers	Smokers	Difference
Verbal performance	109.7	104.6	5.1*
Full scale	109.9	105.9	4.0*
Vocal encoding	−0.50	−0.73	−0.23*

[1] Calculated from authors' data, assuming rate of birth <2,041 g birthweight = 4%.
[2] Bender Gestalt, Knox cube, sentence repetition and draw a person all nonsignificant.
  * $p < 0.05$.
  ** $p < 0.01$.
  *** $p < 0.001$.

Comments:
Vocabulary one of three significant differences on eight subscales of verbal IQ, suggesting SES difference between subject and control children.

Results minimally controlled for SES differences.

Test states "sons of smokers showed consistently greater misbehavior (on Haggerty-Olson-Wickman Behavior Rating Schedules) than the sons of nonsmoking mothers," but the tabulated differences in behavior problems were not shown as significant; significant differences in cognition, physical traits, social development, and temperament.

Author:
Saxon [33]

Population studied:
Fifteen 4-6 day old infants of mothers in Dundee, Scotland who smoked 15+ cigarettes/day, compared to infants of seventeen nonsmokers.

Results:
Four of twenty items on Brazelton neonatal assessment scale were significantly different: infants of smokers had greater response decrement to a bell, had lower inanimate and animate auditory orientation and were less easily consolable.

No difference in initial or predominant states.

Comments:
Subjects and controls said to be "matched for maternal age, social class and parity" but no explanation of unequal numbers of subjects and controls.

Apgar scores not different between subjects and controls.

No mention whether observer was blinded to sampling status.

Not clear whether difference in response decrement adverse or favorable; interpreted in text opposite to direction of score.

Authors:
Hingson *et al.*[34]

Population studied:
Boston City Hospital, 2/78 to 10/79. Low income population.
1,670 (out of 1,709) mother-child pairs with one and five minute Apgar scores, and postpartum maternal interviews.

Results:
"No significant univariate relationship between amount of current cigarette smoking or number of years that respondents smoked and low 1-minute and 5-minute Apgar scores."

In stepwise multiple regression analysis (controlling for many possible confounding factors), amount of smoking was not significantly related to Apgar scores.

Comments:
Actual results not presented.
Relatively few subjects with high levels of smoking (*i.e.,* may not have been large enough to test issue).

Authors:
Picone *et al.*[35]

Population studied:
Sixty pregnant women and offspring. Sampling method (whether serial births, or stratified), racial composition, and distribution of independent variables (smoking, low weight gain) not specified.

Results:
"Apgar scores were not significantly related to any of the independent variables." Brazelton exams were done at 2.3 and 14 days postpartum. Maternal smoking was related to more rapid auditory habituation, but less good auditory orientation, autonomic regulation, and regulation of state. Performance scores abnormal at 2 and 3 days, but not at two weeks.

Comments:
Description of analytic methods leaves unclear whether maternal low weight gain and smoking might have been confounded by sampling design and analytic methods. What, and how, possible confounding factors were approached was not specified.

Authors:
Jacobson *et al.*[36]

Population studied:
173 infants (91 M and 82 F) of predominantly white, middle class mothers.

Results:
Bazelton exam on day 3 and/or 4, smoking was associated with *lower* irritability ($0.05 < p < 0.10$) and less good auditory orientation ($0.05 < p < 0.10$). The latter ("disappeared") after adjusting for socioeconomic status and caffeine use.

Comments:
Careful attention was paid to potential confounding and colinearity between smoking, alcohol, and caffeine use by mother.

Author:
Rantakallio[7]

Population studied:
Cohort of 14 year old children in northern Finland born to 12,068 mothers. Offspring of the 1,819 whose mothers smoked during pregnancy were matched by maternal marital status, age, parity, and place of residence with nonsmoking controls. 1,763 children of smokers and 1,781 control children contacted at age 14.

Results:
Height[1] (cm)

	Cigarettes/Day during Pregnancy		
	0	< 10	10+
	161.5	160.9	160.6
Difference from nonsmokers	—	−0.6	−0.9

[1] Adjusted for maternal height and age, no. of older and younger sibs, fathers social class, and sex of child. Results approximate: taken from published graph. ($p = 0.013$ by analysis of covariance). After further adjustment for adverse maternal factors (see comments below) effect of maternal smoking no longer significant (Analysis probably overcontrolled by inclusion of paternal smoking).

School performance:
Mean ability on theoretical subjects (on arbitrary 6 point scale) significantly depressed among children of smokers ($p = 0.000$).[1] After further control for adverse maternal factors, maternal smoking still significantly related to lower score ($p = 0.004$).

Comments:
"In each social class of the husband, the smoking mother was in a less favorable situation in terms of (unemployment, sick leave or sick pension, not living with the family, or having died) than her nonsmoking counterpart, with the exception of sick leave and pension in the highest classes and unemployment among the class of farmers."

"Smoking on the part of the father carried about as strong an association with retardation in mental and physical development as did maternal smoking in this series."

Authors:
Kolvin et al.[37] Newcastle, England, Maternity Study.

Population Studied: Maternal Smoking during Pregnancy

	Cigarettes/Day			
	0	1-5	> 5	Total
Groups				
(1) Random controls	114	18	54	186
(2) Short gestation[1]	20	4	35	59
Light for Dates:				
(3) 6-10th percentile	23	8	35	66
(4) < 5th percentile	21	7	45	73

[1] Not defined.

Results: Differences in Scores of 5-7 Year Old Children of Mothers Smoking > 5 Cigarettes/ Day vs Others, within Groups[1]

	Groups			
	(1)	(2)	(3)	(4)
Language quotient	−3.1	0.7	−6.3	−5.7
IQ	−0.8	−1.6	−5.4	−0.1
Rutter behavior score	0.8	4.0	−1.3	1.0

[1] No statistical tests reported.

Number of Items Significantly Correlated with Maternal Smoking Controlling for:

	Social Class and Maternal Neuroticism	Plus Birthweight
Behavior and temperament	11/72	11/72
Height, weight and neurological exam	13/24	0.24
Cognitive function	6/25	2.25

Comments:
Among behavioral dimensions, acting out, and hyperactivity related to smoking ($p < 0.001$), with effects undiminished by control for social factors and birthweight [contributed entirely by groups (2) and (4)] misconduct and shyness (negatively) related to smoking ($p < 0.01$) in group (4), unaffected by adjusting for same covariates.

Picone *et al.*[36] studied sixty pregnant women and their offspring. They found that Apgar scores were not significantly related to smoking, but that maternal smoking was related to more rapid auditory habituation, and less good auditory orientation, autonomic regulation and regulation of state, by Brazelton examinations performed at two, three and fourteen days of age. Performance scores were abnormal at two and three days of age but not at two weeks. The description of the analytic methods left unclear whether maternal weight and smoking might not have been confounded either by the sampling design or in analysis. What and how possible confounding was addressed was not specified.

Rantakallio[7] compared 1763 fourteen year old children whose mothers had smoked during pregnancy to 1781 children whose mothers had not smoked, and were matched by maternal marital status, age, parity, and place of residence. Results for height in TABLE 5 were abstracted from her graphic presentation. The children whose mothers smoked under ten cigarettes a day during pregnancy were 0.6 centimeters shorter than children of nonsmokers, and those of women who smoked ten or more cigarettes a day, 0.9 centimeters shorter. These results were reported to be significant with value of $p = 0.013$, by analysis of covariance. This result was adjusted for maternal height and age, number of older and younger sibs, father's social class, and sex of child. After further adjustment for several adverse maternal factors, as well as paternal smoking, the difference was no longer significant, but control for paternal smoking may have caused the relationship with maternal smoking to be an underestimate.

Ability on theoretical school subjects was significantly depressed among smokers, and remained significantly depressed even after further adjustment for the adverse maternal factors and paternal smoking.

Jacobson *et al.*[36] performed the Brazelton examination on days three and/or four of life on 173 infants of predominantly white middle class mothers. In this study smoking was associated with lower irritability ($0.05 < p < 0.10$) and less good auditory orientation ($0.05 < p < 0.10$). This latter result was entirely accounted for by adjusting for socioeconomic status and caffeine use. This project was impressive for the careful attention that was paid to potential confounding between smoking, alcohol, and caffeine use of the mother.

Kolvin *et al.*[37] studied 59 children of short gestation (the criterion was not stated), 139 of whom were light for dates, and 186 children of normal gestation and birthweight, at five to seven years of age, in Newcastle, England. In three of four subgroups, children of smokers ($5+$ cigs/day) had lower language quotient, and in one of four, IQ or Rutter behavior scores more than two units worse than control children. No statistical tests of these differences were reported. After controlling for social class and maternal neuroticism, children of smokers did significantly worse on 11 of 72 items measuring behavior and temperament, six of 25 indices of cognitive function, and 13 of 24 "physical" measures (height, weight, neurological indices). (Which indices were not specified.) With further control for birthweight, there was no change in the number of significant behavioral and temperamental differences, but only two cognitive measures and no physical measures remained significant. Thus, the associations with behavior were not mediated by prenatal growth retardation, the associations with cognitive function were in part, and the physical measures, entirely. Some of the behavioral dimensions were identified, and acting out and hyperactivity were significantly related to maternal smoking (both $p < 0.001$), and effects were undiminished by statistical control for social class or maternal neuroticism. The effects were entirely contributed by the children of short gestation or by those who were extremely (< 5th percentile) small for dates. Also, among the very small for dates, smoking was significantly related to misconduct, and negatively to shyness, and these differences were again unaffected by the same control variables.

Physical Stature and Postnatal Parental Smoking (TABLE 6)

Rona *et al.*[38] graphically related height among primary school children to the number of adult smokers in the child's household, separately for England and Scotland, from the National Study of Health and Growth. Smoking in pregnancy was accounted for in analysis by adjusting for reported birthweight. The results in TABLE 6 are approximate, since they are our extrapolations from the author's graphic presentation. There were significant relationships between the number of adult smokers in the household and childhood stature in England, which were reduced but not eliminated, by adjustment for birthweight and social class; differences in Scotland were not significant after such adjustment.

DISCUSSION AND SUMMARY

Somatic development and maternal smoking during pregnancy (TABLE 7)

The relationship of children's stature to the mother's smoking during pregnancy is summarized in TABLE 7. There is a consistent decrement of around one to two centimeters in child's height associated with maternal smoking during pregnancy, with the possible exception of the study of Fried and O'Connell,[26] which reported no significant relationship (this was a small series and the magnitude of difference was not reported). In the NCDS, adjustment for social status (and several other variables) accounted for about 40% of the difference in height between children of smokers and

TABLE 6. Stature in Childhood and Passive Exposure to Cigarette Smoke

Authors:
Rona et al.[38]

Source of information:
National Study of Health and Growth (UK), primary school children

Results:
Standardized Height,[1] Primary School Children

| | No. of Smokers in Household | | | |
	0	1	2+	
England				
Unadjusted	0.16	0.01	−0.10	***
+ adj for bw	0.14	0.02	−0.06	***
+ adj for SES, no. sibs, parents[1] height	0.10	0.04	0.01	*
Scotland				
Unadjusted	0.22	0.09	0.00	**
+ adj for bw	0.18	0.09	0.04	
+ adj. for SES, no. sibs, parents[1] height	0.14	0.09	0.07	

[1] $\frac{Ht - Ht}{SD^{ht}}$; Ht derived by age, sex, country.

* $p < 0.05$.
** $p < 0.01$.
*** $p < 0.001$.

Comments:
Results approximate (taken from published graph). No. of subjects not given. Effect of smoking during pregnancy accounted for by adjusting for birthweight.

Adult smoker = 5+ cigarettes/day.

nonsmokers before controlling for birthweight. The exact extent to which the remaining deficit was due to smoking remains problematical, but the consistency and persistence of these findings after statistical adjustment for possible confounding variables suggests a causal relationship. Whether such depressed stature has functional consequences is an open question.

TABLE 7. Summary: Height Decrements (cm) Associated with Maternal Smoking during Pregnancy, Compared to Children of Nonsmokers

					Study						
	Ref. 29		Ref. 15	Refs. 32, 33	Refs. 10-12		Ref. 18			Ref. 7	
					Cigarettes/Day						
Age (yrs)	<15	15+	10+	1+	<10	10+	+1	<20	20+	<10	10+
1			−0.13(0.32)	−0.92							
4			−0.70(0.15)	−1.68							
5	−0.40	−0.90									
7					−0.6 (−0.4)	−1.0 (−0.7)	−1.7[1]	−1.1[2]	−2.1[2]		
11					−0.6	−1.0					
14										−0.59[3]	−0.92[3]
16					boys: (−0.57)[4]	(−0.89)[4]				−0.28[3]	−0.47[3]
					girls: (−0.19)[4]	(−0.33)[4]					

( ) = value after controlling for birthweight.

[1] 140 intrapair comparisons; mothers smoked in one pregnancy and not other. No mention whether adjusted for sex of child, or birth order.

[2] Calculated from author's data, assuming n at seven years identical to n at birth; 4,497 pregnancies. Not adjusted for any social or other disparities between smokers and nonsmokers.

[3] Adjusted for SES, sex, mother's height.

[4] Dose categories: 10 cigarettes/day and > 10 cigarettes/day.

Comments:

Kolvin et al.[37] found 13/24 "physical measures" (height, weight, neurological exam, etc.) significantly depressed in 384 five to seven year old children of mothers who smoked > 5 cigarettes/day in pregnancy, after controlling for SES, maternal neuroticism, and no significant differences after also controlling for birthweight. (Nonrepresentative sample: children of bw <2,500 grams overrepresented approximately 20-fold.)

Mental Development, Neurologic Status and Behavior, and Maternal Smoking—Neonatal Effects

The case for a relationship between maternal smoking during pregnancy and neonatal neurological status and behavior is mixed. It is reviewed here because of possible implications for later cognition and behavior.

The only studies in which Apgar scores appeared related to maternal smoking during pregnancy were those of Garn et al.[13,14] The effect appeared limited to the few infants whose mothers smoked over two packs of cigarettes a day. It is therefore not surprising that other investigators have not observed a positive relationship between maternal smoking during pregnancy and Apgar score: it would be unusual to have enough very heavy smokers to replicate this observation.

There appear to be fairly consistent relationships between maternal smoking during pregnancy and abnormalities in the Brazelton neonatal behavioral assessment. Generally, neonates of smoking mothers habituated more rapidly to auditory stimuli, but oriented less well. Other findings were inconsistent. Saxon[33] found infants of smoking mothers less easily consolable, but did not note any state difference associated with maternal smoking. Picone et al.[35] observed poor autonomic regulation and regulation of state among infants of smokers. On the other hand, performance scores, which were depressed at two and three days of age, were normal by two weeks. Possibly the early abnormalities on the Brazelton exam were associated with effects of withdrawal from toxic cigarette products and may or may not have long-term implications. Fried and Makin[26] found significantly reduced habituation to sound among infants of smokers (as well as increased tremulousness).

In contrast, Jacobson et al.[36] noted *lower* irritability among infants of smoking mothers (at the margins of statistical significance) as well as less good auditory orientation, consistent with most other studies.

Thus, there do appear to be real and consistent behavioral effects on the neonate from the smoking of their mothers. It is entirely unclear whether these are associated with any long-term or permanent deficit.

Infant Behavior and Cognition (Primarily Assessed by the Bayley Examination)

The evidence for any infant deficits using Bayley exams is inconsistent. Garn et al.[13,14] showed weak trends in low Bayley scores among whites with increased amounts of smoking, but the highest rates of abnormality were among the few infants of mothers who had smoked more than two packs of cigarettes a day. There was little or no relationship of smoking among black mothers with the Bayley motor scores of their infants, and a possible weak relationship with the Bayley mental score. Streissguth et al.[21] could not demonstrate a relationship between prenatal maternal smoking and either the Bayley mental or psychomotor developmental indices in the Seattle longitudinal study. Gusella and Fried[25] found nonsignificant relationships between cigarette smoking during pregnancy and either the Bayley mental or psychomotor index at thirteen months of age. However, there was a strong and highly significant relationship between the psychomotor developmental index and the amount of cigarette smoking prior to pregnancy. The record is thus by no means consistent, and does not show a regular and strong pattern of deficit of the Bayley exam among infants of smoking mothers.

Cognitive Development and School Achievement in Childhood and Maternal Smoking in Pregnancy

There is a consistent pattern of depressed cognitive development and tests of school achievement associated with maternal smoking during pregnancy. The one possible exception is the study of Streissguth et al.[24] who implied that there was probably no significant relationship of prenatal cigarette smoking to performance on a laboratory vigilance task at ages six and a half to eight and a half, in contrast to significant findings on a vigilance task among much the same children at age four and $\frac{3}{12}$ years.[25] In all other studies, even very small ones, in which differences might not have reached statistical significance, there was a regular and consistent pattern of lower IQ and ability, and less advanced verbal, reading, and mathematical skills associated with maternal smoking during pregnancy. On the other hand, it appears beyond current knowledge to conclude that these associations were causally related.

Much the same problem arises in attempting to relate starvation in early life to later behavior and function.[39] One insult cannot be presumed to exist independent of a web of other contingent and powerful influences on the child. When social class has been taken into account, differences between children of smokers and of nonsmokers are markedly attenuated; for instance, differences were about halved among 11 year olds in the NCDS with social class adjustment.[11] Thus, we must withhold any secure judgment on these issues, and await further research. The sibling comparisons of Naeye and Peters[19] represent the strongest attempt to overcome these inherent methodologic problems.

Behavior, Temperament, Hyperactivity, etc.

There appear to be consistent characterological, temperamental, and behavioral difficulties among children whose mothers smoked during pregnancy.

Denson et al.[30] found that mothers of hyperactive children smoked much more than controls both during pregnancy, and later. Dunn et al.[32] found that children of smokers, especially males, were judged worse by teachers on all components of the Haggerty-Olson-Wickman Behavior Rating, having more frequent misbehavior (n.s.), worse cognition, social development, and temperament, and more abnormal physical traits. Streissguth et al.[23] found maternal nicotine dose in pregnancy significantly related to poor performance by four year olds on a vigilance task. It is not clear that the ratings reported by Naeye and Peters[19] represented abnormal levels of activity or inattention, since the scales used were pathological at both extremes. Kolvin et al.[37] found 11 of 72 behavioral and temperamental indices significantly different (presumably worse) and these differences appeared to be unaffected by adjusting for the disparity in birthweight between children of smokers and nonsmokers.

Davie et al.[10] found social adjustment significantly worse at age seven. Nichols and Chen[17] demonstrated marked association of maternal smoking with all three components of what they termed minimal brain damage at age seven: learning difficulties, hyperactivity-impulsivity, and neurological soft signs.

In sum, the reported differences are consistent, particularly for hyperactivity, but not entirely convincing that maternal smoking during pregnancy is causally related to abnormal behavior. Are the abnormalities caused by smoking, or do they reflect other differences in the lives of children of smokers? In the sibling comparisons, did smoking reflect stresses present around the time of one pregnancy, but not the other? That maternal smoking during pregnancy causes later behavioral abnormality in the child remains an important and intriguing hypothesis, but a causal relationship cannot be posited from the available data.

SUMMARY

Past studies relating smoking during pregnancy (and afterwards) and later child development are critically reviewed. There are consistent deficits among offspring of smokers in stature, cognitive development and educational achievement, as well as more frequent problems of temperament, adjustment, and behavior, particularly abnormally high levels of activity and inattention.

The meaning of these relationships remains obscure, since it cannot be assumed that these abnormalities of child development are caused by parental cigarette smoking. In most studies there has been relatively little attention paid to the potential confounding by social, demographic, and psychological differences between smokers and nonsmokers. It is thus essential to carefully balance the comparative impact of social and environmental influences that may be different between families of smokers and nonsmokers, versus the toxic effects of tobacco.

REFERENCES

1. Rush, D. & E. H. Kass. 1972. Maternal smoking: A reassessment of the association with perinatal mortality. Am. J. Epidemiol. **96:** 183-196.
2. Heath, C. W. 1958. Differences between smokers and nonsmokers. Arch. Intern. Med. **101:** 377-388.
3. Lilienfeld, A. M. 1959. Emotional and other selected characteristics of cigarette smokers and nonsmokers as related to epidemiological studies of lung cancer and other diseases. J. Natl. Cancer Inst. **22:** 259-282.
4. Harrison, R. H. & E. H. Kass. 1967. Differences between Negro and white pregnant women on the MMPI. J. Consult. Clin. Psychol. **31:** 454-463.
5. Reiter, H. H. 1970. Some EPPS differences between smokers and nonsmokers. Percept. Mot. Skills **30:** 253.
6. Schneider, N. G. & J. P. Houston. 1970. Smoking and anxiety. Psychol. Rep. **26:** 941.
7. Rantakallio, P. 1983. A follow-up study up to the age of 14 of children whose mothers smoked during pregnancy. Acta Paediatr. Scand. **72:** 747-753.
8. Butler, N. R. & D. G. Bonham. 1963. Perinatal Mortality: The First Report of the 1958 British Perinatal Mortality Survey. Livingstone. Edinburgh.
9. Butler, N. R. & E. D. Alberman. 1969. Perinatal Problems: The Second Report of the 1958 British Perinatal Mortality Survey. Livingstone. Edinburgh.
10. Davie, R., N. R. Butler & H. Goldstein. 1972. From birth to seven: A report of the National Child Development Study. Longman. London.

11. BUTLER, N. R. & H. GOLDSTEIN. 1973. Smoking in pregnancy and subsequent child development. Br. Med. J. **4:** 573-575.
12. FOGELMAN, K. 1980. Smoking in pregnancy and subsequent development of the child. Child Care Health Dev. **6:** 233-249.
13. GARN, S. M., A. S. PETZOLD, S. A. RIDELLA *et al.* 1980. Effect of smoking during pregnancy on Apgar and Bayley scores. Lancet **II:** 912-913.
14. GARN, S. M., M. JOHNSTON, S. A. RIDELLA *et al.* 1981. Effect of maternal cigarette smoking on Apgar scores. Am. J. Dis. Child. **135:** 503-506.
15. HARDY, J. B. & E. D. MELLITS. 1972. Does maternal smoking during pregnancy have a long-term effect on the child? Lancet **II:** 1332-1336.
16. BROMAN, S. H., P. L. NICHOLS & W. A. KENNEDY. 1975. Preschool IQ: Prenatal and Early Developmental Correlates. Lawrence Erlbaum Associates. Hillsdale, NJ.
17. NICHOLS, P. L. & T. C. CHEN. 1981. Minimal Brain Dysfunction: A Prospective Study. Lawrence Erlbaum Associates. Hillsdale, NJ.
18. NAEYE, R. L. 1981. Influence of maternal cigarette smoking during pregnancy on fetal and childhood growth. Obstet. Gynecol. **57:** 18-21.
19. NAEYE, R. L. & E. C. PETERS. 1984. Mental development of children whose mothers smoked during pregnancy. J. Am. Coll. Obstet. Gynecol. **64:** 601-607.
20. MARTIN, J., D. C. MARTIN & C. A. LUND *et al.* 1977. Maternal alcohol ingestion and cigarette smoking and their effects on newborn conditioning. Alcohol. Clin. Exp. Res. **1:** 243-247.
21. STREISSGUTH, A. P., H. M. BARR & D. C. MARTIN *et al.* 1980. Effects of maternal alcohol, nicotine, and caffeine use during pregnancy on infant mental and motor development at eight months. Alcohol. Clin. Exp. Res. **4:** 152-164.
22. LANDESMAN-DWYER, S. & A. S. RAGOZIN. 1981. Behavioral correlates of prenatal alcohol exposure: A four year follow-up study. Neurobehav. Toxicol. Teratol. **3:** 187-193.
23. STREISSGUTH, A. P., D. C. MARTIN, H. M. BARR *et al.* 1984. Intrauterine alcohol and nicotine exposure: Attention and reaction time in 4-year-old children. Dev. Psychol. **20:** 533-541.
24. STREISSGUTH, A. P., H. M. BARR & P. D. SAMPSON *et al.* 1986. Attention, distraction and reaction time at age 7 years and prenatal alcohol exposure. Neurobehav. Toxicol. Teratol. **8:** 717-725.
25. GUSELLA, J. L. & P. A. FRIED. 1983. Effects of maternal social drinking and smoking on offspring at 13 months. Neurobehav. Toxicol. Teratol. **6:** 13-17.
26. FRIED, P. A. & J. E. MAKIN. 1987. Neonatal behavioural correlates of prenatal exposure to marihuana, cigarettes and alcohol in a low risk population. Neurotoxicol. Teratol. **9:** 1-7.
27. FRIED, P. A., B. WATKINSON, R. F. DILLON *et al.* 1987. Neonatal neurological status in a low-risk population after prenatal exposure to cigarettes, marijuana, and alcohol. Dev. Behav. Pediatr. **8:** 318-326.
28. FRIED, P. A. & C. M. O'CONNELL. 1987. A comparison of the effects of prenatal exposure to tobacco, alcohol, cannabis and caffeine on birth size and subsequent growth. Neurotoxicol. Teratol. **9:** 79-85.
29. WINGERD, J. & E. J. SCHOEN. 1974. Factors influencing length at birth and height at five years. Pediatrics **53:** 737-741.
30. DENSON, R., J. L. NANSO & R. N. McWATTERS. 1975. Hyperkinesis and maternal smoking. Can. Psychiatr. Assoc. J. **20:** 183-187.
31. DUNN, H. G., A. K. McBURNEY, S. INGRAM *et al.* 1976. Maternal cigarette smoking during pregnancy and the child's subsequent development: I. Physical growth to the age of 6 ½ years. Can. J. Public Health **67:** 499-505.
32. DUNN, H. G., S. K. McBURNEY, S. INGRAM *et al.* 1977. Maternal cigarette smoking during pregnancy and the child's subsequent development: II. Neurological and intellectual maturation to the age of 6½ years. Can. J. Public Health **68:** 43-50.
33. SAXON, D. W. 1978. The behaviour of infants whose mothers smoke in pregnancy. Early Hum. Dev. **2:** 363-369.
34. HINGSON, R., J. B. GOULD, S. MORELOCK *et al.* 1982. Maternal cigarette smoking, psychoactive substance use, and infant Apgar scores. Am. J. Obstet. Gyncol. **144:** 959-966.

35. PICONE, T. A., L. H. ALLEN, P. N. OLSEN *et al.* 1982. Pregnancy outcome in North American women. II. Effects of diet, cigarette smoking, stress, and weight gain on placentas, and on neonatal physical and behavioral characteristics. Am. J. Clin. Nutr. **36:** 1214-1224.
36. JACOBSON, S. W., G. G. FEIN, J. L. JACOBSON *et al.* 1984. Neonatal correlates of prenatal exposure to smoking, caffeine, and alcohol. Infant Behav. Dev. **7:** 253-265.
37. KOLVIN, I., R. F. GARSIDE, I. M. LEITCH *et al.* Smoking in pregnancy and child behaviour. Unpublished report.
38. RONA, R. J., C. D. FLOREY, G. C. CLARKE *et al.* 1981. Parental smoking at home and height of children. Br. Med. J. **23:** 1363.
39. RUSH, D. 1984. The behavioral consequences of protein-energy deprivation and supplementation in early life: An epidemiologic perspective. *In* Human Nutrition: A Comprehensive Treatise. Vol. 5. Nutrition and Behavior. J. R. Galler, Ed.: 119-158. Plenum Press. New York, NY.

Mothers Who Smoke and the Lungs of Their Offspring[a]

ADRIEN C. MOESSINGER

Divisions of Perinatal Medicine and Developmental Pathology
Departments of Pediatrics and Pathology
College of Physicians and Surgeons of Columbia University
Babies Hospital, Box 34
3959 Broadway
New York, New York 10032

INTRODUCTION

The multiple adverse effects of maternal smoking during pregnancy have been clearly documented in a number of studies published over the last thirty years.[1] These include an increased incidence of spontaneous abortions, impaired fetal growth and excess perinatal mortality as well as increased long-term morbidity. The Sudden Infant Death Syndrome is also significantly associated with maternal smoking.

Since the early seventies several studies have reported an association between parental smoking and pulmonary morbidity of their children.[2-6] Harlap and Davies,[2] for instance, found that the prevalence of hospital admission for infants with the diagnoses of bronchitis or pneumonia was twice as common for infants of smokers (> 24 cigarettes/day) than for infants of nonsmokers. Tager *et al.*,[5] using pulmonary function studies, documented decreased lung growth during childhood and adolescence in association with parental smoking. While not all studies documented significant associations, it is fair to say that the majority of studies not only found the association to be present but also that its strength correlated with the number of cigarettes smoked, supporting the concept of a causal link.

In studies where it was looked for, the effect on respiratory morbidity appeared to be more, if not exclusively related to maternal rather than paternal smoking. Likewise, most studies that have provided the data have found a larger effect of maternal smoking on female rather than male children's pulmonary functions. As reviewed recently by Tager,[7] a number of explanations for the predominance of the maternal rather than paternal smoking effect seem possible. The explanation most often given is that because mothers spend more time with their children, they are the predominant source of exposure to postnatal passive smoking. The fact that female children have been observed to show larger effects of maternal smoking than male children can be interpreted to support this explanation if one envisions that girls may share more activities with their mothers than boys. Another explanation is the possibility that maternal smoking during pregnancy produces effects on fetal lung de-

[a] This work was supported by National Institute of Child Health and Human Development Grant HD-13063.

velopment that parallel the subtle and general growth retarding effects of smoking during pregnancy.

Evidence for a Prenatal Effect

We presented five years ago an animal model supporting the hypothesis that maternal smoking during pregnancy alters fetal lung development and could, at least in part, explain the increased pulmonary morbidity in the offspring of smokers by a prenatal in-utero effect.[8,9] The results of a recent study in the human lend support to this hypothesis.[10]

Animal Model

Bassi et al.[8] developed a rat model of maternal smoking and demonstrated, while controlling for caloric intake and litter size, that the fetuses suffered from a disproportionate type of fetal growth retardation with a predominant impact on lung growth. Collins et al.[9] demonstrated reduced lung volume, lower internal surface area, and fewer and larger alveoli in the offspring of rats exposed to cigarette smoke. Also, the proportion of the lung occupied by interstitial tissue and its outgrowths (septae), which are necessary for airspace formation, was reduced. The total length of a component of the interstitium, parenchymal elastic tissue, was severely diminished. Singh et al.[11] documented that while total phospholipid contents and phosphatidyl choline levels were not significantly decreased, there was a significant decrease (i.e., 27-28%) in both disaturated phosphatidyl choline and phosphatidyl glycerol.

These data show that fetal lung growth and maturation are impaired as a consequence of maternal smoke exposure in the rat model. Unfortunately fetal gender was not consistently recorded in these studies. Quantitative reduction of interstitial tissue is part of the lung maturation process; however, deficient formation of airspace septae suggests that fetal lung connective tissue growth may have been impaired through gestation. Diminution of elastic tissue growth may have reduced septal growth since elastic tissue appears to be critical for the septation process. The substrates for surfactant production are not reduced; there appears therefore to be a block in surfactant synthesis. The functional sequelae of the structural abnormalities need to be explored: it is not known if the lung can recover postnatally from the structural alterations that occur antenatally as a result of maternal smoking in the animal model.

Human Studies

Both direct and indirect support for the concept of a prenatal insult can be found in studies of human subjects.[5,7,12] Morgan et al.[13] provided evidence for dysanaptic lung growth in young infants born to mothers who smoked during pregnancy. The most convincing support for this concept is the study of Taylor and Wadsworth.[10] Using the British Births Survey, they first confirmed that maternal, but not paternal, smoking was significantly associated with the reported incidence of bronchitis and hospital admission for lower respiratory tract illness in early life. They were then able to identify subsets of women who either smoked during pregnancy but not after delivery (n = 493) and of women who smoked only after their child was born (n = 353). Reported rates of admission to hospital for lower respiratory tract diseases were found to be as high in children born to mothers who stopped smoking during pregnancy as in those whose mothers smoked continuously both during and after pregnancy. It is of interest that no difference in the rate of hospital admission was found for children whose mothers started to smoke only after delivery as compared to children of mothers who never smoked. These findings support the concept that maternal smoking influences the incidence of respiratory illnesses in children mainly through a congenital effect, and only to a lesser extent (for bronchitis) through passive exposure after birth.

SUMMARY

Maternal smoking is associated with an increased prevalence of respiratory morbidity in children. It had been widely assumed in the past that this effect was the result of postnatal environment tobacco smoke exposure (passive smoking). There is mounting evidence, based on studies in humans and in animal models to suggest that maternal smoking during pregnancy adversely affects fetal lung development. The pathogenesis for this lesion is unclear and it is not known if the insult is the same in the human and the animal model.

REFERENCES

1. JAMES, L. S., A. C. MOESSINGER, H. REY & H. E. FOX. 1986. Maternal smoking and the outcome of pregnancy. In Recent Advances in Perinatology. K. Maeda, K. Okuyama & Y. Takeda, Eds.: 3-14. Elsevier. Amsterdam.
2. HARLAP, S. & A. M. DAVIES. 1974. Infant admissions to hospital and maternal smoking. Lancet ii: 529-532.
3. COLLEY, J. R. T., W. W. HOLLAND & R. T. CORKHILL. 1974. Influence of passive smoking and parental phlegm on pneumonia and bronchitis in early childhood. Lancet ii: 1031-1034.
4. RANTAKALLIO, P. 1978. Relationship of maternal smoking to morbidity and mortality of the child up to age of five. Acta Paediatr. Scand. 67: 621-631.
5. TAGER, I. B., S. T. WEISS, A. MUNOZ, B. ROSNER & F. R. SPEIZER. 1983. Longitudinal study of the effects of maternal smoking on pulmonary function in children. N. Engl. J. Med. 309: 699-703.
6. FERGUSSON, D. M. & L. J. HORWOOD. 1985. Parental smoking and respiratory during early childhood: A six year longitudinal study. Pediatr. Pulmonol. 1: 99-106.
7. TAGER, I. B. 1986. "Passive smoking" and respiratory health in children—Sophistry or cause for concern? (Editorial) Am. Rev. Respir. Dis. 133: 959-961.
8. BASSI, J. A., P. ROSSO, A. C. MOESSINGER, W. A. BLANC & L. S. JAMES. 1984. Fetal growth retardation due to maternal tobacco smoke exposure in the rat. Pediatr. Res. 18: 127-130.
9. COLLINS, M. H., A. C. MOESSINGER, J. KLEINERMAN, J. A. BASSI, P. ROSSO, A. M. COLLINS, L. S. JAMES & W. A. BLANC. 1985. Fetal lung hypoplasia associated with maternal smoking: A morphometric analysis. Pediatr. Res. 19: 408-412.

Developmental Neurotoxicity of Nicotine, Carbon Monoxide, and Other Tobacco Smoke Constituents

CHARLES F. MACTUTUS [a]

Jefferson Medical College
Philadelphia, Pennsylvania 19107

INTRODUCTION

Animal models of the developmental neurotoxicity of tobacco smoke constituents provide a particularly advantageous context in which to examine the consequences of tobacco (ab)use under rigorous experimental control. The major emphasis of the present overview is on the identification of conceptual and practical issues which pervade the literature on animal models of tobacco (ab)use during pregnancy. The major aim is to facilitate our further development of valid animal models and to highlight those studies of the last decade which have focused on the development and functional integrity of the central nervous system.

Cigarette Smoking: Prospective on Scope

The costs of cigarette smoking are substantial and well-documented both in terms of adverse health effects and medical care costs.[1] It is encouraging that there has been a 25% decrease from the peak per capita consumption of cigarettes in the early to mid-1960's.[2–4] However, if we remove the bias from this statistic due to the increase in the U.S. population, we learn that total domestic cigarette consumption has risen 11.5% over this same period (FIG. 1). It should be emphasized that the 25% per capita decrease is averaged over active smokers, former smokers, and nonsmokers. Among persons who are current smokers, consumption per adult smoker has increased from 27.6 to 30.2 cigarettes/day.

For potentially susceptible subpopulations, such as the fetus, there appears more than ever great reason for concern regarding the adverse health effects of cigarette smoking (FIG. 2). First, the primary cause for the 25% per capita cigarette decrease is due to a marked reduction from 52% to 33% by adult males.[5] In contrast, the rate among women has only decreased from 34% to 28% over that same period. Second, considering the comparable increases in rate of quitting for both males and females

[a] Address correspondence to: Charles F. Mactutus, Ph.D., 1905 Winding Ridge Road, Winston-Salem, NC 27127-5772.

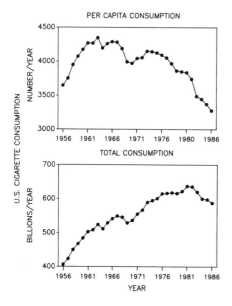

FIGURE 1. Average per capita cigarette consumption for persons 18 years and older as a function of year (*top panel*). Total cigarette consumption in the U.S. as a function year (*bottom panel*). (Derived from U.S.D.A.[2–4])

FIGURE 2. Percent of adults (> 20 yr) who are *former* smokers shown as a function of gender over a recent 20-yr period (*top panel*). Percent of adults (> 20 yr) who are *current* smokers as a function of gender over a recent 20-yr period (*bottom panel*). (Derived from N.C.H.S.[5])

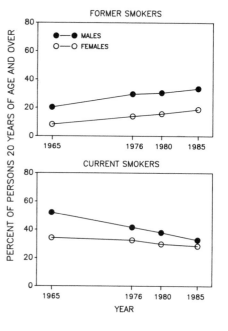

(FIG. 2) along with this relative lack of change in prevalence of smoking among women suggests that there continues to be a differential recruitment of female smokers. Third, the health significance of any reduction in number of smokers may be offset by shifts in intake of the remaining smokers (FIG. 3). Indeed, the latest statistics available indicate that for both males and females the percent of heavy smokers (25 or more/day) has increased steadily since the mid-1960's (males 24.1% to 33.6%; females 13.0% to 20.6%).[5] Finally, despite the extensive efforts promoting an aware-

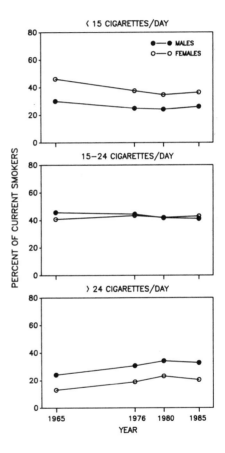

FIGURE 3. Changes in the percent of current men and women (> 20 yr) who are *light* (< 15 cigarettes/day), *moderate* (15-24 cigarettes/day) or *heavy* (> 24 cigarettes/day) smokers across a recent 20-yr period. (Derived from N.C.H.S.[5])

ness of the effects of smoking during pregnancy, it is disturbing that the greatest smoking prevalence rates among females are for those of child-bearing age (20-34 years; 32.3%). Collectively, these factors suggest that today's unborn child not only remains, but may more likely be, in grave danger from the adverse health effects of cigarette smoking.

Tobacco Smoke Constituents

The complex and variable composition of tobacco smoke represents a primary conceptual issue in developing any animal model of smoking. The generation of tobacco smoke from a cigarette is the result of a number of physical and chemical processes occurring in an oxygen deficient, hydrogen-rich environment with a steep temperature gradient (over 900°C). More than 3,800 products are formed[6] in the smoke of a single cigarette with the majority originating just behind the heat generating combustion zone.[7] FIGURE 4 displays the 10 major components of mainstream cigarette smoke which are biologically active.[8] Nicotine is the primary component of the particulate phase of tobacco smoke, while carbon monoxide is the primary component of the vapor phase. The data portrayed are derived from machine-smoking under standard laboratory conditions for analysis of mainstream smoke: one 35 ml puff drawn over a 2 sec period, once per min, until a butt length of 23 mm or filter plus overwrap plus 3 mm is attained.

Standard laboratory methods of determining particulate yields provide invaluable information for comparisons of various brands and designs; however, they have limited

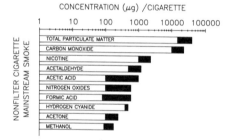

FIGURE 4. The 10 biologically active components of greatest concentration in the mainstream smoke of a nonfilter cigarette burned under standard laboratory conditions. (Derived from the IARC.[8])

applicability to specific human dosage, *i.e.,* they do not reflect the idiosyncratic habits of a smoker. Indeed, plasma nicotine and alveolar carbon monoxide levels in smokers using various low-tar brands correlated poorly with reported tar and nicotine yields.[9] Moreover, smokers appear to compensate for reduced yields by altering their smoking methods so that the amount of tar, nicotine, and carbon monoxide they receive actually bears little relation to reported yields.[10]

Animal Model Assumptions

The animal models that have been employed to study the consequences of tobacco (ab)use during pregnancy may be organized according to their apparent underlying strategy. The prominent strategy chosen is based on a **primary component** assumption—the biological agents of highest concentration in tobacco smoke are the most likely responsible for adverse effects on the fetus. Thus, the majority of studies have employed prenatal nicotine exposure or prenatal carbon monoxide exposure. The alternative strategy which has been employed is based on a **composite effluent** assumption, *i.e.,* the adverse effects of tobacco smoke are a complex function of the interaction of its many diverse constituents. Accordingly, prenatal inhalation exposure to cigarette smoke has been used. A third, presently unexplored strategy is proposed based on an **interactive component** assumption.

Primary Component Exposure: Nicotine

Animal models of tobacco (ab)use during pregnancy which have studied the consequences of prenatal nicotine exposure for potential neurotoxicity have employed one of three different exposure models. These models may be distinguished by the route of nicotine administration: sc injection (TABLE 1), ingestion via drinking water (TABLE 2), and infusion via osmotic pump (TABLE 3). It should be emphasized, however, that the choice among these models reflects much more than the practical concern of ease of administration. Indeed, each harbors a clear conceptual bias regarding the most appropriate pharmacological factor(s) involved in providing a "smoking dose" of nicotine. It would appear from relevant clinical observations that at least three pharmacological factors must be considered with respect to developing an animal model for prenatal nicotine exposure.

Dose Level. Tobacco smoking provides a rare form of drug administration in that nicotine enters the circulation through the pulmonary system—this produces nicotine delivery no less rapid than by iv injection. Smokers absorb approximately 1 mg nicotine/cigarette.[11,12] The increment in blood nicotine levels after a single cigarette range from 16 to 48 ng/ml depending upon how the cigarette is smoked.[13] Average plasma concentrations of nicotine in cigarette smokers during mid-afternoon are approximately 30-40 ng/ml.[14]

Dose Regimen. Smoking provides a dosing regimen which is characterized by a marked waxing and waning of nicotine levels from cigarette to cigarette as well as a net accumulation over the first few hr of the day while a "steady state" is achieved.[13] This pulsed dosing is readily apparent under conditions of smoking approximately 1/cigarette hr; smoking several cigarettes/hr not only yields a higher steady state nicotine level, but also tends to moderate this peak to trough variation. A clear circadian profile of nicotine levels has also been shown, although potential biologically active concentrations nicotine may remain present throughout the night for habitual smokers of approximately 30 or more cigarettes/day.[15]

Half-Life. Half-life estimates of nicotine in blood following the smoking of a single cigarette or an iv infusion of nicotine are in the order of 3 to 9 min. If concentrations of nicotine are followed over a longer period of time or subsequent to multiple doses, a two-compartment elimination model is noted—the terminal half-life averaging 2 hr.[12,16] Nicotine is primarily metabolized in the liver, but also in the lung and kidney.[17] Neither of the major metabolites, cotinine and nicotine-N-oxide, appear to have appreciable pharmacological activity. Cotinine, which has a blood half-life of approximately 20 hr,[18] is particularly useful as a marker of nicotine intake/cigarette smoking.

Critique. What is the relevance of these pharmacological factors to each of these exposure models in rodents? In the rat, sc injections of nicotine provide peak blood levels within several min after injection and their return close to baseline levels by 160 min.[19] The sc route thus provides a clear bolus dose of nicotine and thus also a spike of nicotine to the brain. As such it appears to be a reasonable alternative route to iv administration—the preferred technique for modeling the blood levels of nicotine

TABLE 1. Neurological and Psychological Effects of Subcutaneous Injection of Nicotine during Pregnancy[a]

Species	Ref.[b]	Experimental Design	Prominent Effects
Rat	58	6.0 mg/kg/day with half the dose given twice daily from GEST D3-20 inclusive; included vehicle control; randomly fostered pups.	Maternal mortality (15%); decreased maternal weight gain (DNS); increased perinatal mortality (15-20%) altered body weight (D1-35, +5% to −16%) as well as decreased brain region (up to 10%) and organ weights (up to 12%); increased levels and turnover of norepinephrine (not dopamine)—greatest in cerebellum; altered development of peripheral sympathetic nervous system.
Rat	59	6.0 mg/kg/day with half the dose given twice daily from GEST D4-20 inclusive; included vehicle control; randomly fostered pups.	Maternal mortality (14%); litter resorptions (13%); decreased maternal weight gain (50%); decreased fetal weight (GEST D13; 25%), birthweight (12%) and early neonatal weight (up until D14); decreased brain weight (8%) and increased RNA concentration (27%) (GEST D18); shifted the developmental profiles of ODC and DNA; greatest effect on cerebellar DNA, RNA and protein.
Mouse	60,61	0.9, 1.8 or 2.7 mg/kg/day with half the dose given twice daily during one trimester; included vehicle control.	Increased incidence of stillbirths (r = 0.78) and neonatal deaths (r = 0.55) correlated with dose; decreased gestation length (5%, 3rd trimester); increased latency, delayed development, and delayed dissolution of audiogenic seizures (3rd trimester).
Rat	62,63	0.68 mg/kg/day with half the dose given twice daily from GEST D1-20; included vehicle controls.	Decreased birthweight (8%); produced a sex-dependent difference in avoidance learning (D60)—mainly an impairment for males.
Rat	64	1.5, 3, or 6 mg/kg/day by single daily dose prior (1 wk) and throughout GEST; included vehicle control.	Sterile matings increased (73%, 6 mg dose); dose-response decrease in dam body weight (1st week); dose-response increase in organ/body and brain/body weight ratios (D2); dose-response increase in brain/body weight ratio and brain protein (D180 females).

TABLE 1. (Continued)

Species	Ref.[b]	Experimental Design	Prominent Effects
Rat	65	6.0 mg/kg/day with half the dose given twice daily from GEST D1-20; included vehicle controls.	Maternal measures, early developmental tests, nighttime activity, and operant behavior unaffected; offspring weights (DNS).
Guinea pig	66	6.0 mg/kg/day with half the dose sc injected twice daily throughout GEST; included vehicle controls.	Decreased birthweight and head diameter; decreased spontaneous alternation (58%, D10-21 and 58%, D60-71); fewer entries into novel alley (67%, D21); increased errors in discrimination learning (120%, D85); more trials required to learn a reversal task (96%), more errors were made (248%), and more perseveration occurred (273%).
Rat	39,40, 41	6.0 mg/kg/day with half the dose given twice daily throughout GEST; included vehicle and uninjected controls.	Lower body weight gain of dams (30%); increased gestation length; decreased litter size (12%); birthweight (14%) and body weight (D7, D14, D21, D28, 7-11%); increased body weight (Mon. 11-16, 54g, 7%); generally increased nighttime activity (Mon. 12-30); organ pathology unaffected.
Rat	67	1.5 mg/kg/day by daily dose throughout GEST; included pair-fed, vehicle, and cross-fostered controls.	Decreased food (13%) and water (10%) consumption of pregnant dams; birthweight unaffected; decreased body weight (7%, D21; 3.5%, D77); higher lung/body weight ratios (24%, D84 females).

[a] Abbreviations: GEST-gestation, DNS-data not shown, ODC-ornithine decarboxylase.
[b] Multiple publications employing the same set of animals are summarized collectively.

produced by tobacco smoke.[20] However, given the rapid elimination of nicotine, the twice daily injection does not provide a sustained titer for a significant portion of the day. Attempts to increase the duration of elevated nicotine by injecting large doses will produce convulsions—a 3 mg/kg dose produces mild convulsions while a 5 mg/kg dose may be expected to produce severe convulsions with temporary apnea.[21] Attempts to provide more frequent nicotine spikes by increasing number of daily injections would only increase the probability that the prenatal stress effects will contribute to or interact with the nicotine treatment.

The use of nicotine via drinking water, has a great advantage in avoiding the stress of repeated daily or twice daily injections. Unfortunately, rats do not readily consume nicotine flavored water, a fact perhaps attributable to the neophobic tendencies of this species. Indeed, the introduction of .02% nicotine into drinking water may produce

TABLE 2. Neurological and Psychological Effects of Nicotine Administration via Drinking Water during Pregnancy[a]

Species	Ref.[b]	Experimental Design	Prominent Effects
Rat	23,24	2.4 or 4.5 mg/kg/day prior (1 wk) and throughout GEST and LACT; included vehicle and cross-fostered controls.	High dose decreased water intake (25%) and body weight of lactating dams; dose-response decrease of litter size (27%), but not birthweight; dose-response decrease in body weight from GEST or LACT exposure (D10-40); decreased tyrosine hydroxylase in striatum from GEST (D20, D40) or LACT exposure (D40); GEST or LACT exposure decreased incidence of vaginal opening (D40) and altered developmental profile of LH (D20-D40).
Rat	25	6 mg/kg/day prior (6 wk) and throughout GEST; included vehicle, cross-fostered and fostered controls.	Decreased male birthweight (3%); increased levels of norepinephrine in hypothalamus (D8) and cortex (D8-36); increased adrenergic receptor binding in cortex (D80).
Rat	68	Same as above	Fewer number of males/litter (22%) and decreased male birthweight (7%); lower 24 hr activity of males (D60, D85); less locomotion and rearing of males (D60); adrenal weight (D45) decreased (males) or increased (females).
Rat	69	1.4 or 2.6 mg/kg/day prior (2 wk) and over GEST D1-20; included vehicle control.	Decreased fetal weight (15%, GEST D20-high dose); increased cell necrosis in brain stem (29-50%).
Rat	70	6 mg/kg/day prior (8 wk) and throughout GEST; included vehicle and cross-fostered controls.	Decreased parent body weight (12%); increased dams' daytime activity and decreased dams' corticosterone stress response (40%); decreased male birthweight (15%); consistent (females) or inconsistent (males) increase of daytime activity (D60-80).

[a] Abbreviations: GEST-gestation, LACT-lactation, LH-luteinizing hormone.
[b] Multiple publications employing the same set of animals are summarized collectively.

smoking once they become pregnant. Given the data that rats ingest in multiple bouts throughout the day, one might expect a rather constant dosing of nicotine. On the other hand, a major disadvantage of the oral route of administration is that one would not expect the nicotine spike characteristic of smoking. Oral ingestion, which would result in the slow release of nicotine into the hepatic portal circulation, might be expected to slow and reduce nicotine levels via a first pass metabolism effect. It does appear that appreciable blood levels of nicotine may be achieved via oral ingestion, but they were obtained with 2.5 times the nicotine dose administered by sc route.[26] The available data on plasma nicotine levels of exposed dams are consistent with this notion of reduced nicotine levels via oral administration. Plasma nicotine levels of 18.4 ng/ml were obtained after at least 4 weeks of oral dosing at a rate of 4.5 mg/kg/day.[24] In contrast, plasma nicotine levels obtained after 3 weeks of dosing at the same rate were 66.6 ng/ml when delivered by osmotic pump.[22]

The use of implanted osmotic pumps represents the most recent approach to providing chronic nicotine exposure during pregnancy. Like the oral ingestion method, this approach precludes the daily handling and stress of injection. By their very nature, these infusion pumps will provide a sustained titer of nicotine, but this is at the expense of providing neither the multiple nicotine spikes nor the circadian nicotine changes characteristic of cigarette smoking. A potentially serious limitation is imposed by the surgical stress required to implant the pump. As the longest-acting commercially available pumps have an effective life of 28 days, surgery must be performed either shortly prior to mating or during pregnancy. Although admittedly neither alternative appears particularly attractive, pump implantation during pregnancy has been successfully employed with the use of a short acting anesthetic.[22,27–29] Unfortunately, this method has promoted the use of nicotine levels even higher than 6 mg/kg/day.[22,28,29]

Based on the current clinical data indicating that smokers absorb about 1 mg of nicotine/cigarette, an average 60 kg adult female would have to smoke 30 cigarettes/day to achieve a dose rate of 0.5 mg/kg/day. Doses this low have been rarely used (TABLES 1-3). In contrast, 11 out of 17 studies have relied exclusively on a daily dose of 6 mg/kg or more. The need for more dose-response studies notwithstanding, this most frequently chosen dose of 6 mg/kg/day theoretically corresponds to smoking an unbelievable 360 cigarettes/day by a 60 kg woman. Clearly such dosing is well beyond the physiological realm.

Effects on the Fetus. Nicotine and cotinine have been detected in the amniotic fluid[30] and in the umbilical vein serum of cigarette smokers.[31] Most recently it has been shown that nicotine levels in placental tissue (first trimester), in amniotic fluid (second trimester), and in placental tissue and fetal serum at parturition were all greater than maternal serum values taken at corresponding time periods.[32] Similarly obtained cotinine levels were all lower than or comparable to corresponding maternal serum levels. Collectively, these data indicate that not only is the fetus exposed to nicotine via maternal smoking, but that it may be exposed to higher concentrations of nicotine than the mother. It is noteworthy that a similar outcome had been previously established in rhesus monkeys[33] and sheep.[34]

With respect to the rat, nicotine and its metabolites may be noted in the fetus within 5 min after iv injection of the dam[35] with the concentration of radioactivity in the fetal plasma exceeding that of maternal plasma from 30 min through 20 hr. While peak fetal brain concentrations were present initially (5 min) after maternal dosing, peak plasma levels in the fetus did not occur until 1 hr. In contrast, placental passage of nicotine in mice was reported to be generally low and delayed.[36] Unfortunately, comparative maternal to fetal plasma levels are not available to more critically evaluate this possible species difference. This latter study did suggest, however, that nicotine concentration may be higher in placental ($3\times$) and fetal ($2\times$) tissue after sc than iv administration. It is generally accepted that little appreciable liver metabolism occurs during the fetal period; the presence of cotinine in the fetus is attributable to transplacental passage from the mother.[37]

Studies of potential nicotine-induced neurotoxicity must also consider the diverse well-documented effects of this agent on early pregnancy. Among the alterations which have been reported are a suppression of conceptus growth, an impairment of uterine decidualization, and a retardation of implantation. A marked reduction in uterine blood flow and intrauterine oxygen tension contributes, at least in part, to each of these effects.[38] Decreases in litter size[24] or birthweight[39-41] and increases in fetal resorptions[28,29] may very well reflect the indirect effects of impaired embryo and fetal oxygenation. Each nicotine exposure model appears to affect at least one of these parameters, particularly at the high 6 mg/kg/day dose. Finally, it is noted that maternal dosing with nicotine during lactation may be expected to produce profound interference with postnatal growth consequent to an inhibitory effect on prolactin.[42]

Conclusions. Each currently employed exposure model has its advantages and disadvantages, but from the prospective of providing a parallel to the conditions of nicotine intake via cigarette smoking, it appears unreasonable to argue that any one technique is best. A more creative protocol will be required to provide an intermittent, bolus delivery of nicotine for approximately half a day over a prolonged period of time. This goal should be achievable with the use of current technology. Advances in the study of subtle effects of nicotine on the developing nervous system are also more likely to be fostered by a more judicious choice of doses, regardless of route, and the frequent use of a dose-response design. The determination of physiological levels of nicotine in plasma is also of critical importance, particularly with respect to comparing results across exposure models and species. At present it would appear difficult to convincingly argue that any of the reported psychological and neurological alterations of offspring following prenatal nicotine exposure will be replicable with models more closely paralleling the physiological conditions of cigarette smoking. A further goal remains the differentiation of mechanisms of potential neurotoxicity: What is attributable to a direct effect of the transmitted nicotine upon the fetus versus impaired placental perfusion (concomitant hypoxia and acidosis)?

Primary Component Exposure: Carbon Monoxide

The use of prenatal carbon monoxide exposure for assessing potential neurotoxicity in an animal model has been less widely studied than use of nicotine. This fact undoubtedly relates to the greater complexities involved in inhalation exposures, the only acceptable exposure route for chronic studies. TABLE 4 highlights those studies of the last decade which have examined the consequences of such early exposure on the nervous system. Several pharmacological factors relevant to cigarette smoking as well as those major physiological mechanisms involved in the susceptibility of the fetus to elevated carbon monoxide levels provide a characterization of this approach.

Dose level. Current clinical studies suggest that the carbon monoxide levels achieved via cigarette smoking by the end of the day (*i.e.,* equilibrium values) are in the range of 8-11% for habitual smokers of an average of 28-30 cigarettes/day.[14] Smokers of an average of 37 cigarettes/day show blood carboxyhemoglobin (HbCO) levels of 9.1% (range, 5.1-13%) 2 min after smoking a cigarette in the afternoon of a day during which they have smoked in their usual manner.[13]

TABLE 4. Neurological and Psychological Effects of Carbon Monoxide Inhalation during Pregnancy[a]

Species	Ref.	Experimental Design	Prominent Effects
Rat	71	75, 150 or 300 ppm exposure from GEST D1-LACT D10; HbCO levels of 11.5%, 18.5%, & 26.8%; included air exposure controls and GEST only exposure dams.	Dose-response decrease in birthweight (up to 13.8%); apparent dose-response decrease in neostriatal DNA (up to 17%, D21, GEST D1-LACT D10 and protein (up to 8.5%); dose-response increase in neostriatal dopamine concentration, with no change in metabolites (up to 20%, D21, GEST D1-LACT D10).
Rat	53	Same as above, but without GEST only exposure dams.	Dose-response decrease in body weight (up to 24.6%, D10, not present at D21); dose-response decrease in cerebellar weight (up to 26%, D10; up to 6.6%, D21); dose-response decrease in GABA uptake (up to 26%, D10; up to 9.5%, D21); fewer cerebellar fissures (14%, 300 ppm, D21) but depth of major fissures comparable; decreased number and density of cerebellar Purkinje cells (10%, 300 ppm, D21).
Rat	51	75, 150 or 300 ppm exposure throughout GEST; HbCO levels of 11.5%, 18.5%, & 26.8%; included air exposure controls.	Dose-response decrease in birthweight (up to 12.5%); dose-response decrease in cerebellar weight (up to 11.4%, D21; up to 8.3%, D42); dose-response decrease in pons/medulla norepinephrine concentration (up to 7%) and serotonin concentration (up to 9.5%, D21); dose-response increase of norepinephrine concentration in neocortex (up to 14%) and hippocampus (up to 22%, D42).
Rat	52	150 ppm exposure throughout GEST; HbCO levels of 10-11%; included air exposure controls.	Increased cerebellar norepinephrine concentration and content, but not cortical values, from D14-42.
Rat	55	150 ppm exposure throughout GEST; HbCO levels of 15.6%; included air exposure controls.	Normal acquisition of two-way avoidance (D120) with moderate or difficult task requirements; minor (24-hr) and severe (28-day) retention impairments; impaired acquisition and (24-hr) retention of two-way avoidance (D300-360).

TABLE 4. (Continued)

Species	Ref.	Experimental Design	Prominent Effects
Rat	54	Same as above.	Decreased birthweight (5%); impaired acquisition and retention (24-hr) of two-way active avoidance (D30); pseudoconditioning controls were not affected, nor was there any detectable evidence of altered activity or reactivity.
Rat	72	10,000 ppm exposure for 2 or 3 hr on GEST D15; HbCO levels of 50%.	Maternal loss of righting reflex followed by coma; decreased preweaning weight (5%); increased (26%, D30) exploratory activity (3-hr exposure); decreased dendritic branching in caudate (D1); 20% (2-hr)-70% (3-hr) ectopic swelling of caudate (D1-D210).
Rat	73	150 ppm exposure throughout GEST; no HbCO levels included cross-fostering air exposure controls.	Decreased birthweight (7.6%) and preweaning weights; impaired negative geotaxis (D3) and homing behavior (D3-5).
Mouse	74	Exposure throughout GEST; HbCO levels of 6-11%; included air exposure controls.	Increased errors in heat-motivated Y-maze (39% males, 69% females, D42); decreased maternal weight gain (10%).
Rat	75	Same as above, but no cross-fostering.	Increased amplitude of N1-P1 and N1-P2 components of females (D78), but not males.

[a] Abbreviations: GEST-gestation, LACT-lactation, HbCO-carboxyhemoglobin.

Dose regimen. The blood levels of HbCO may be roughly estimated on the basis of ambient carbon monoxide concentration in ppm and exposure time.[43] The absorption half-time for 50 ppm carbon monoxide, producing an HbCO level of 8% at equilibrium, is approximately 2 hr. As smoking does not represent a continuous source of inspired carbon monoxide, an increase of HbCO levels to a steady state may continue over many hr of the day. A clear circadian profile has also been reported, although above background levels of HbCO may remain present through the night.[15]

Half-life. It is commonly held that the decline in blood HbCO levels follows a biphasic function, presumably reflecting a rapid distribution (20-30 min) followed by a slower linear decline. Half-time estimates for HbCO at levels relevant to cigarette smoking (5-16%) are in the range of 3-4 hr.

Critique. A 24 hr/day exposure of carbon monoxide throughout the gestational period was employed by nine of the ten reported studies. This procedure importantly minimizes handling and its associated stress during pregnancy. On the other hand, humans do not typically smoke cigarettes 24 hr/day. There has only been one experiment published which has employed a partial daily exposure through a significant portion of gestation—this was a teratology study with no postnatal measures recorded.[44] The "tenth" study employed a severe 2- or 3-hr carbon monoxide exposure on gestational day 15. Such an acute high-dose exposure provides little information regarding an animal model of smoking. Two of the nine chronic exposures provided at least some litters for whom the exposure continued through postnatal day 10. While this is of potential interest (re: exposure via passive smoking) on the assumption that smokers who maintain their habit during pregnancy are not likely to suddenly stop smoking once their infant is born, this issue has yet to be purposefully addressed. The rationale for continuing exposure through the early postnatal period was to maintain exposure of the rat pup to carbon monoxide until the maturation of its cerebellum approximated that of the human's at birth. This is an instance of a specific mechanistic hypothesis underlying the design of the study, and it reveals a limitation of prenatal studies with rats.

With respect to dose levels, the majority of studies have employed at least one dose which approximates the HbCO levels of heavy cigarette smokers. It must be emphasized, however, that because the animal studies have employed 24 hr/day dosing, there is no opportunity for HbCO levels to decrease during sleep. Consequently, the lower dosage levels employed more closely approximate peak HbCO levels of cigarette smokers. Either a further reduction in dosage levels or an accommodation of dosing schedule will help provide a more appropriate analogy.

Effects on the Fetus. There are several reasons which predict greater susceptibility of the fetus to carbon monoxide in comparison to the mother. The first reason derives from the fact that the oxygen dissociation curve of the fetus lies to the left of the maternal oxygen dissociation curve. When carbon monoxide binds to hemoglobin, it does so more tightly than oxygen by a factor of 210 to 250, and produces a conformational change in oxyhemoglobin that results in further shift of the oxygen dissociation curve to the left.[45] This means that oxygen is held more tightly to hemoglobin and is less likely to be given up to tissues at a given oxygen tension. It follows that fetal oxygen tension must then be reduced to very low levels to provide adequate tissue oxygenation. A second consequence of these alterations is that fetal HbCO levels are higher than those seen in maternal circulation at equilibrium. For the human the ratio of fetal to maternal HbCO levels is 1.1:1; but this value varies for other mammals.[46] Third, it has been demonstrated in sheep that both the absorption and elimination half-times for the fetus are about three times longer than those for the mother.[47]

Although the fetus is not unprotected in defense against elevated carbon monoxide levels,[48] the extent and conditions of such compensation are not well understood. For example, redistribution of blood flow in the fetus may help protect the brain under conditions of hypoxia; nevertheless, the bulk of this flow is shifted to brainstem areas rather than to higher subcortical and cortical areas.[49] Other adaptive mechanisms which function in the adult in response to hypoxia, such as an increase in cardiac output, do not occur to any appreciable extent in the fetus—the output of its heart normally functions at two to three times that of an adult on a per weight basis.[50]

Conclusions. An improvement in the carbon monoxide model of prenatal tobacco (ab)use may be fostered by the implementation of a circadian cycle on the dosing schedule. This goal appears readily achievable. It remains an open question as to whether the challenge of adapting daily to elevations in HbCO levels would have a more deleterious effect on the fetus than adapting to a sustained elevation of HbCO levels. The increasing use of dose-response studies in this model should continue to yield informative relationships between the effects of carbon monoxide and the developing nervous system. The majority of studies have recorded physiological levels of carbon monoxide exposure (HbCO levels at equilibrium); this is of particular value in interpretation of the data. Evaluations of HbCO levels of the fetus would be an important further advance for this model. Additional long-term goals include determining the basis for the vulnerability of the cerebellum to carbon monoxide[51–53] as well as assessing the replicability and basis of the apparently permanent deficits in memory processes induced by prenatally elevated HbCO levels.[54,55]

Composite Exposure: Cigarette Smoke Inhalation

The use of a composite effluent strategy has the distinct advantage of studying the specific agent that those employing the primary component strategy are attempting to model. Similar to the use of the carbon monoxide model, the complexities of

TABLE 5. Neurological and Psychological Effects of Cigarette Smoke Inhalation during Pregnancy[a]

Species	Ref.	Experimental Design	Prominent Effects
Rat	63	Two 15-min exposures a day from GEST D1-20; 2.1% nicotine/cigarette; 16.3% HbCO at end of exposure.	Decreased maternal weight gain (25.4%); decreased birthweight (87%); increased rate of avoidance acquisition (22.7%, D60).
Mouse	76	Two 15-min exposures a day throughout GEST; 2 mg nicotine/cigarette; 500 ppm carbon monoxide.	Decreased fertility (44%, high active strain; 22% low active strain); decreased survival to weaning (25.2%); depressed open-field activity (58%, D28); trend of decreased activity in hole board (D50, DNS); increased liver weight (11.9%, D62).

[a] Abbreviations: GEST-gestation, HbCO-carboxyhemoglobin, DNS-data not shown.

inhalation exposures are inherent. Obviously, one must also deal with the fact that animals do not inhale smoke like humans—some criticize such exposures as more akin to asphyxiation than to smoking. The irritant properties of the smoke may also add a prenatal stress factor to this approach.

Despite the potential attractiveness of the basic strategy, it appears these practical and interpretative concerns have stopped all but a few investigators from employing prenatal cigarette smoke exposure as a model for investigations of potential neurotoxicity of tobacco (ab)use during pregnancy. The data for the two relevant experiments published during the last decade are presented in TABLE 5. Both have made some attempt at specifying the exposure conditions which were provided by the cigarette smoke, but physiological levels of both nicotine and HbCO would be ideally desired. It does appear that the smoke conditions employed produced maternal toxicity as well as altered the behavior of the offspring. Striking decreases in maternal weight gain have been reported in several other studies[56,57] with concomitant decreases in fetal growth. Perhaps the use of an adaptation period to the daily smoking treatment, similar to that required with oral consumption of nicotine, might help mitigate the severity of the maternal toxicity and permit a more direct assessment of fetal susceptibility.

Interactive Component Exposure: Nicotine and Carbon Monoxide

The advantage of looking at a combination of components, as in cigarette smoke exposure, may be coupled with the strengths of investigating individual primary components via an interactive component model. The investigation of such joint effects should be more manageable in the absence of the myriad particulate and gaseous phase substances conferring the irritant properties of tobacco smoke. Whether joint effects of exposure to nicotine and carbon monoxide would be greater than either alone, strictly additive, or synergistic remains an unexplored, but readily testable concern. One might also reasonably consider superimposing a circadian pattern on this interactive component strategy. The promise of greater clinical relevance with this interactive component strategy is obvious (the framework it offers is more integrative), but at present one may only anticipate that it will provide a more comprehensive understanding of the neurotoxic potential of tobacco (ab)use during pregnancy.

REFERENCES

1. U.S. DEPARTMENT OF HEALTH, EDUCATION AND WELFARE. 1979. Smoking and Health: A Report of the Surgeon General. U.S. Government Printing Office. Washington, DC.
2. U.S. DEPARTMENT OF AGRICULTURE. 1964. Agricultural Statistics, 1964. U.S. Government Printing Office. Washington, DC.
3. U.S. DEPARTMENT OF AGRICULTURE. 1975. Agricultural Statistics, 1975. U.S. Government Printing Office. Washington, DC.
4. U.S. DEPARTMENT OF AGRICULTURE. 1987. Agricultural Statistics, 1987. U.S. Government Printing Office. Washington, DC.
5. NATIONAL CENTER FOR HEALTH STATISTICS. 1988. Health, United States, 1987. U.S. Government Printing Office. Washington, DC.
6. DUBE, M. F. & C. R. GREEN. 1982. Recent Adv. Tob. Sci. 8: 42-102.
7. BAKER, R. R. 1981. Prog. Energy Combustion Sci. 7: 135-153.
8. INTERNATIONAL AGENCY FOR RESEARCH ON CANCER (IARC). 1986. IARC Monographs on the Evaluation of the Carcinogenic Risk of Chemicals to Humans, Vol. 38. Tobacco Smoking. IARC, Lyon, France.
9. RUSSELL, M. A. H., M. JARVIS, E. IYER & C. FEYERABEND. 1980. Br. Med. J. 280: 972-976.
10. BENOWITZ, N. L., P. JACOB III, L. T. KOZLOWSKI & L. YU. 1986. N. Engl. J. Med. 315: 1310-1313.
11. BENOWITZ, N. L. & P. JACOB III. 1984. Clin. Pharmacol. Ther. 35: 499-504.
12. FEYERABEND, C., R. M. J. INGS & M. A. H. RUSSELL. 1985. Br. J. Clin. Pharmacol. 19: 239-247.
13. RUSSELL, M. A. H., C. FEYERABEND & P. V. COLE. 1976. Br. Med. J. 1: 1043-1046.
14. BENOWITZ, N. L., F. KUYT & P. JACOB III. 1984. Clin. Pharmacol. Ther. 36: 74-81.
15. BENOWITZ, N. L., F. KUYT & P. JACOB III. 1982. Clin. Pharmacol. Ther. 32: 758-764.
16. BENOWITZ, N. L., P. JACOB III., R. T. JONES & J. ROSENBERG. 1982. J. Pharmacol. Exp. Ther. 221: 368-372.

17. VOLLE, R. L. & G. B. KOELLE. 1970. Ganglionic stimulating and blocking agents. *In* The Pharmacological Basis of Therapeutics. L. S. Goodman & A. Gilman, Eds., Macmillan. New York, NY.
18. BENOWITZ, N. L., F. KUYT, P. JACOB III, R. T. JONES & A. L. OSMAN. 1983. Clin. Pharmacol. Ther. **34**: 604-611.
19. PRATT, J. A., I. P. STOLERMAN, H. S. GARCHA, V. GIARDINI & C. FEYERABEND. 1983. Psychopharmacology **81**: 54-60.
20. ARMITAGE, A. K., C. T. DOLLERY, C. F. GEORGE, T. H. HOUSEMAN, P. J. LEWIS & D. M. TURNER. 1975. Br. Med. J. **4**: 313-316.
21. BECKER, R. F., C. R. LITTLE & J. E. KING. 1968. Am. J. Obstet. Gynecol. **100**: 957-968.
22. MURRIN, L. C., J. R. FERRER, W. Y. ZENG & N. J. HALEY. 1987. Life Sci. **40**: 1699-1708.
23. MEYER, D. C. & L. A. CARR. 1987. Neurotoxicol. Teratol. **9**: 95-98.
24. CARR, L. A., D. E. WALTERS & D. C. MEYER. 1985. Res. Commun. Subst. Abuse **6**: 151-164.
25. PETERS, D. A. V. 1984. Res. Commun. Chem. Pathol. Pharmacol. **46**: 307-317.
26. TURNER, D. M. 1975. Xenobiotica **9**: 553-561.
27. LICHTENSTEIGER, W. & M. SCHLUMPF. 1985. Pharmacol. Biochem. Behav. **23**: 439-444.
28. SLOTKIN, T. A., L. ORBAND-MILLER & K. L. QUEEN. 1987. J. Pharmacol. Exp. Ther. **242**: 232-237.
29. SLOTKIN, T. A., L. ORBAND-MILLER, K. L. QUEEN, W. L. WHITMORE & F. J. SEIDLER. 1987. J. Pharmacol. Exp. Ther. **240**: 602-611.
30. VAN VUNAKIS, H., J. J. LANGONE & A. MILUNSKY. 1974. Am. J. Obstet. Gynecol. **120**: 64-66.
31. LANGONE, J. & H. VAN VUNAKIS. 1975. Res. Commun. Chem. Pathol. Pharmacol. **10**: 21-30.
32. LUCK, W., H. NAU, R. HANSEN & R. STELDINGER. 1985. Dev. Pharmacol. Ther. **8**: 384-395.
33. SUZUKI, K., T. HORIGUCHI, A. C. COMAS-URRUTIA, E. MUELLER-HEUBACH, H. O. MORISHIMA & K. ADAMSONS. 1974. Am. J. Obstet. Gynecol. **119**: 253-262.
34. MANNING, F. A., D. WALKER & C. FEYERABEND. 1978. Obstet. Gynecol. **52**: 563-568.
35. MOSIER, H. D., JR. & R. A. JANSONS. 1972. Teratology **6**: 303-311.
36. TJÄLVE, H., E. HANSSON & C. G. SCHMITERLÖW. 1968. Acta Pharmacol Toxicol. **26**: 539-555.
37. STÅLHANDSKE, T., P. SLANINA, E. TJÄLVE, E. HANSSON & C. G. SCHMITERLÖW. 1969. Acta Pharmacol. Toxicol. **27**: 363-380.
38. MITCHELL, J. A., R. E. HAMMER & H. GOLDMAN. 1983. Adv. Exp. Biol. Med. **159**: 231-241.
39. MARTIN, J. C. & D. C. MARTIN. 1981. Neurobehav. Toxicol. Teratol. **3**: 261-264.
40. MARTIN, J. C., D. C. MARTIN, B. RADOW & G. SIGMAN. 1976. Exp. Aging Res. **2**: 235-251.
41. MARTIN, J. C., D. D. MARTIN, B. RADOW & H. E. DAY. 1979. Exp. Aging Res. **5**: 509-522.
42. TERKEL, J., C. A. BLAKE, V. HOOVER & C. H. SAWYER. 1973. Proc. Soc. Exp. Biol. Med. **143**: 1131-1135.
43. PETERSON, J. E. & R. D. STEWART. 1970. Arch. Environ. Health **21**: 165-171.
44. SCHWETZ, B. A., F. A. SMITH, B. K. J. LEONG & R. E. STAPLES. 1979. Teratology **19**: 385-392.
45. LONGO, L. D. 1970. Ann. N. Y. Acad. Sci. **174**: 312-341.
46. LONGO, L. D. 1977. Am. J. Obstet. Gynecol. **129**: 69-103.
47. LONGO, L. D. & E. P. HILL. 1977. Am. J. Physiol. **232**: H324-H330.
48. HARNED, H. S., JR. 1978. Respiration and the respiratory system. *In* Perinatal Physiology. U. Stave, Ed. Plenum Press. New York, NY.
49. ASHWAL, S., J. S. MAJCHER & L. D. LONGO. 1981. Am. J. Obstet. Gynecol. **139**: 365-372.
50. POWER, G. G. & L. D. LONGO. 1975. Gynecol. Invest. **6**: 342-355.
51. STORM, J. E. & L. D. FECHTER. 1985. Toxicol. Appl. Pharmacol. **81**: 139-146.
52. STORM, J. E. & L. D. FECHTER. 1985. J. Neurochem. **45**: 965-969.
53. STORM, J. E., J. J. VALDES & L. D. FECHTER. 1986. Dev. Neurosci. **8**: 251-261.
54. MACTUTUS, C. F. & L. D. FECHTER. 1984. Science **223**: 409-411.

55. MACTUTUS, C. F. & L. D. FECHTER. 1985. Teratology **31**: 1-12.
56. TACHI, N. & M. AOYAMA. 1983. Bull. Environ. Contam. Toxicol. **31**: 85-92.
57. TACHI, N. & M. AOYAMA. 1986. Bull. Environ, Contam. Toxicol. **37**: 877-882.
58. SLOTKIN, T. A., H. CHO & W. L. WHITMORE, 1987. Brain Res. Bull. **18**: 601-611.
59. SLOTKIN, T. A., N. GREER, J. FAUST, H. CHO & F. J. SEIDLER. 1986. Brain Res. Bull. **17**: 41-50.
60. NASRAT, H. A., G. M. AL-HACHIM & F. A. MAHMOOD. 1986. Biol. Neonate **49**: 8-14.
61. AL-HACHIM, G. M. & F. A. MAHMOUD. 1985. **26**: 661-665.
62. GENEDANI, S., M. BERNARDI & A. BERTOLINI. 1983. Psychopharmacology **80**: 93-95.
63. BERTOLINI, A., M. BERNARDI & S. GENEDANI. 1982. Neurobehav. Toxicol. Teratol. **4**: 545-548.
64. PETERS, M. A. & L. L. NGAN. 1982. Arch. Int. Pharmacodyn. Ther. **257**: 155-167.
65. MARTIN, J. C., D. C. MARTIN, S. CHAO & P. SHORES. 1982. Neurobehav. Toxicol. Teratol **4**: 293-298.
66. JOHNS, J. M., T. M. LOUIS, R. F. BECKER & L. W. MEANS. 1982. Neurobehav. Toxicol. Teratol. **4**: 365-369.
67. ABEL, E. L., B. A. DINTCHEFF & N. DAY. 1979. Neurobehav. Toxicol. **1**: 153-159.
68. PETERS, D. A. V. & S. TANG. 1982. Pharmacol. Biochem. Behav. **17**: 1077-1082.
69. KROUS, H. F., G. A. CAMPBELL, M. W. FOWLER, A. C. CATRON & J. P. FARBER. 1981. Am. J. Obstet. Gynecol. **140**: 743-746.
70. PETERS, D. A. V., H. TAUB & S. TANG. 1979. Neurobehav. Toxicol. **1**: 221-225.
71. FECHTER, L. D., M. D. KARPA, B. PROCTOR, A. G. LEE & J. E. STORM. 1987. Neurotoxicol. Teratol. **9**: 277-281.
72. DAUGHTREY, W. C. & S. NORTON. 1983. Exp. Neurol. **80**: 265-278.
73. FECHTER, L. D. & Z. ANNAU. 1980. Neurobehav. Toxicol. **2**: 7-11.
74. ABBATIELLO, E. R. & K. MOHRMANN. 1979. Clin. Toxicol. **14**: 401-406.
75. DYER, R. S., C. U. ECCLES, H. S. SWARTZWELDER, L. D. FECHTER & Z. ANNAU. 1979. J. Environ. Sci. Health **13**: 107-120.
76. BAER, D. S., G. E. MCCLEARN & J. R. WILSON. 1980. Dev. Psychobiol. **13**: 643-652.

Postnatal Consequences of Maternal Marijuana Use in Humans[a]

PETER A. FRIED

Department of Psychology
Carleton University
Colonel By Drive
Ottawa, Ontario, Canada K1S 5B6

Perhaps the only definitive statement to be made about marijuana use during pregnancy and its consequences upon the offspring is that, although there is no lack of individuals willing to state strong opinions, there is a surprising paucity of objective information. The term *surprising* is appropriate for at least two reasons. Marijuana is not a drug that has just arrived on the scene. Abel's[1] title of his engaging book says everything—"Marihuana: The First Twelve Thousand Years." A second reason for being taken somewhat aback by the lack of data is that marijuana use is not limited to a small or select group of women of reproductive age. The extent of marijuana smoking among pregnant women has been examined by several investigators with a variety of populations and has been reviewed elsewhere.[2] Later in this report is described what has been found among a predominantly middle-class population in the Ottawa, Canada region.

The focus of this report is on the postnatal consequences of maternal marijuana use. Data describing the postnatal effects of cannabis beyond the neonatal period are limited to a report by Tennes[3] describing one year old babies (with essentially no drug effect being found) and a series of reports based on our Ottawa sample. Because much of the data reported below is based upon the latter work, the protocol and the limitations of the Ottawa work is described in some detail. Additional procedural information can be found in an earlier report.[4]

The Ottawa Prenatal Prospective Study (OPPS)

Prior to the late seventies, the only information pertaining to the role marijuana might play on the course of human pregnancy and pregnancy outcome were two polydrug case reports. This dearth of objective information, the results of animal work (reviewed in REF. 5), the relatively widespread use of marijuana by women of reproductive age, and the cooperation of the major teaching hospitals in the Ottawa area combined to serve as the impetus for the Ottawa Prenatal Prospective Study

[a] Fried's research described in this report was supported by grants from the National Research Council of Canada and the Canadian Department of Health & Welfare and is currently being supported by a National Institute on Drug Abuse Grant.

(OPPS). TABLE 1 outlines the general testing and information gathering procedures that have been, are being and will be followed in this work.

The OPPS started in 1978 and between 1979 and 1985 pregnancy data was collected, in a prospective fashion, from approximately 700 women residing in the Ottawa, Canada region. The study was brought to the mothers-to-be attention by their obstetricians and/or by notices in waiting rooms or prenatal clinics. Any information that was disseminated at this point did not mention marijuana but rather, in general terms, discussed how lifestyle habits during pregnancy may affect the unborn child both immediately and in the future. Upon contacting our research facility at Carleton University, the prospective subject was given further details about the "particular" habits that we would be focussing upon, namely, alcohol, cigarettes, and marijuana. At the time of this conversation it was also emphasized that, for the purposes of comparison, we were very interested in women who had not used any of these substances during pregnancy. If, at this point the woman was interested in volunteering, a time was arranged for a one-on-one meeting at which an informed consent was signed and an interview took place. Each subject was interviewed once during each of the trimesters remaining in her pregnancy with the interviews typically taking place at the home of the mother-to-be.

Ethical and practical considerations were the primary factors in dictating the method of recruiting subjects. This volunteer method has both negative and positive consequences that pervade the entire OPPS. The self-selection procedure puts considerable limitation on the degree of generalization that can be made in terms of the epidemiological information that is collected. The possibility of selection bias is obvious. However, as reported elsewhere,[3,4] on a number of key demographic factors (*e.g.*, parity, age, income, etc.), the sample participating in the OPPS is quite similar to nonparticipating women living in the Ottawa area giving birth in the hospitals involved in our study.

The recruiting procedures employed in our study have decidedly positive consequences in a number of ways. As elaborated below, the reliability of self-report was seemingly enhanced by the procedure. Further, the volunteer recruiting served to increase the long-term commitment of the women to the study. Aside from subjects who have moved away from the Ottawa area (32 percent) there has been a continued participation rate of over 95 percent during the past seven years with a substantial number of women having more than one child in the study.

During each of the approximately two hour interviews during the pregnancy, information was collected pertained to a host of variables. These included socioeconomic status, mother's health (both current and prior to pregnancy), the health history of the father, obstetrical history of previous pregnancies, a 24 hour dietary recall (including assessment of caffeine intake) and past and present drug use with particular emphasis upon marijuana, alcohol and cigarette use. Drug use data involved collecting information for both the year preceding the pregnancy and for each trimester of the pregnancy. Although the focus of the work was upon marijuana, the use of alcohol and cigarettes was also carefully monitored, as it was anticipated that these drugs would be used relatively extensively by the marijuana users and thus, in order to disassociate the various drug effects, detailed information about all three substances would be needed.

When interviewed during pregnancy and asked about marijuana usage in the year before pregnancy, 80 percent of the women reported no use, 12 percent had used it irregularly and/or were exposed to the drug passively, three percent smoked two to five joints per week and five percent smoked six or more joints per week.[6] With the recognition of pregnancy, women reported significantly less use of marijuana but within each of the trimesters the extent of use remained relatively constant. Six percent reported irregular use and/or passive exposure, one percent stated that they had smoked two to five joints per week and three percent reported smoking six or more joints per week.[6] In this same report[6] alcohol and cigarette use was also monitored and some interesting differences were noted between the three drugs in terms of changes during and even after pregnancy. Compared to alcohol and cigarette use, heavy marijuana smoking was the least reduced with the recognition of pregnancy. This

TABLE 1. Protocol Followed in the Ottawa Prenatal Prospective Study (OPPS)

Birth Date	Postnatal Questionnaire (one after child's first birthday)	Tactile Form Recognition Test (48, 60, 72 months)
Brazelton Neonatal Assessment Scale (day 4)		
	Physical Anomaly Assessment (one examination between 18 months and 4 years)	Peabody Picture Vocabulary Test (48, 60, 72 months)
Prechtl Neurological Test (day 9, 30)		
	Reynell Expressive Language and Verbal Comprehensive Scale (18, 24, 36, 48 months)	Conner's Parent Rating Scale (48 months)
Neonatal Perception Inventory (day 9, 30)		
	HOME Inventory (24, 48 months)	Gordon Diagnostic System (Vigilance & Impulsivity) (60, 72 months)
Bayley Scales of Infant Development (6, 12, 18, 24 months)		
	McCarthy Scales of Children's Abilities (36, 48, 60, 72 months)	Neuropsychological Battery (60, 72 months)
Visual and Auditory Sensory Assessment (one year at 3-5 years)	Pegboard Fine Motor Coordination Test (48, 60, 72 months)	Wide Range Achievement Test (60, 72 months)

may reflect the concerted governmental campaign to reduce cigarettes and alcohol during pregnancy coupled with virtually no public information with respect to marijuana use during pregnancy.

When interviewed a year after the birth of the baby, women reported further differences between the usage patterns of marijuana, alcohol and cigarettes.[7] The women who were categorized as heavy social drinkers in the year before pregnancy, typically reduced their drinking during pregnancy and this reduction was still evident one year after birth of the baby. In a parallel fashion, cigarette smoking which declined during pregnancy continued at the lower level one year postpartum. However, heavy marijuana use, which was the least reduced of the three drugs during pregnancy, returned to prepregnancy levels a year after the birth of the child.

The range of marijuana use was considerable and the drug was not used by a similar number of subjects across the levels of usage. As a result, for descriptive and for some statistical purposes, marijuana data were treated in a categorical fashion. The groups were designated nonusers, irregular users (one joint or less per week or regular exposure to the exhaled smoke of others), moderate users (two to five joints per week) and heavy users (six or more joints per week).

On a number of factors that could be associated with negative effects on the course of pregnancy and on the development of the offspring, many of the regular marijuana users differed from the remainder of the sample. Such potential confounding factors included a lower socioeconomic level, less formal education and increased cigarette smoking. Heavy marijuana use was also associated with increased alcohol consumption but not as strongly as was cigarette smoking. There was no difference in terms of parity between the heavy marijuana users and the nonusers, but there was a difference in terms of age with the heavy marijuana users, they being a significant 3.2 years younger. Nutritional adequacy, as determined by comparisons with recommended governmental dietary standards, revealed no differences between the nonusers and those in the three categories of marijuana use.

The procedures employed in the OPPS rely on the use of self-report to assess such variables as nutrition and drug habits. Despite the obvious potential shortcomings of such a procedure—perhaps chief of which are the critical issues of validity and reliability—there is no practical alternative to ascertain drug use. A number of procedures have been implemented in the OPPS in order to enhance the likelihood of accurate data collection. A comfortable relationship in a congenial environment between the interviewer and the individual being interviewed is one aspect which has been emphasized in the OPPS. This has been accomplished by carrying out the interview in the location of choice of the subject (typically the home of the mother-to-be) and having the same female interviewer "follow" the mother-to-be during her entire pregnancy. A second aspect of the procedures employed in the study that plays a role in enhancing the accuracy of the drug self-report is the number of times the same drug related questions are asked. The questionnaire was administered once during each trimester. During each of these interviews, the questions pertaining to drug use for each three month period of the pregnancy that had passed and for the year before pregnancy were repeated permitting a test-retest reliability measure.

Marijuana Interacting with Other Risk Factors

Although this report will focus upon postnatal consequences of maternal marijuana use there is one aspect of marijuana's influence on the course of pregnancy that has particular relevance for the interpretation of the drug's effect upon the developing offspring. Data from the OPPS[8,9] revealed no differences between marijuana users and control subjects who were matched in terms of alcohol consumption, cigarette use and family income when considering a variety of birth outcome measures. These measures included miscarriage rates, type of presentation at birth, Apgar status and the frequency of complications or major physical anomalies at birth. No evidence of increased meconium staining was noted among any of the groups of marijuana users. This observation is inconsistent with the first of two reports by Greenland and his associates[10] but agrees with a second report by the same researchers.[11] In the second of these reports, there was a higher level of health and living standards among the participating sample as compared to the earlier work of Greenland et al.[10] The women in the later report[11] who, like the Ottawa sample, showed no association between meconium staining and marijuana use, were more similar to the Ottawa subjects in terms of ethnicity, education and general health.

The interactive role that overall lifestyle may have with the teratogenic effects of marijuana has ramifications for interpreting some of the literature describing the postnatal consequences of maternal cannabis use. A report from the animal literature also has a bearing on this topic.

Pregnant rats were exposed to one of three drug conditions and one of three diet conditions.[12] The drug manipulation included marijuana smoke, placebo smoke (cannabis material with the cannabinoids removed) or no smoke. The diet manipulation included a low protein diet, a standard laboratory diet or an enriched protein diet. In this three by three design, the drug plus diet manipulation commenced 20 days prior to conception and continued throughout gestation. The results revealed a striking interaction between the drug and diet variables. Outcomes such as stillbirths, litter destruction, and postnatal deaths were significantly potentiated by the combination of the low protein diet and marijuana smoke. Conversely, some of the physiological and developmental milestones that were delayed in the offspring of animals receiving normal diet plus marijuana smoke were attenuated in the rat pups born to dams exposed to the high protein plus marijuana smoke. These results are consistent with the interpretation given earlier with respect to Greenland's work[10,11] suggesting that marijuana's potential teratogenic effects are more likely to manifest themselves in an environmental circumstance in which the drug is just one of many risk factors. Further, the results of the high protein/marijuana condition in the rats in which the drug effects were attenuated raises the possibility that, in a low risk population such as the Ottawa sample, the fetus may actually be protected from some of marijuana's consequences.

Physical Anomalies and Prenatal Marijuana Exposure

The interaction of nonmarijuana risk factors and cannabis on outcome variables may have a bearing on the issue of the relationship between physical anomalies and prenatal marijuana exposure. In the OPPS, major physical anomalies were not found to be related to drug exposure prenatally. A study was also undertaken with offspring ranging in age from six months to four years in order to determine whether maternal use of cannabis increased the risk of minor physical anomalies.[13] The children of 25 marijuana using women and the offspring of 25 matched controls were examined for the presence of over 40 types of minor physical anomalies. Neither the total number of anomalies nor the frequency of particular clusters of anomalies or individual anomalies were significantly different between the two groups of children. Although no specific pattern of anomalies was seen among the offspring of the marijuana users, two anomalies associated with the visual system were noted uniquely among the children of the heavy users of the drug. One anomaly was the presence of severe epicanthal folds (unusual amount of skin covering the nasal portion of the eye). The other minor malformation found uniquely among three other children born to the same group of marijuana users was true ocular hypertelorism (unusually wide separation of the eyes). It may be more than coincidental that in four day old neonates visual behavior was found to be altered in the babies born to marijuana users.[14] This and other behavioral observations are described later in this report.

The lack of a clear, statistically significant relationship between minor physical anomalies and maternal marijuana use is consistent with several other recent reports in the literature.[3,15,16] There are, however, two apparent exceptions. One is a large study using a mixed prospective and retrospective design,[17] and the other comprises two reports of five cases.[18,19]

In those instances in which anomalies were associated with prenatal marijuana use, the described physical effects are ones that are part of the diagnostic criteria for the fetal alcohol syndrome (FAS). In the large study[17] women who smoked marijuana during pregnancy were found to be five times more likely to have a baby with FAS type physical anomalies than nonusers of the drug.

In the case studies[18,19] four of the five patients with infants with FAS physical anomalies reported regular use of marijuana during pregnancy but no use of either alcohol or any other psychoactive substances. The denial of alcohol consumption by 80 percent of the marijuana using women appears questionable as virtually all reports in both the marijuana and alcohol literature have noted a moderately high correlation between these two substances.

The absence of a significant association in the OPPS between prenatal marijuana use and minor physical anomalies in the offspring may arise for a number of reasons. It may represent the true picture, there may be a type 2 statistical error, the age of the children may obscure some anomalies and, as discussed earlier, the low 'risk status' of the women in the OPPS may attenuate this outcome variable.

The relatively small size of the Ottawa sample serves to decrease the likelihood of finding a significant relationship between maternal use of marijuana and anomalies in the offspring. In the study in which anomalies were found,[17] the rate of occurrence among the marijuana offspring was two percent. Applying that figure to the OPPS sample, only one child would be expected to meet the criteria.

A second contributing factor that may be of importance in the different observations between the OPPS and the Hingson[17] study is the timing of the assessment of the children. In the Hingson work the infants were examined within a week of birth whereas in the Ottawa study the average age of the child at the time of the examination was 29 months. Some minor physical anomalies have been shown to be transient,[20] and European workers have noted that physical abnormalities associated with FAS normalize with age.[21] Both of these observations emphasize the importance of the variable of age in the interpretation of minor physical anomalies.

As described earlier, there is reason to consider that maternal nutrition may interact with prenatal marijuana use. If maternal weight gain is used as an indicator of nutrition during pregnancy the Ottawa sample with an average gain of 16.02 kilograms appear better nourished than the sample of Hingson who averaged 13.64 kilograms. Additionally, the sample of Hingson were of lower socioeconomic status and reported many more chronic illnesses during pregnancy. Variables such as these may play a critical role in determining the dysmorphologic effects of marijuana.

Neurobehavioral Effects and Prenatal Marijuana Exposure

In the OPPS, using a sample of 250 babies of whom 47 were exposed to marijuana during fetal development, the relationships between that drug and performance on the Brazelton Neonatal Assessment Scale was explored.[14] The infants were less than one week of age when tested. Prenatal exposure to marijuana was associated with increased fine tremors typically accompanied by exaggerated and prolonged startles, both spontaneous and in response to mild stimuli. Although these indicators of central nervous system excitation or jitteriness are consistent with signs of neonatal withdrawal, other symptoms of withdrawal, such as hyperactivity or constant signs of distress were not observed. There was, however, a marginal trend towards increased irritability associated with maternal marijuana usage.

Prenatal cannabis exposure was also found to be associated with poorer habituation to visual stimuli although not poorer habituation in the auditory modality. Habituation in infants is used as an indicator of nervous system functioning and integrity. However, the level at which the altered behavior is occurring and why the visual system appears particularly vulnerable to marijuana remains unanswered at this time. It may be noteworthy that the animal literature also suggests a particular vulnerability of the visual system to prenatal marijuana exposure. In a primate study[22] the behavior of the offspring of rhesus monkeys who had been exposed daily to cannabinoids prior to and during pregnancy and throughout lactation was examined. The behavior that distinguished the marijuana offspring from control subjects was that the experimental monkeys failed to visually habituate to novel visual stimuli. In rodents, visual developmental milestones have been found to be delayed in the offspring of cannabis or cannabis constituent exposed animals.[12,23,24]

In the OPPS work cited above[14] in which the Brazelton scale was used, the implicit assumption was that the behavior was a reflection of the neurological status of the infant. This unstated, underlying assumption was examined in a somewhat more direct fashion when the infants were slightly older (9 and 30 days) using the Prechtl neurological examination.[25] Of the 250 babies examined, 32 were born to women who had used marijuana regularly during pregnancy. Factors such as birth weight, socioeconomic status, nicotine, alcohol, caffeine, maternal weight gain, nutrition and maternal age were statistically controlled.

Maternal marijuana use was associated with relatively similar observations in the 9 and 30 day old infant. At both ages increased fine tremors, tremors associated with the Moro reflex, and startles were more pronounced. A number of motor reflexes were also more marked among the marijuana offspring. At the younger age, hand-to-mouth behavior was associated with marijuana use during pregnancy. Overall, these observations are consistent with, but milder in degree, than those reported among infants undergoing opioid withdrawal. The heightened tremors and startles among the offspring of the marijuana users are consistent with the observations made using the Brazelton behavioral assessment as described above[14] when the infants were less than one week old. At 9 and 30 days of age, however, no statistical associations were apparent between marijuana use and a number of variables associated with the visual system in the Prechtl test. This lack of association included such variables as pupil dilation, doll's eye, nystagmus, and acoustic blink. Compared to the remainder of the sample, more marijuana babies demonstrated strabismus and a lack of optical blink and habituation but the increased incidence did not reach statistical significance.

Possible Interpretation of Infant Findings

Both the data derived from the newborn and that obtained from the 9 and 30 day old infants may be interpreted as indicating that prenatal marijuana exposure might subtly depress the normal rate of development of the central nervous system. Manifestations of a slowing in the rate of maturation would most likely be functionally evident in complex, interactive systems. Because of the behavioral observations in the newborn[14] and the somewhat suggestive trends in the dysmorphology study[13] and the Prechtl assessment,[25] the visual system was chosen as the target for examining the developmental course of the nervous system in the children of marijuana users. It was presumed that the visual system is dependent upon the interaction of a large number of components and each component has its own characteristic rate of maturation. The hypothesis being considered was that there would be a relatively greater degree of "normal" variability in an immature, complex system. As maturation is reached by each of the components the variability in the total system would be expected to decrease.

This hypothesis was tested by using a transient pattern that evoked visual cortical potential.[26] This variable was chosen as parameters within it—amplitude and latency—systematically change from infancy to adulthood. A reversing checkerboard pattern was used as the stimulus under both monocular and binocular conditions for 101 children averaging four years of age. Approximately a third of these children had been prenatally exposed to marijuana.

The marijuana offspring tended to have slightly longer latencies for the major wave-form component of the evoked potential—a sign of immaturity in the system. More robust however, was a significantly greater degree of variability in the marijuana group compared to matched (in terms of age, alcohol and nicotine) controls. These data are consistent with the interpretation of fetal exposure to marijuana retarding the rate of maturation of visual components of the human nervous system.

Are There Longer-Term Effects of Prenatal Exposure to Marijuana?

The offspring of the participating mothers in the OPPS have been assessed with a multitude of tests designed to examine behavioral and cognitive functioning at one year of age and beyond (TABLE 1). At this time analysis has been completed on 12 and 24 month old children.[27] At these ages an assessment of mental development, motor development and general behavior was undertaken. Additionally, at 24 months, expressive and comprehensive language was examined as was the home environment.

Using a multiple regression analysis, the variable of prenatal exposure to marijuana was not found to significantly contribute in a unique fashion to either mental, motor or language outcome variables. Further, maternal marijuana use was not related to a visual composite score derived from the infant's behavior. Items that were considered in this created variable included responsiveness to objects, manipulation of objects and sights-looking.

Where to Next?

The failure to find effects at one and two years of age are in contrast to the neonatal observations, and this discrepancy is open to a multitude of interpretations. It may be that the drug's effects are transitory and, using the notion of nervous system immaturity discussed earlier, the nervous system has "caught up" sufficiently in the marijuana offspring to be undifferentiated at a behavioral level from control subjects.

An alternative possibility is that the long-term effects of maternal marijuana use are very subtle and the facets of behavior that are affected manifest themselves under more complex situations than can be examined in a very young child. As indicated in TABLE 1, in the OPPS, as the children are getting older, they are being assessed with an extensive battery of age appropriate neuropsychological tests. Subtle deviations and nonoptimal performance, not testable or visible at an earlier age may now be revealed. From a pragmatic point of view, the children in the OPPS are now entering school age. The consequential demands of this new environment emphasizes the need to ascertain the potential long-term neurobehavioral teratogenic effects of prenatal marijuana exposure.

REFERENCES

1. ABEL, E. 1980. Marihuana: The First Twelve Thousand Years. Plenum Press. New York, NY.
2. DALTERIO, S. & P. A. FRIED. Marijuana. In Perinatal Substance Abuse: Research Findings and Clinical Implications. T. B. Sonderegger, Ed. Johns Hopkins University Press. Baltimore, MD. In press.
3. TENNES, K., N. AVITABLE, C. BLACKARD, C. BOYLES, B. HOUSSOUN, L. HOLMES & M. KREYE. 1985. Marijuana: Prenatal and postnatal exposure in the human. In Current Research on the Consequences of Maternal Drug Abuse. T. M. Pinkert, Ed.: 48-60. NIDA Research Monograph 59. U.S. Government Printing Office. Washington, DC.
4. FRIED, P. A., B. WATKINSON, A. GRANT & R. K. KNIGHTS. 1980. Changing patterns of soft drug use prior to and during pregnancy. Drug Alcohol Depend. 6: 323-343.
5. FRIED, P. A. 1984. Prenatal and postnatal consequences of marihuana use during pregnancy. In Neurobehavioral Teratology. J. Yanai, Ed.: 275-285. Elsevier. Amsterdam.
6. FRIED, P. A., K. S. INNES & M. V. BARNES. 1984. Soft drug use prior to and during pregnancy: A comparison of samples over a four-year period. Drug Alcohol Depend. 13: 161-176.
7. FRIED, P. A., M. V. BARNES & E. R. DRAKE. 1985. Soft drug usage after pregnancy compared to use before and during pregnancy. Am. J. Obstet. Gynecol. 151: 787-792.
8. FRIED, P. A., M. BUCKINGHAM & P. VON KULMIZ. 1983. Marijuana use during pregnancy and perinatal risk factors. Am. J. Obstet. Gynecol. 144: 922-924.
9. FRIED, P. A., B. WATKINSON & A. WILLAN. 1984. Marijuana use during pregnancy and decreased length of gestation. Am. J. Obstet. Gynecol. 150: 23-27.
10. GREENLAND, S., K. STAISCH, N. BROWN & S. GROSS. 1982. The effects of marijuana use during pregnancy. I. A preliminary epidemiologic study. Am. J. Obstet. Gynecol. 143: 408-413.
11. GREENLAND, S., K. STAISCH, N. BROWN & S. GROSS. 1983. Effects of marijuana on human pregnancy, labor, and delivery. Neurobehav. Toxicol. Teratol. 4: 447-450.
12. CHARLEBOIS, A. T. & P. A. FRIED. 1980. The interactive effects of nutrition and cannabis upon rat perinatal development. Dev. Psychobiol. 13: 591-605.
13. O'CONNELL, C. M. & P. A. FRIED. 1984. An investigation of prenatal cannabis exposure and minor physical anomalies in a low risk population. Neurobehav. Toxicol. Teratol. 6: 345-350.
14. FRIED, P. A. & J. E. MAKIN. 1987. Neonatal behavioral correlates of prenatal exposure to marijuana, cigarettes and alcohol in a low risk population. Neurotoxicol. Teratol. 9: 1-7.
15. LINN, S., S. C. SCHOENBAUM, R. R. MONSON, R. ROSNER, P. C. STUBBLEFIELD & K. J. RYAN. 1983. The association of marijuana use with outcome of pregnancy. Am. J. Public Health 73: 1161-1164.
16. ROSETT, H. L., L. WEINER, A. LEE, B. ZUCKERMAN, E. DOOLING & E. OPPENHEIMER. 1983. Patterns of alcohol consumption and fetal development. Obstet. Gynecol. 61: 539-546.

17. HINGSON, R., J. ALPERT, N. DAY, E. DOOLING, H. KAYNE, S. MORELOCK, E. OPPEN-HEIMER & B. ZUCKERMAN. 1982. Effects of maternal drinking and marijuana use on fetal growth and development. Pediatrics **70:** 539-546.
18. QAZI, Q. H., E. MARIANO, E. BELLER, D. MILMAN & W. CRUMBLEHOLME. 1982. Is marijuana smoking fetotoxic? Pediatr. Res. **16:** 272A.
19. QAZI, Q. H., E. MARIANO, E. BELLER, D. MILMAN, W. CRUMBLEHOLME & M. BUENDIA. 1983. Abnormalities in offspring associated with prenatal marijuana exposure. Pediatr. Res. **17:** 1534.
20. SMITH, D. W. 1974. Recognizable Patterns of Human Malformation. W. B. Saunders. Philadelphia, PA.
21. MAJEWSKI, F. 1981. Alcohol embryopathy: Some facts and speculations about pathogenesis. Neurobehav. Toxicol. Teratol. **3:** 129-144.
22. GOLUB, M. S., E. N. SASSENRATH & C. F. CHAPMAN. 1981. Regulation of visual attention in offspring of female monkeys treated chronically with delta-9-tetrahydrocannabinol. Dev. Psychobiol. **14:** 507-512.
23. BORGEN, L. A., W. M. DAVIS & H. B. PACE. 1973. Effects of prenatal THC on the development of the rat offspring. Pharmacol. Biochem. Behav. **1:** 203-206.
24. FRIED, P. A. 1976. Short and long term-effects of pre-natal cannabis inhalation upon rat offspring. Psychopharmacologia **6:** 285-296.
25. FRIED, P. A., B. WATKINSON, R. F. DILLON & C. S. DULBERG. 1987. Neonatal neurological status in a low-risk population after prenatal exposure to cigarettes, marijuana, and alcohol. J. Dev. Behav. Pediatr. **8:** 318-326.
26. TANSLEY, B. W., P. A. FRIED & H. T. J. MOUNT. 1986. Visual processing in children exposed prenatally to marihuana and nicotine. Can. J. Public Health **77:** 72-78.
27. FRIED, P. A. & B. WATKINSON. 1988. 12 and 24-month neurobehavioral follow-up of children prenatally exposed to marihuana, cigarettes and alcohol. Neurotoxicol. Teratol. **10:** 305-313.

Animal Studies of Prenatal Delta-9-Tetrahydrocannabinol: Female Embryolethality and Effects on Somatic and Brain Growth[a]

DONALD E. HUTCHINGS, STEPHEN C. BRAKE, AND
BRIAN MORGAN[b]

New York State Psychiatric Institute
Department of Developmental Psychobiology
722 West 168th Street
New York, New York 10032
and
[b] *Institute of Human Nutrition*
Columbia University
College of Physicians and Surgeons
New York, New York 10032

INTRODUCTION

When we began our developmental research with delta-9-tetrahydrocannabinol (delta-9-THC) some four years ago, our laboratory had just concluded 12 years of research with the synthetic opioid, methadone. When that work was initiated in 1973, except for the observation that methadone did not appear to be teratogenic in humans, little else was known of its developmental toxicity in either humans or laboratory animals. This experience with methadone was in stark contrast to what confronted us when we turned our attention to cannabis and delta-9-THC. Instead of beginning a research effort in a near scientific vacuum, we suddenly found ourselves overwhelmed with a history of marijuana that spanned thousands of years and an American medical literature dating back to 1843.[1] In fact, by the late 1970s, the literature had exceeded well over 5,000 articles with more than a thousand of these related to human health consequences.[2]. In our brief research experience with cannabis, we have come to regard it as the most intractably complex of all the major abuse compounds. And while our understanding of its effects has increased enormously in the past 20 years, many aspects of its health consequences continue to baffle researchers.

A reader of the scientific marijuana literature invariably encounters two unrelated pieces of information that appear in nearly ever contemporary article—first, that marijuana is the most widely used of all illicit drugs available in the United States and second, that delta-9-THC is the major psychoactive ingredient. The first of these—the popularity of marijuana—remains a guiding impetus to continue studies

[a] Supported by Grant DA3544 from the National Institute on Drug Abuse.

133

of its health-related effects. But it is the second fact—the role of delta-9-THC—that requires some additional comment.

Indeed, delta-9-THC is the principle active ingredient in marijuana, producing almost all of the characteristic pharmacological effects. But the term has become so inextricably associated with marijuana that it has come to be viewed by some as nearly synonymous with marijuana or erroneously misperceived as "synthetic" marijuana. Given the intricate complexity of marijuana botany, chemistry and pharmacology, the confusion is understandable. But prerequisite to a meaningful discussion is some familiarity with basic terms and definitions of marijuana-related products and discussion of a few interpretive problems related to human and animal studies of its developmental toxicity.

First, a brief list of commonly used terms in the cannabis literature: *Cannabis* is the crude material from the plant *Cannabis sativa*. *Marijuana* is usually a mixture of crushed leaves, twigs, seeds and sometimes flowers. *Sinsemilla* is a seedless variety of high potency marijuana originally grown in northern California. *Hashish* is a resin obtained by pressing, scraping and shaking the plant and *hash oil*, a very potent solvent extract.[3]

Plant Chemistry. Cannabis contains more than 400 chemicals, many common to all plants. Sixty-one of these are unique to cannablis and are collectively referred to as *cannabinoids*. Because of its potent pharmacological activity, *delta-9-tetrahydrocannabinol* has been the most extensively studied. It is important to appreciate, however, that other cannabinoids, for example, *cannabidiol* (CBD) and *cannabinol* (CBN), though exerting little or no psychoactive effects, do have biological activity. CBD is an anticonvulsant and appears, at least under some conditions, to attenuate the effects of delta-9-THC, whereas CBN appears to exert weak cannabinoid activity (for review, see REFS. 4,5).

Smoke Chemistry. In the United States, most cannabis is consumed by smoking marijuana, a mode of administration that, by virtue of the products produced by pyrolosis, complicates an understanding of its pharmacology and toxicity. Marijuana smoke shares certain chemical characteristics with tobacco smoke; both contain hundreds of chemicals of known or potential biological activity in a mixture of very small particles and a gas-vapor phase. The amounts of a few constituents in tobacco and marijuana cigarette smoke are compared in TABLE 1. How much active material is actually absorbed by the smoker depends on the manner in which the cigarette is smoked. In the U.S., a common marijuana smoking technique is to inhale deeply and hold the smoke for as long as possible; the more "efficient" the technique, the higher the tissue concentrations of absorbed material.

While the dose of delta-9-THC can be accurately specified in human laboratory studies by the use of prepared experimental material, with "street" marijuana, variations in the content of just delta-9-THC alone shows extreme variation from 0% or trace amounts to levels as potent as 18%. Parenthetically, throughout the 1970s, delta-9-THC concentrations of cannabis confiscated by the Drug Enforcement Agency in the U.S. averaged around 1-2%. More recently, however, averages have increased to 3-5% and potency appears to be on the rise.[6] Moreover, cannabis from different sources also differs widely in the proportion of other chemicals including cannabinoids.

These considerations pose a number of dilemmas for both human and animal researchers interested in the developmental toxicity of cannabis: First, basic to an understanding of the pharmacology and toxicity of a compound is knowing how much active substance is delivered to biological tissues. A major advantage of animal studies is the ability to administer specified quantities of a compound in order to precisely describe dose-response effects. Nearly all of the developmental animal studies, because of practical advantages, have investigated delta-9-THC; it is a biologically active,

TABLE 1. Marijuana and Tobacco Reference Cigarette Analysis of Mainstream Smoke[a]
(Abbreviated List[b])

Mainstream Smoke	Marijuana Cigarette	Tobacco Cigarette
Gas phase		
Carbon monoxide, vol %	3.99	4.58
mg	17.6	20.2
Carbon dioxide, vol %	8.27	9.38
mg	57.3	65.0
Acetaldehyde, μg	1200	980
Acetone, μg	443	587
Benzene, μg	76	67
Toluene, μg	112	108
Vinyl chloride, ng[c]	5.4	12.4
Particulate phase		
Cannabidiol, μg	190	—
Delta-9-THC, μg	820	—
Cannabinol, μg	190	—
Nicotine, μg	—	2850
Benz (a) anthracene, ng[c]	75	43
Benzo (a) pyrene, ng[c]	31	21

[a] Data from REFERENCE 3.
[b] Some 150 compounds identified in marijuana smoke.
[c] Known carcinogen.

quantifiable chemical constituent of cannabis and clearly exerts some degree of dose-related embryotoxicity. But it is important to emphasize that delta-9-THC represents only one ingredient of the natural material, and effects produced by other cannabinoids and cannabis-related products and their interactions may also prove important. Though an obvious remedy would be to expose rats to marijuana smoke, the amount of delta-9-THC delivered in smoke can only be approximated and only small amounts are actually absorbed.[7]

By contrast, human reproductive studies typically investigate the effects of smoked marijuana. In order to approximate dose response, experimental groups are usually defined with respect to usage pattern, for example number of marijuana "joints" smoked per day or per week. But since the potency of the material being used by a particular study population is seldom reported—probably because it is un-known—specifying usage, for example, as "low," "moderate" or "high" represents more a rank ordering of the locally available illicit cannabis than a reliable estimate of actual potency. Thus, problems of interpretation arise, especially when findings between laboratories are in disagreement. If, for example, one research group finds evidence of dysmorphogenesis or neurobehavioral deficits and another does not, there is no way of knowing whether or not quantitative as well as qualitative difference in the smoked material may be contributing to different outcomes.

One could reasonably argue that a lack of complete information about the nature and potency of the maternally abused substance is certainly not unique to marijuana. But with the other major abuse compounds—alcohol, opioids, cocaine and phency-clidine—we have far more assurance in human studies that it is primarily these compounds, possibly along with some adulterants, that are being used, and it is these compounds, without the adulterants, that are administered to laboratory animals.

These issues are raised, not to imply that marijuana research can only yield chaotic and uninterpretable results but rather that we need to appreciate certain constraints in the interpretation, comparison and extrapolation of cannabis research data. Animal studies of delta-9-THC, though of demonstrated value, are not studies of marijuana. And by the same token, human studies would be greatly enhanced if more information were provided about the nature of the cannabis being used as well as the amount of cannabinoids actually entering the body.

Delta-9-THC during Pregnancy in the Rat

Methods

Animal studies of the developmental toxicity of delta-9hyTHC administered prenatally have often yielded ambiguous results. A major problem shared by many of these studies is that adverse effects observed in the offspring may not have been produced by direct drug effects on the embryo and fetus but rather, were secondary to delta-9-THC-induced maternal toxicity (for review, see REF. 8). For example, one potent effect of delta-9-THC administration in rats is a substantial inhibition of food and water intake with consequent maternal undernutrition and dehydration. Also, delta-9-THC can disrupt normal maternal care at parturition and inhibit milk production and let-down, all with possible negative consequences for the neurobehavioral development of the offspring (e.g., see REF. 9).

The studies reported here from our laboratory[10,11] used essentially the same design: Two dose levels of delta-9-THC, 15 or 50 mg/kg/day, were administered to pregnant rats. The compound was dissolved in sesame oil and administered by gastric intubation. To study potential effects on major developmental events, exposure was initiated on Day 8 of gestation, the beginning of organogenesis, and continued through fetogenesis to term. To control for the effects of reduced food and water intake among delta-9-THC-exposed dams, pair-fed controls were administered the vehicle alone and allowed to eat and drink only the amount consumed by the 50-mg/kg group on the same gestation days. A group of nontreated controls, except for weighing, were left undisturbed throughout pregnancy. In addition, to obviate possible postnatal effects of being reared by a drug-treated dam, all experimental and control litters were reared by surrogate dams. The results of these first studies were derived from a total of some 73 dams and their 940 offspring and are summarized as follows:

Maternal Nutrition and Embryotoxicity

Among the dams receiving 50 mg/kg of delta-9-THC, food and water intake, as shown in FIGURE 1, was initially reduced to 75-80% of nontreated controls but then recovered over 3-4 days to approximately a 15-20% reduction until term. compared with the nontreated dams, both dose-level drug groups and pair-fed controls gained significantly less bodyweight from conception to term. Offspring mortality did not differ between the nontreated and pair-fed controls; significant dose-related increases in offspring mortality were observed among the delta-9-THC groups.

Of particular interest was the observation of a dose-related increase in the sex-ratio of live male-to-female offspring. In many studies carried out in our laboratory over several years, we have typically found a sex-ratio of 50%, ±5%, for both nontreated and pair-fed controls. Among litters from dams receiving 50 mg/kg of delta-9-THC, we have consistently found a significant dose-related increase in the proportion of male offspring ranging from 57%[10] to 61%.[15] The data have further indicated that this has resulted from a selective lethal effect on female embryos. Interestingly, Tennes *et al.*[12] found in a study of women who smoked marijuana during pregnancy, that heavy use was similarly associated with a significant increase in male over female births. But because the women had been recruited into the study well into their pregnancy, spontaneous abortion or early loss of female conceptuses could not explain their sex-ratio effects.

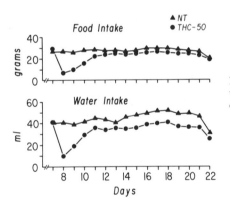

FIGURE 1. Mean food and water intake for the nontreated controls and THC-50-treated dams from Gestation Days 7 through 22.

Offspring Growth

Although birthweights were reduced among the drug-exposed offspring, this appeared to result largely from the reduced maternal food and water intake rather than the drug. Soon after birth, however, an interesting effect on growth was observed: Whereas the bodyweights of the pair-fed caught up to the nontreated controls by Day 2 of life, bodyweights of both treated groups remained significantly lower. In fact, as shown in FIGURE 2, during the first five days of life, male pups in both dose-level groups grew at a slower rate than the controls. But beginning on Day 5, the 15-mg/kg pups grew faster than the other groups so that by Day 11, they had caught up to the controls. By comparison, the 50-mg/kg pups still weighed less than all of the other groups on Days 5-11 and did not entirely catch up in bodyweight until a month of life. By 32 days of age, there were no weight differences between any of the groups.

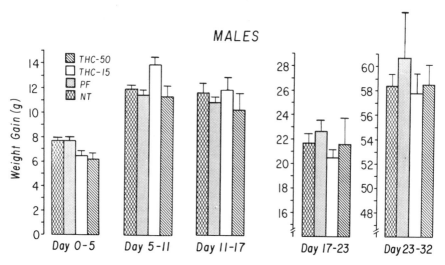

FIGURE 2. Mean weight gained by THC-exposed and control male offspring from birth to 32 days of age.

The growth data of the female offspring are not shown here but were virtually identical to the males. Abel[8] reviewed several rats studies from his laboratory of postnatal growth following prenatal exposure to cannabinoids and concluded that the results were inconsistent. But within the context of the effects found here, all suggest differential dose-response effects on growth rate: Low doses produce relatively short-term growth inhibition followed by rapid catch-up whereas high doses produce a more prolonged period of delayed growth with relatively slow catch-up.

Offspring Behavior

Intact litters from each of the treated and control groups were tested at three-day intervals from birth to 32 days of age for difference in activity level. We had previously reported that prenatally administered methadone[13] and more recently, cocaine,[14] produces effects in the offspring on this measure. None of the delta-9-THC-treated or control litters, however, showed any differences in activity level.

Pups were also tested for their ability to nipple-attach on Days 2, 5, 8, 11 and 14 of age.[11] For this, a test dam was anesthetized and placed in a test cage, and 2-3 littermates per five-minute test period were placed in proximity to her ventrum. Each pup's latency to attach was measured; group means are shown in FIGURE 3. This shows that the 50-mg/kg pups took considerably longer to attach to the test dam's nipples on Days 5 and 8. It is unlikely, however, that the drug treatment contributed to this effect, as the pair-fed pups also took longer to nipple-attach on the same days. This suggests that the poor attachment behavior of the 50-mg/kg pups was probably due to the secondary effects of reduced food and water intake in the dams, particularly the severe reduction that occurred during early organogenesis.

Brain DNA, RNA and Protein

To extend the studies of prenatal delta-9-THC on somatic growth to possible effects on postnatal brain growth, we analyzed offspring brains at 7, 14 and 21 days of age for DNA, RNA and protein content.[15]

A second problem addressed in this study is the severe inhibition of both food and water intake produced by THC administration in the rat. In our previous studies described above we initiated THC administration on Gestation Day (G) 8 so that the maximal inhibition of food and water intake occurred during the earliest development of embryonic CNS, on G9-11. In this study, drug treatment was initiated on the day after conception so that the severe THC-induced undernutrition/dehydration would be confined to the preimplantation period (*i.e.*, Day 1 to approximately Day 6), a period generally found to be refractory to teratogenic effects (for discussion, see REF. 16).

Except for beginning treatment earlier, treated and control groups were prepared and fostered as described above. On Postnatal Days (PND) 7, 14, and 21, 3 treated and control pups were decapitated, brains excised and using standard procedures, analyzed for total protein, DNA, and RNA.

FIGURE 4 shows that there was an increase in brain DNA, RNA and protein with increasing age in all groups. There were no differences among groups at any time for values of DNA or RNA. However, the brains of the nontreated, 15-mg/kg and pair-fed groups all had significantly greater amounts of total protein than the 50-mg/kg group. The difference disappeared with age so that by PND21, all of the treated and control groups yielded the same brain protein content.

In this study no differences were observed among the nontreated and the pair-fed pups with respect to DNA and RNA indicating that the reduced food intake of the mother during gestation had no effect on nucleic acid synthesis in the brain. Furthermore, that there were no differences in RNA and DNA levels between the THC-

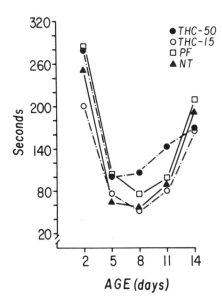

FIGURE 3. Mean latency to attach to a nipple for THC-exposed and control pups from 2 through 14 days of age.

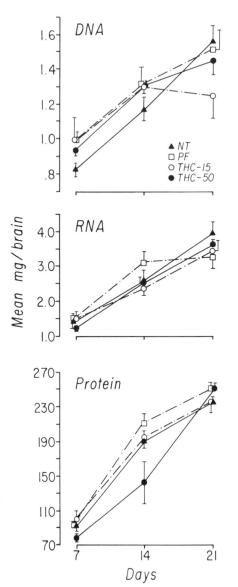

FIGURE 4. Mean DNA, RNA, and protein values for THC-exposed and control offspring. The number of pools of tissues ranged from 4 to 8 for each of the brain measures.

treated pups and the pair-fed group, suggests that RNA or DNA synthesis was not affected by THC.

Protein, however, was affected by THC. As with the nucleic acids, there were no differences between the values for pair-fed and nontreated animals indicating that the nutritional deficit in the dam was not great enough to impair protein synthesis. Neither was the 15-mg/kg dose of THC sufficient to affect protein synthesis as pups in this group showed similar protein accumulation to the nontreated and pair-fed groups.

However, the THC-50 pups were significantly affected. Brain protein levels were significantly lower than in the other groups at PND7 and 14 suggesting that the higher dose reduced protein synthesis for at least the first 14 days of life. Subsequently, THC-50 pups rapidly caught up, increasing their brain protein by 43% in the next seven days compared with only 18% in the pair-fed controls.

Protein synthesis in the brain correlates with growth of axons and dendrites and the formation of synoptic connections between cells. Thus, the 50-mg/kg dose of THC appears to have inhibited proliferation of neural processes in those animals during the first 14 days of life. Subsequently, however, they caught up to the controls by Day 21.

In our findings for somatic growth, we described a dose-response relationship for THC; 15 mg/kg produced short-term growth inhibition followed by rapid catch-up whereas 50 mg/kg produced a prolonged period of delayed growth followed by gradual catch-up. Here, the 15-mg/kg dose had no observable effect on brain growth. That the lower dose was without effect on the brain parallels similar studies of maternal undernutrition that find offspring CNS to be more resistant to growth deficits than other developing organ systems.[17]

The observation that there were no differences in RNA, DNA and protein between the nontreated and pair-fed controls suggests that confining the severe maternal nutrition/dehydration to the preimplantation period spared offspring brain from growth inhibition. The decreased brain protein synthesis among the 50-mg/kg animals followed by catch-up parallels the delayed rate of somatic growth described above and suggests a transitory rather than a permanent effect of delta-9-THC on both somatic and brain growth.

Delta-9-THC Plasma Concentrations

Because of the reported slow clearance of delta-9-THC in several species (see REF. 3) we suggested that these effects might be related to the prenatal accumulation of delta-9-THC in dams and fetuses followed by its postnatal persistence and slow clearance in the offspring. To study this possibility, delta-9hyTHC was administered to pregnant dams either multiply (MULT) throughout pregnancy or acutely (ACUTE), as a single dose on the last day of gestation.[18]

For the multiple exposure, beginning on G2, either 15 or 50 mg/kg of delta-9-THC suspended in sesame oil was administered to two groups of gravid dams (MULT THC-15; MULT THC-50) once daily by gastric intubation. Both MULT dose-level groups received daily drug administration through G22. For the acute exposure, the same doses, vehicle and route were used but the dams received delta-9-THC only once on G22 (ACUTE THC-15; ACUTE THC-50).

Sixty min after the last drug administration on G22, all dams and their offspring were decapitated, blood collected and quantitative measurement of delta-9-THC carried out using capillary column gas chromatography negative ion chemical ionization mass spectrometry.

The mean plasma concentrations of delta-9-THC found in dams and fetuses following either acute or multiple exposure are shown in TABLE 2. Among the dams, plasma concentrations covaried with dose and multiple dosing produced higher concentrations than acute. Although the MULT-50 dams yielded a mean plasma concentration that was nearly three times higher than the other groups, the dose $\times$ treatment statistical interaction was not significant.

Among the fetuses, plasma concentrations were approximately 10% of those found for the dams and differed significantly as a function of dose and treatment. In addition, the high plasma concentration found for the MULT-50 fetuses yielded a significant dose × treatment interaction.

It is well documented that radioactivity appears in the fetus following an acute administration of ^{3}H-delta-9-THC to maternal mice,[19] rats[20] and dogs.[21] Greater than 60% of the radioactivity in fetal dog brain corresponded to unchanged ^{3}H-delta-9-THC, demonstrating placental transfer.[21] Bailey et al.[22] reported that delta-9-THC administered during late pregnancy in the rhesus monkey resulted in the rapid transfer of parent compound but not 11-nor-9-carboxy-THC to fetal tissues. All of these studies demonstrated that the placenta acted to partially limit the exposure of the fetus to delta-9-THC and its metabolites. The findings reported here similarly show that the concentrations of delta-9-THC in fetal plasma were 10 and 7 times less than those in the plasma of dams receiving the low and high dose of delta-9-THC, respectively.

Multiple dosing of delta-9-THC to the dams resulted in an insignificant increase in the maternal plasma concentrations of the 15-mg/kg-treatment group but in a significant twofold increase in the 50-mg/kg group. A similar profile of delta-9-THC

TABLE 2. Mean (±SEM) Concentration of Plasma Delta-9-THC (ng/ml)

	Acute	Multiple
Dams		
15 mg/kg	(N = 8) 99 ± 20[a]	(N = 01) 134 ± 38[a,b]
50 mg/kg	(N = 8) 132 ± 36	(N = 9) 309 ± 59[b]
Fetuses		
15 mg/kg	(N = 9) 10 ± 2[a]	(N = 10) 12 ± 4[a]
50 mg/kg	(N = 8) 19 ± 5	(N = 9) 41 ± 6[b]

[a] $p < 0.05$ compared to respective 50-mg/kg group.
[b] $p < 0.05$ compared to respective acute group.

concentrations in fetal plasma suggests that the maternal plasma concentration rather than fetal tissue depots, serves as the primary source for fetal plasma levels. These findings are particularly relevant given the paucity of information regarding fetal concentrations of cannabinoids following repeated exposure to dams. Additionally, most previous studies have been concerned with measurement of placental transfer of undifferentiated radioactivity following exposure to radiolabeled delta-9-THC rather than the direct measurement of parent compound.

CONCLUSION

Our laboratory has described three dose-related effects in the offspring following maternal administration of delta-9-THC in the rat: at birth, we have consistently found a dose-related increase in the sex-ratio of live male-to-female offspring suggesting that female conceptuses have greater susceptibility to delta-9hyTHC lethality. During the postnatal period, we found a dose-related inhibition of both somatic growth and brain protein synthesis. These effects were transitory, however, and the delta-9-THC-exposed animals caught up to the controls by weaning. Although confirming studies are needed, both the accumulation of delta-9-THC in the 50-mg/kg-treatment group and the possibility that delta-9-THC is persisting in pharmacologically active concentrations into the postnatal period may be important elements underlying the transitory inhibition of both body growth and brain protein synthesis. And though our research remains in progress, as yet, we have not found any evidence of neurobehavioral deficits in the offspring independent of maternal toxicity, findings that are consistent with other well-controlled animal studies.[8]

REFERENCES

1. ABEL, E. 1980. Marijuana, the First Twelve Thousand Years. Plenum Press. New York, NY.
2. JONES, R. T. 1980. Human Effects: An Overview. *In* Marijuana Research Findings. R. C. Petersen, Ed.:54-80. National Institute on Drug Abuse Series. DHHS Publication No. (ADM) 80-1001. U.S. Government Printing Office. Washington, DC.
3. Marijuana and Health. 1982. Report of a Study by the Committee of the Institute of Medicine, Div. of Health Sciences Policy. National Academy Press. Washington, DC.
4. DEWEY, W. L. 1986. Cannabinoid Pharmacology. Pharmacol. Rev. **38:** 151-178.
5. MARTIN, B. R. 1986. Cellular effects of cannabinoids. Pharmacol. Rev. **38:** 45-74.
6. Quarterly Report: Potency Monitoring Project. Report #26. April 1, 1988 - June 30, 1988. NIDA Marijuana Project. Research Institute of Pharmaceutical Sciences. The University of Mississippi. University (Lafayette Co.), MS.
7. FRIED, P.A. 1976. Short and long-term effects of prenatal inhalation upon rat offspring. Psychopharmacology **50:** 285-291.
8. ABEL, E. L. 1985. Effects of prenatal exposure to cannabinoids. *In* Current Research on the Consequences of Maternal Drug Use. T. M. Pinkert, Ed.:20-35. National Institute on Drug Abuse Series. DHHS Publication No. (ADM) 85-1400. U.S. Government Printing Office. Washington, DC.
9. HUTCHINGS, D. E. 1985. Issues of methodology and interpretation in clinical and animal behavioral teratology studies. Neurobehav. Toxicol. Teratol. **7:** 639-642.
10. HUTCHINGS, D. E., S. C. BRAKE, T. SHI & E. LASALLE. 1987. Delta-9-tetrahydrocannabinol during pregnancy in the rat: I. Differential effects on maternal nutrition, embryotoxicity and growth in the offspring. Neurotoxicol. Teratol. **9:** 39-43.
11. BRAKE, S. C., D. E. HUTCHINGS, B. MORGAN, E. LASALLE & T. SHI. 1987. Delta-9-tetrahydrocannabinol during pregnancy in the rat. II. Effects on ontogeny of locomotor activity and nipple attachment in the offspring. Neurotoxicol. Teratol. **9:** 45-49.
12. TENNES, K., N. AVITABLE, C. BLACKARD *et al.* 1985. Marijuana during pregnancy. *In* Current Research on the Consequences Maternal Drug Use. T. M. Pinkert, Ed.:48-60. National Institute on Drug Abuse Series. DHHS Publication No. (ADM) 85-1400. U.S. Government Printing Office. Washington D.C.
13. HUTCHINGS, D. E., J. P. TOWEY & S. R. BODNARENKO. 1980. Effects of prenatal methadone on activity level in the preweanling rat. Neurobehav. Toxicol. **2:** 231-235.
14. HUTCHINGS, D. E., T. A. FICO & D. L. DOW-EDWARDS. Prenatal cocaine: Maternal toxicity, fetal effects and motor activity in the offspring. Neurotoxicol. Teratol. In press.
15. MORGAN, B., S. C. BRAKE, D. E. HUTCHINGS, N. MILLER & Z. GAMAGARIS. 1988. Delta-9-tetrahydrocannabinol during pregnancy in the rat: Effects on development of RNA, DNA, and protein in offspring brain. Pharmacol. Biochem. Behav. **31:** 365-369.
16. HUTCHINGS, D. E. 1987. Drug abuse druing pregnancy: Embryopathic and neurobehavioral effects. *In* Genetic and Perinatal Effects of Abused Substances. M. C. Braude & A. M. Zimmerman, Eds.:131-151. Academic Press. New York, NY.

17. WINICK, M. 1976. Malnutrition and prenatal growth. *In* Malnutrition and Brain Development. 98-127. Oxford University Press. New York, NY.

18. HUTCHINGS, D. E., B. R. MARTIN, Z. GAMAGARIS, N. MILLER & T. FICO. 1989. Plasma concentrations of delta-9-tetrahydrocannabinol in dams and fetuses following acute or multiple prenatal dosing in rats. Life Sci. **44:** 697-701.

19. KENNEDY, J. S. & W. J. WADDELL. 1972. Whole-body autoradiography of the pregnant mouse after administration of ^{14}C-delta-9-THC. Toxicol. Appl. Pharmacol. **22:** 252-258.

20. HARBISON, R. D. & B. MANTILLA-PLATA. 1972. Prenatal toxicity, maternal distribution and placental transfer of tetrahydrocannabinol. J. Pharmacol. Exp. Ther. **180:** 446-453.

21. MARTIN, B. R., W. L. DEWEY, L. S. HARRIS & J. S. BECKNER. 1977. ^{3}H-delta-9-tetrahydrocannabinol distribution in pregnant dogs and their fetuses. Res. Commun. Chem. Pathol. Pharmacol. **17:** 457-470.

22. BAILEY, J. R., H. C. CUNNY, M. G. PAULE & W. SLIKKER, JR. 1987. Fetal disposition of delta-9-tetrahydrocannabinol (THC) during late pregnancy in the rhesus monkey. Toxicol. Appl. Pharmacol. **90:** 315-321.

Neurobehavioral Dose-Response Effects of Prenatal Alcohol Exposure in Humans from Infancy to Adulthood[a]

ANN P. STREISSGUTH,[a,d,e] PAUL D. SAMPSON,[c] AND
HELEN M. BARR[b]

[b] *Department of Psychiatry and Behavioral Sciences*
[c] *Department of Statistics*
[d] *Alcoholism and Drug Abuse Institute*
[e] *Child Development Mental Retardation Center*
University of Washington School of Medicine
2707 N. E. Blakeley Street
Seattle, Washington 98105

Alcohol has been well established as a teratogenic agent in that prenatal exposure can cause a variety of adverse pregnancy outcomes depending on the dose, timing and conditions of exposure. Although alcohol, like many other teratogens, can cause alterations in morphology, growth, and neurobehavioral outcomes, this report focuses primarily on the latter effects.

As with other teratogens causing neurobehavioral aberrations, the neurobehavioral effects of prenatal alcohol are produced at lower exposure levels than the morphologic or growth effects,[1] and except in extreme cases, they are more devastating to the offspring. Neurobehavioral effects are difficult to measure, however, because their manifestations change with the age of the offspring, and because at the current state of the art, their measurement involves outcomes that can be exacerbated or ameliorated by postnatal experience.

This report describes two separate studies which have been ongoing in our laboratory for many years, both of which concern the long-term developmental and behavioral consequences of prenatal alcohol exposure. By comparing the results of the two studies, we can observe the contributions of dose to the teratogenic effects of alcohol.

The first is a clinical study in that all subjects were originally referred because they were suspected of having some clinical manifestations of fetal alcohol exposure. Those described in the present report were all diagnosed either Fetal Alcohol Syndrome or Fetal Alcohol Effects and they were examined psychologically as adolescents or adults. All of their mothers were known to be alcoholic or clearly abusing alcohol

[a] This work was partially supported by the National Institute on Alcohol Abuse and Alcoholism (AA01455-1-13); the Indian Health Service (Contract #243-87-0047); and the University of Washington Alcoholism and Drug Abuse Institute.

during pregnancy. Other offspring of such mothers, who were exposed but not affected, are not included in this sample.

The second is a longitudinal prospective study in which a large unselected group of pregnant women were interviewed during pregnancy regarding their alcohol use. A follow-up cohort was selected on the basis of exposure alone, and this cohort of 500 offspring, variably exposed to alcohol *in utero,* was examined at several key developmental ages between birth and 7 years.

Utilizing these two studies we can learn about the neurobehavioral dose-response effects of prenatal alcohol exposure in humans if we conceptualize alcohol as having increasingly severe effects depending on the level of exposure. Together, these two studies demonstrate the continuum of alcohol related birth defects. FIGURE 1 displays the exposure histories of subjects in the two studies.

DEFINITIONS: FAS, FAE

Fetal Alcohol Syndrome (FAS) is a birth defect consisting of three types of features: growth deficiency, dysmorphic characteristics, and central nervous system (CNS) manifestations. The growth deficiency is of prenatal origin for height and/or weight, and continues postnatally. The dysmorphic characteristics include short palpebral fissures, flat midface, flat and/or long philtrum, thin upper lip and/or small chin as well as other anomalies of the face and limbs. The CNS problems include microcephaly, tremulousness, seizures, slow development, hyperactivity, learning problems, attentional deficits, and/or memory problems. To be diagnosed FAS, it is necessary to have some manifestations from each of the three categories and a history of heavy *in utero* alcohol exposure. Patients who do not have enough characteristics for a diagnosis of FAS are often called possible or probable FAS or possible or probable Fetal Alcohol Effects (FAE). We refer the reader to Clarren and Smith,[2] Clarren,[3] Jones and Smith,[4] and Hanson and Jones,[5] for more definitive explanations of FAS and FAE. As the facial characteristics are particularly useful in differentiating FAS, FIGURE 2 presents some of the relevant facial characteristics.

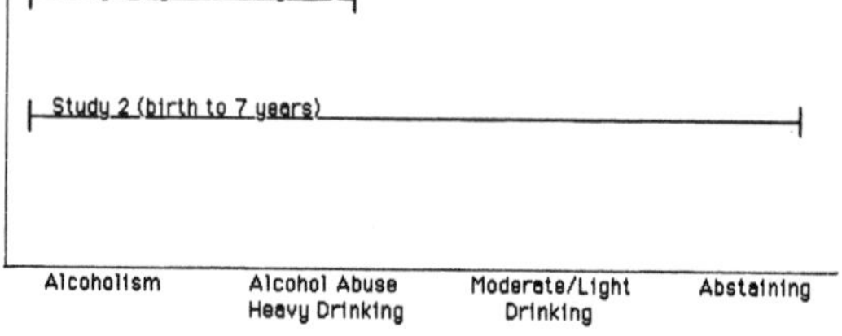

FIGURE 1. Schematic diagram of the composition of the two study samples in terms of prenatal alcohol exposure.

| Study 1 (ages 12-38 years) |

| Study 2 (birth to 7 years) |

| Alcoholism | Alcohol Abuse / Heavy Drinking | Moderate/Light Drinking | Abstaining |

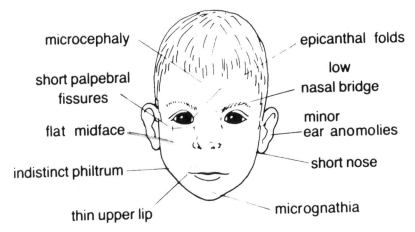

microcephaly

short palpebral
fissures

flat midface

indistinct philtrum

thin upper lip

epicanthal folds

low
nasal bridge

minor
ear anomolies

short nose

micrognathia

FIGURE 2. This figure describes the typical facial features in fetal alcohol syndrome. The features on the *left* are those that are the most characteristic and delineating; those on the *right* are less frequently observed and are not as differentiating. (From Little and Streissguth.[6] Reprinted by permission from Dartmouth Medical School.)

METHODS

Study 1

The 92 subjects in this sample were referred either from four Indian reservations of the southwest United States as part of an FAS prevalence study[7,8] or were referred to our clinic in Seattle, Washington or the clinic of Dr. D. W. Smith in Vancouver, BC for suspected FAS. All diagnoses were confirmed by examination of pediatric dysmorphologists experienced in diagnosing FAS; the prenatal exposure history was established by clinical report. All patients with FAS or FAE who met these criteria and who were 12 years old or older were included in this study.

The sample for Study 1 includes 92 patients, 58 with FAS, and 34 with FAE. These figures do not represent the relative prevalence of FAS vs FAE, but rather reflect the constraints of the referral and follow-up procedures. Subjects ranged in age from 12 to 42 years, mean age 18.4 years. Males constituted 61% of the sample; reservation Indians 55%, nonreservation Indians 22%, and non-Indians 23%. Statistical analyses contrasting these three racial/residence groups do not suggest that the findings are unduly influenced by the composition of the sample.[9]

The following tests were administered under standardized conditions: an age-appropriate IQ test: the Wechsler Intelligence Scale for Children-Revised (WISC-R) or the Wechsler Adult Intelligence Scale-Revised (WAIS-R); a test of academic achievement: the Wide Range Achievement Test-Revised (WRAT-R); a test of auditory receptive ability: the Peabody Picture Vocabulary Test (PPVT); a test of adaptive and maladaptive behavior: the Vineland Adaptive Behavior Scales (VABS), and the Symptom Checklist (SC) developed for this study. Not all test data were available on all patients.

Study 2

The cohort of approximately 500 children in this study was selected for participation based on maternal reports of alcohol use during pregnancy or prior to pregnancy recognition. Full details of the Seattle Longitudinal Prospective Study on Alcohol and Pregnancy have been previously presented.[10–12] An unselected sample of 1,500 pregnant women was interviewed during the fifth month of pregnancy regarding use of alcohol, cigarettes, caffeine and other drugs. A stratified sample was selected which included all the heavier drinkers from the interview sample and a proportion of moderate, light, and infrequent drinkers and nondrinkers. The sample was primarily white (87%), married (86%), middle class (80%) and well educated (58% had some college).

Maternal alcohol use was measured with a quantity-frequency-variability interview[13] and scored according to 25 different alcohol scores described elsewhere.[10,14] Some of the most useful alcohol scores in predicting later offspring effects were the "AA" score (ounces of absolute alcohol per day)[15] and a "Binge ≥ 5" score (a dichotomous score of whether or not the woman reported ever drinking 5 or more drinks at a time during the designated period). Alcohol scores were obtained for two time periods: (1) the "during pregnancy" (D) scores reflected self-reported alcohol use during midpregnancy, while (2) the "prior to pregnancy" (P) scores reflected self-reported use in the month or so prior to pregnancy. This latter period, which was designed to measure exposure during the very earliest part of pregnancy before the woman was aware of being pregnant, is extremely important in teratology research, because it represents the period of organogenesis when the fetus is most vulnerable to toxic exposures.

Because alcohol use is often associated with use of cigarettes, caffeine and other drugs, the mothers were also queried about these potentially confounding variables and these data were quantified and used in multiple regression analyses in studying the long-term effects of alcohol. Additional covariates which could affect the development of the children (major life changes in the household, mother-child interactions, age of siblings, injuries and illnesses, and so forth) were obtained postnatally from parental interview and observation. The Caldwell HOME scale measuring the general level of the homes in terms of intellectual stimulation, was administered to a subset of the sample when the children were one year old. In this basically middle class sample, maternal alcohol use was not significantly related to differences in the stimulation level of the homes.[16] The full list of the approximately 150 covariates examined in this study has been presented elsewhere.[12]

Outcome (dependent) variables were assessed on days 1 and 2, at 8 and 18 months, and at 4 and 7 years of age. A diagram of the study design and the primary dependent variables appears in FIGURE 3, along with the relevant sample sizes at each examination. Additional subjects from the screening sample were occasionally added to the follow-up cohort to keep the sample size around 500.

Follow-up of this cohort across time has been excellent, 86% overall.[17] At 7 years we examined 95% of the children seen at 4 years. At 7 years the overall attrition rate was the same for heavier drinkers as for the rest of the sample (14%).

RESULTS

In this section we summarize the main results from the two studies in order to answer questions about the dose response effects and the effects of prenatal alcohol exposure across the lifetime.

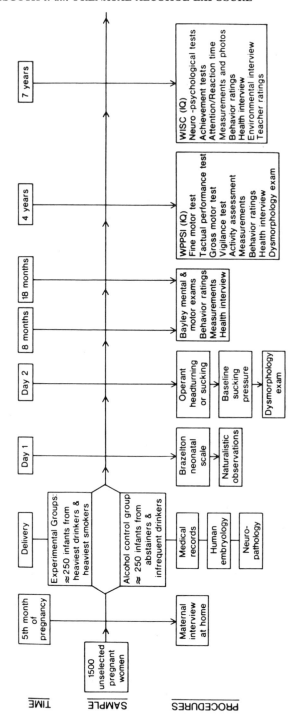

FIGURE 3. The experimental design for the Seattle Longitudinal Prospective Study on Alcohol and Pregnancy (Study 2). Sample sizes for substudies: Brazelton, 469; naturalistic observation, 124; operant head-turning, 225; operant sucking, 80; base-line sucking study, 151; neonatal dysmorphology, 163; eight-month follow-up, 468; 18-month follow-up, 496; four-year follow-up, 465; seven-year follow-up, 486.

Intelligence

We begin with IQ scores because subjects in both studies have been given the same IQ tests. From a subset of 8 patients from Study 1 who have been studied across a 10 year period,[18] we note that IQ scores of patients with FAS remain quite stable across time, revealing that for patients with this diagnosis, the long-term teratogenic effects of alcohol as measured by low IQ, are predictable for the most part from preschool IQ tests. However, one of the 8 patients showed a large systematic increase in IQ across this 10 year period from 50 to 80 points. As no clear environmental manipulations accompanied this improvement, it appears to be associated with a marked decrease in hyperactivity which enabled a better response to the test situation at later evaluations.

Further indication of the lifelong impact of alcohol teratogenesis is found in the 82 patients previously diagnosed FAS/FAE who were tested as adolescents and adults.[9] Their mean IQ was (70 ± 17), reflecting overall intellectual functioning in the mildly retarded range. However, their range of IQ scores was considerable, from a minimum of 20 to a maximum of 108. Patients with FAS had a significantly lower IQ than those with FAE (mean IQ of 65 vs 80), but both groups had an exceptionally broad range of IQ scores, as TABLE 1 indicates.

From these statistics we note several points. Intellectual impairment is observed into maturity in patients with FAS/FAE. Those with more physical manifestations of alcohol teratogenesis have a poorer intellectual outcome, in general, than those with fewer physical manifestations: the mean IQ of patients with FAS is significantly lower than those with FAE. However, the range of IQ for patients with both FAS and FAE is broad enough to argue against prediction in the individual case, based on diagnosis alone. While the physical manifestations can serve as markers for offspring affected by alcohol teratogenesis, the degree of brain damage sustained in the individual patient is variable and not always directly proportional to the degree of physical manifestations. Although we caution against overgeneralization of the test scores in Study 1 (because sample selection bias can be a factor in clinical studies), we nevertheless note that in this group of children with features of fetal alcohol effects, who experienced heavy ethanol exposure *in utero,* the intellectual handicaps last well into adolescence and adulthood.

In Study 2, we administered IQ tests to our cohort of nearly 500 children at two ages, 4 and 7 years. In this study, which is *unselected* for alcohol teratogenesis, and which involves offspring of primarily low-risk light/moderate drinkers, we do not anticipate individually debilitating effects of prenatal alcohol exposure on offspring IQ. Rather, we look for significant group decrements in IQ, attributable to alcohol, after other factors significantly related to alcohol and IQ have been statistically adjusted for. Using multiple regression techniques we find that prenatal alcohol exposure is related to significantly lower IQ scores even though the mean IQ for the cohort was well within the normal range. A robust estimate of this net alcohol effect at 4 years of age is a decrement of one IQ point per maternal drink per day.[19] In estimating the public health impact, we note that a 5 IQ point decrement is equivalent to tripling the risk of low IQ attributable to alcohol, as FIGURE 4 demonstrates.[19] In analyses of the 7 year exam data from this cohort, we find that two particular IQ subtests were more highly correlated with prenatal alcohol exposure than the full-scale IQ score, which includes subtests not apparently as sensitive to prenatal alcohol.[20] These two subtests are Arithmetic and Digit Span. For these analyses of the 7 year data we used a relatively new method of statistical analyses called "latent variable modeling," or "partial least squares," which is particularly well suited to the complex multidi-

TABLE 1. Mean IQ and Achievement Scores for Adolescents and Adults with FAS and FAE[a]

	Full Sample Mean (SD) Min-Max	FAS Mean (SD) Min-Max	FAE Mean (SD) Min-Max	Difference F	FAS/FAE p
IQ	70 (17) 20-108	65 (15) 20-91	80 (17) 39-108	16.426	0.0001
Reading	71 (18) 39-116	68 (16) 39-103	75 (20) 45-116	2.215	0.1415
Spelling	72 (14) 45-104	71 (13) 46-104	74 (15) 45-99	0.883	0.3507
Arithmetic	64 (14) 26-103	62 (11) 39-97	67 (18) 26-103	1.854	0.1779

[a] Sample size for IQ: FAS: n = 56; FAE: n = 26. Sample size for Achievement Test Standard Scores: FAS: n = 67 (Reading); 68 (Spelling) and 68 (Arithmetic); FAE = 22.

mensional data sets we deal with in behavioral teratology studies. This method allows us to deal effectively with multiple alcohol predictor scores and multiple outcome scores. Through these analyses we learn that some of the important aspects of maternal drinking that affect offspring are binge drinking and drinking prior to recognition of pregnancy.

Thus, from these two studies we see that the effects of alcohol teratogenesis last well into adolescence and adulthood in patients with FAS/FAE who are heavily exposed by virtue of having alcoholic or alcohol abusing mothers (Study 1); and we see that for moderate levels of exposure the effects of alcohol teratogenesis are less dramatic, but nevertheless statistically significant, and measurable at both 4 and 7 years (Study 2). (Further studies of this cohort at older ages are planned but have not yet been carried out.)

Academic Achievement

In Study 1 we found that patients with FAS/FAE had long-term deficits in academic achievement, even into adolescence and adulthood.[9] With a median age of 15 years, the 70 patients tested were functioning at the 4th grade level for Word Recognition, the 3rd grade level for Spelling, and the 3rd grade level for Arithmetic.

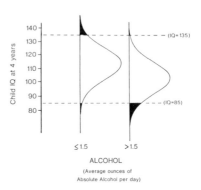

FIGURE 4. Normal distributions picturing the effect of a 5-point mean IQ decrement at the overall average profile of the Seattle, Washington sample described in Study 2 (primarily a white, middle class, well-educated, low risk group of mothers). The standard deviation of the normal distributions is the standard error of the regression model described in TABLE 2. (From Streissguth *et al.*[19] Reprinted by permission from *Developmental Psychology.*)

Their mean standard scores on Word Recognition and Spelling were 71 and 72, respectively, as would be predicted from their mean IQ of 70. Their mean standard score of 64 on Arithmetic was lower than would be predicted by their mean IQ. Furthermore, we found that despite significantly higher IQ scores, the patients with FAE did *not* perform significantly better than the patients with FAS on these achievement tests (see TABLE 1). Thus we see that for academic achievement, patients both with and without the full manifestations of FAS are at risk for severe functional deficits. We must ask if other cognitive processes not necessarily correlated with IQ, such as attention and memory, may be impaired regardless of diagnosis and thus affect the ability to learn. On the other hand, educational opportunities differentially available to low IQ students may have facilitated their educational attainment. If we consider that only children with an IQ score below 70 would have easy access to special education (as stated in the guidelines of many school districts) then we see that 52% of the patients with FAS but only 35% of those with FAE would be eligible for special education by these criteria.

In Study 2 the WRAT-R was administered to 482 subjects when they were between 6 1/2 and 8 1/2 years of age, usually just after finishing the first grade of school. As TABLE 2 indicates, both arithmetic and reading deficits were significantly associated with prenatal alcohol exposure, even though the mean scores were within the normal range for the age and grade of the subjects.

From the preceding two studies of academic achievement, we see that prenatal alcohol exposure at the heaviest end (alcoholism and maternal alcohol abuse) is associated with severe and prolonged impairment in mastery of basic educational skills, and these last into adolescence and adulthood in patients with characteristics of FAS/FAE. We note that even in more moderately exposed offspring, statistically significant group decrements in arithmetic and reading skills were observed at 7 years of age. These studies suggest that the cognitive processes required for the acquisition of arithmetic skills are more vulnerable to prenatal alcohol exposure than those required for early word recognition or spelling. These deficits may have more subtle manifestations in other aspects of daily life such as judgment, problem solving, memory, and so forth.

Other Effects of Maternal Alcoholism and Alcohol Abuse on Adolescents and Adult Offspring

As the patients in Study 1 were evaluated on many other dimensions besides IQ and achievement, it is clear that the psychosocial manifestations of FAS/FAE are also important in assessing the long-term impact of alcohol teratogenesis. As adolescents and adults, these patients had a variety of behavioral problems that appear to derive from the cognitive insults sustained *in utero,* but cannot be fully separated from their often difficult rearing environments.

On the Vineland Adaptive Behavior Scales (VABS), 58% of the adolescents and adults with FAS/FAE were classified as having "significant" levels of maladaptive behavior. Some of the specific behaviors that were characteristic of these patients include: poor concentration and attention (77%); social withdrawal (62%); impulsivity (57%); dependency (53%); teasing/bullying behavior (53%); periods of high anxiety (51%); stubborn or sullen (50%); lies, cheats, steals (49%); negative or defiant (43%); cries or laughs too easily (42%); shows lack of consideration (42%); poor eye contact (40%); and overly active (40%).

These data demonstrate the high level of psychosocial problems that persist into adolescence and adulthood, at least in this sample of patients with FAS/FAE. As the environmental problems associated with parental alcoholism are well documented,[21] we would anticipate that this high proportion of maladaptive behaviors represents the combined effects of prenatally-induced brain damage and postnatal rearing in high risk environments. Nevertheless, many of these patients were reared in foster or adoptive homes throughout much of their lives. Further evaluation of the long-term psychosocial consequences of alcohol teratogenesis are clearly needed.

TABLE 2. Major Behavioral Findings of the Seattle Longitudinal Study on Alcohol and Pregnancy to Date

Outcome	Test Procedure	Age Assessed	R	F Test for Alcohol[a] F(df)	p
1. Habituation	Brazelton	day 1	0.32	7.07(1,323)	0.008
Low arousal		day 1	0.27	6.75(1,297)	0.010
2. Opened eyes				4.15(1,115)	0.044
Body tremors	naturalistic	day 1		4.21(1,115)	0.042
Head to left	observations			4.00(1,115)	0.048
High level body activity				5.43(1,115)	0.022
Hand to face				5.16(1,115)	0.025
3. Sucking pressure	pressure	day 2	0.25	4.62(1,147)	0.033
Latency to suck	transducer	day 2	0.23	2.90(1,147)	0.091
4. Mental Dev. Index	Bayley scales	8 months	0.33	3.22(2,452)	0.041
Psychomotor Dev. Index		8 months	0.28	5.15(1,453)	0.024
5. Attention					
Errors of omission		4 years	0.23	6.32(1,351)	0.012
Errors of commission	vigilance task	4 years	0.26	5.35(1,351)	0.021
Ratio correct	with	4 years	0.33	7.98(1,351)	0.005
Trials oriented	microcomputer	4 years	0.23	.01(1,276)	0.936
Reaction time		4 years	0.57	11.71(1,066)	0.001
6. Time in movement	motion detector	4 years	0.15	.00(1,362)	0.984
7. Balance	gross motor	4 years	0.27	5.00(1,434)	0.026
8. Errors	fine motor	4 years	0.34	6.47(1,415)	0.011
Latency to correct		4 years	0.42	15.25(1,415)	0.000
Time to complete		4 years	0.32	5.68(1,437)	0.018
9. IQ	WPPSI	4 years	0.62	7.02(1,408)	0.008
10. Word reading	Stroop	7 years	0.80	4.59(1,216)	0.033
Color naming		7 years	0.51	4.08(1,216)	0.045
11. Attention					
Errors of omission-X task		7 years	0.27	5.09(1,444)	0.025
Errors of omission-AX task	Vigilance task	7 years	0.32	4.35(1,443)	0.037
Errors of commission-X task	with	7 years	0.40	4.06(1,444)	0.044
Errors of commission-AX task	microcomputer	7 years	0.45	9.68(1,442)	0.002
Reaction time		7 years	0.38	7.22(1,443)	0.007

[a] The F statistic presented here is for the effect of alcohol after adjusting for all the other variables in the multiple regression model.

Regression models were developed individually for each set of outcomes: nicotine is adjusted for in each analysis. All models except the sucking variables and naturalistic observations also adjust for caffeine, mother's diet during pregnancy, and mother's education. Other covariates were included as appropriate for each set of outcomes.

The alcohol measures and the parameterizations are as follows:

Habituation (day 1): average ounces of absolute alcohol per day: linear in midpregnancy exposure.

Naturalistic observations (day 1): 5-point ordinal alcohol scale defined by *a priori* hypothesized risk to the fetus. It combines amount, timing, and pattern of drinking.

Stroop (7 years): binary indicator of highest risk exposure from the 5-point scale described above.

Reaction time (7 years): average number of drinks per drinking occasion (early pregnancy).

All other results report various parameterizations of exposure described by average ounces of absolute alcohol per day before pregnancy recognition:

(1) Mental development index (8 months) and errors of omission (4 years): quadratic.
(2) Errors of omission (X and AX task: 7 years): linear above 1.5 ounces.
(3) Errors (4 years: fine motor) and IQ (4 years): step function at 1.5 ounces.
(4) Time to complete (4 years: fine motor): step function at 0.5 ounces.
(5) Errors of commission (X task: 7 years): step function at 2.0 ounces.
(6) All else: linear in log ounces.

Other Effects of Moderate Prenatal Alcohol Exposure from Birth to 7 Years

As the cohort from Study 2 has been examined at various points in time, as shown in FIGURE 3, we will now summarize the main findings from the Seattle Longitudinal Study on Alcohol and Pregnancy. TABLE 2 presents the main outcomes examined at each age and the relationship of these outcomes to the generally moderate levels of prenatal alcohol exposure characterizing this sample.

On days 1 and 2 of life, we already see significant neurobehavioral effects of prenatal alcohol exposure, even after statistically adjusting for a wide variety of potentially confounding covariates. The alcohol effects were generally monotone with a greater effect associated with greater exposure. The neonatal findings are particularly important because they reflect alcohol-related performance decrements even prior to the impact of the postnatal home environment. Offspring effects significantly associated with prenatal alcohol exposure include: poor habituation (the ability to tune out redundant stimuli); poor state control; poor sucking pressure and longer latency to suck after contact with the nipple; and increased frequency of body tremors, hand to face activity, head turns to left, opened eyes and a high level of activity.[22–24] Although the above findings all remained significant even after adjustment for maternal smoking and other potential covariates, there was an alcohol by smoking interaction for one study, which found poorer operant learning in both a head-turning and a sucking paradigm, for only those infants whose mothers were both heavy drinkers *and* heavy smokers.[25]

At 8 months of age, prenatal alcohol exposure was associated with small decrements in mental and motor development as measured with the Bayley Scales of Infant Development, even after statistical adjustment for other relevant covariates.

At 4 years of age, prenatal alcohol exposure in this cohort was associated with three classes of variables: IQ scores, which were discussed earlier in this paper,[19] attentional variables[26] and motor performance.[27] The attentional variables were measured with a laboratory vigilance procedure which assessed the child's ability to maintain sustained attention to an infrequently appearing stimulus. Three types of scores were recorded: Errors of Omission (times when the stimulus appeared and the child failed to press the button); Errors of Commission (times when the child pressed the button in the absence of the stimulus); and Ratio Correct (ratio of Errors of Omission to Errors of Commission). In addition, a Reaction Time score was obtained which was the child's latency to button press after the onset of the stimulus. Subtle response decrements on laboratory vigilance tests such as these have been associated with later attention deficit disorders and classroom learning problems in other studies.

At 4 years of age, fine and gross motor behaviors were assessed with the Wisconsin Fine Motor Steadiness Battery and a gross motor battery. Prenatal alcohol exposure was significantly related to the following fine motor items: time to complete the grooved peg board; errors on the grooved form boards (reflecting unsteadiness or tremulousness in fine motor activity); and latency to self-correct (which is a response speed dimension similar to reaction time, but on a fine motor task). Prenatal alcohol exposure was also associated with a balance dimension assessed on a variety of gross motor tasks and with examiner ratings of poor fine motor behavior.

At the 7 year exam, in addition to the IQ and achievement effect discussed earlier,[20] prenatal alcohol exposure was also related to the same type of attentional decrements observed at 4 years, using a vigilance CPT task.[28] The 7 year exam also involved a group of neuropsychologic tests including the Seashore Rhythm Test, a Children's Memory Test and others. Use of latent variable modeling techniques for data analysis revealed a pattern of neurobehavioral deficits significantly related to prenatal alcohol exposure. This pattern includes memory and attentional deficits across both verbal and visual modalities as well as a variety of "process" variables reflecting poor integration and quality of responses. The alcohol-related pattern of neuropsychologic deficits observed in the cohort at 7 years includes characteristics often described clinically as "minimal brain damage."

We also used examiner ratings and the classroom teacher ratings of behavior at the 7 year evaluation, and found a high relationship between the two sets. Prenatal alcohol exposure was significantly related to distractibility, poor organization and cooperation, and a rigid approach to problem solving. The association of these problem behaviors to later learning disabilities has been frequently noted in other studies in the literature.

SUMMARY AND DISCUSSION

The comparison of findings from these two studies results in a broader realization of the impact of prenatal alcohol exposure on the offspring. From Study 1 we learn that patients with FAS/FAE sustain major handicaps into adolescence and adulthood. The serious consequences of prenatal alcohol exposure at the level of maternal alcoholism and alcohol abuse remain throughout the lifetime in most affected children. The long-term consequences of more moderate levels of exposure have not yet been evaluated.

On the other hand, the effects of more moderate levels of exposure (*i.e.,* social drinking) are measurable on the first day of life (even before significant postnatal environmental impact) and continue to be observed during infancy and into childhood.

Prenatal alcohol exposure produces a wide variety of effects on offspring including intellectual decrements, learning problems, attentional and memory problems, fine and gross motor problems, and difficulty with organization and problem solving. In patients with FAS/FAE, psychosocial problems are observable in adolescence and adulthood that may have their roots in early cognitive deficits. Psychosocial problems associated with moderate exposure levels have not yet been evaluated.

The neurobehavioral effects of prenatal alcohol exposure show, in general, a dose response relationship—high levels of exposure are associated with large magnitude effects, while moderate levels of exposure are associated with more subtle effects. With our latent variable models, we can essentially determine the most relevant combination of alcohol scores for predicting offspring effects. Some of the strongest predictors of later neurobehavioral deficits are self-reported binge drinking (reporting *ever* using 5 drinks or more on an occasion in the designated time period) and self-reported drinking in the period prior to pregnancy recognition. However, many outcomes appear to be affected by maternal ingestion of alcohol regardless of timing or pattern.

There is no indication that these effects are due to a small group of outliers or that they are due to confounding with other drugs. The alcoholic women in Study 1 were pregnant between 12 and 40 years ago and most were thought to have abused only alcohol. The mothers in Study 2 reported a very low rate of heroin, methadone, speed, amphetamines and cocaine (19 out of 1,529). Other more frequently used drugs, including caffeine, aspirin, acetaminophen, nicotine, marijuana, antibiotics and/or Valium, were adjusted for or examined in the statistical analyses.

The findings reported here are in general agreement with those found in animal studies where tight laboratory controls can be obtained.[29,30] The comparable findings from the clinical study (Study 1), the epidemiologic study (Study 2), and the animal literature present convincing evidence of the neuroteratogenicity of alcohol and the long-lasting effects on prenatally-exposed offspring.

ACKNOWLEDGMENTS

The collaboration on this paper of Sandra P. Randels, Robin LaDue, Fred Bookstein, Sterling K. Clarren, Pam Phipps, and Meg Bridewell is greatly appreciated.

REFERENCES

1. RILEY, E. P. & C. V. VORHEES. 1986. Handbook of Behavioral Teratology. Plenum Press. New York, NY.
2. CLARREN, S. K. & D. W. SMITH. 1978. The Fetal Alcohol Syndrome. N. Engl. J. Med. **2998:** 1063-1067.
3. CLARREN, S. K. 1981. Recognition of Fetal Alcohol Syndrome. J. Am. Med. Assoc. **245**(23): 2436-2439.
4. JONES, K. L. & D. W. SMITH. 1973. Recognition of the Fetal Alcohol Syndrome in early infancy. Lancet **2:** 999-1001.
5. HANSON, J. W., K. L. JONES & D. W. SMITH. 1976. Fetal Alcohol Syndrome: Experience with 41 patients. J. Am. Med. Assoc. **235**(14): 1458-1460.
6. LITTLE, R. E. & A. P. STREISSGUTH. 1982. Alcohol, pregnancy, and the Fetal Alcohol Syndrome. *In* Alcohol Use and its Medical Consequences: A Comprehensive Teaching Program for Biomedical Education. Project Cork. Dartmouth Medical School. Hanover, NH.
7. MAY, P. A. & K. J. HYMBAUGH. 1982. A pilot project on Fetal Alcohol Syndrome among American Indians. Alc. H. Res. Wld. **7**(2): 3-9.
8. MAY, P. A., K. J. HYMBAUGH, J. M. AASE & J. M. SAMET. 1983. Epidemiology of Fetal Alcohol Syndrome among American Indians of the Southwest. Soc. Biol. **30:** 374-387.
9. STREISSGUTH, A. P. & S. P. RANDELS. 1987. Physical, intellectual, academic, and psychosocial manifestations of Fetal Alcohol Syndrome and Fetal Alcohol Effects in adolescence and adulthood (report to Indian Health Service). Pregnancy and Health Study. University of Washington. Seattle, WA.
10. STREISSGUTH, A. P., D. C. MARTIN, J. C. MARTIN & H. M. BARR. 1981. The Seattle longitudinal prospective study on alcohol and pregnancy. Neurobehav. Toxicol. Teratol. **3:** 223-233.

11. STREISSGUTH, A. P., H. M. BARR & D. C. MARTIN. 1984. Alcohol exposure *in utero* and functional deficits in children during the first four years of life. *In* Mechanisms of Alcohol Damage *in Utero*. R. Porter, M. O'Connor & J. Whelan, Eds.: 176-196. CIBA Found. Symp. 105. Pitman Publishing. London.

12. STREISSGUTH, A. P., P. D. SAMPSON, H. M. BARR, S. K. CLARREN & D. C. MARTIN. 1986. Studying alcohol teratogenesis from the perspective of the Fetal Alcohol Syndrome: Methodological and statistical issues. *In* Mental Retardation: Research, Education, & Technology Transfer. H. M. Wisniewski & D. A. Snider, Eds.: 63-86. N.Y. Acad. Sci. New York, NY.

13. CAHALAN, D., I. H. CISSIN & H. M. CROSSLEY, Eds. 1969. American Drinking Practices: A National Study of Drinking Behavior and Attitudes. Rutgers Center of Alcohol Studies Publications. New Brunswick, NJ.

14. STREISSGUTH, A. P., H. M. BARR, P. D. SAMPSON, F. L. BOOKSTEIN & B. L. DARBY. Neurobehavioral effects of prenatal alcohol: Part I. Literature review and research strategy. Neurotoxicol. Teratol. In press.

15. JESSOR, R., T. D. GRAVES, R. C. HANSON & S. L. JESSOR. 1968. Society, Personality and Deviant Behavior: A Study of a Tri-ethnic Community. Holt, Rinehart & Winston. New York, NY.

16. RAGOZIN, A. S., S. LANDESMAN-DWYER & A. P. STREISSGUTH. 1978. The relationship between mothers' drinking habits and children's home environments. *In* Currents in Alcoholism. F. A. Seixas, Ed. Vol. 4: 39-49.

17. GIUNTA, C. T., H. M. BARR, J. M. GILLESPIE & A. P. STREISSGUTH. 1987. Techniques for minimizing subject attrition in longitudinal research (Tech. Rep. No. 87-01). Pregnancy and Health Study. University of Washington. Seattle, WA.

18. STREISSGUTH, A. P., S. K. CLARREN & K. L. JONES. 1985. Natural history of the Fetal Alcohol Syndrome: A ten-year follow-up of eleven patients. Lancet **2**: 85-92.

19. STREISSGUTH, A. P., H. M. BARR, P. D. SAMPSON, B. L. DARBY & D. C. MARTIN. 1989. IQ at age four in relation to maternal alcohol use and smoking during pregnancy. Dev. Psychol. **25**(1): 3-11.

20. SAMPSON, P. D., A. P. STREISSGUTH, H. M. BARR & F. L. BOOKSTEIN. Neurobehaviroal effects of prenatal alcohol: Part II. Partial least squares analysis. Neurotoxicol. Teratol. In press.

21. Children of Alcoholics. 1985. Children of Alcoholics: A Review of the Literature. Children of Alcoholics Foundation. New York, NY.

22. STREISSGUTH, A. P., H. M. BARR & D. C. MARTIN. 1983. Maternal alcohol use and neonatal habituation assessed with the Brazelton Scale. Child Dev. **54**: 1109-1118.

23. MARTIN, D. C., J. C. MARTIN, A. P. STREISSGUTH & C. A. LUND. 1979. Sucking frequency and amplitude in newborns as a function of maternal drinking and smoking. *In* Currents in Alcoholism. M. Galanter, Ed. Vol. 5: 359-366. Grune & Stratton. New York, NY.

24. LANDESMAN-DWYER, S., L. KELLER & A. P. STREISSGUTH. 1978. Naturalistic observations of newborns: Effects of maternal alcohol intake. Alcohol. Clin. Exp. Res. **2**: 171-177.

25. MARTIN, J. C., D. C. MARTIN, C. A. LUND & A. P. STREISSGUTH. 1977. Maternal alcohol ingestion and cigarette smoking and their effects on newborn conditioning. Alcohol. Clin. Exp. Res. **1**: 243-247.

26. STREISSGUTH, A. P., D. C. MARTIN, H. M. BARR, B. M. SANDMAN, G. L. KIRCHNER & B. L. DARBY. 1984. Intrauterine alcohol and nicotine exposure: Attention and reaction time in 4-year-old children. Dev. Psychol. **20**: 533-541.

27. STREISSGUTH, A. P., H. M. BARR, B. L. DARBY & P. D. SAMPSON. 1988. Prenatal exposure to alcohol, caffeine, and tobacco: Effects on neuropsychological, fine motor, and gross motor function in 4-year-old children (Tech. Rep. No. 88-06). Pregnancy & Health Study. University of Washington. Seattle, WA.

28. STREISSGUTH, A. P., H. M. BARR, P. D. SAMPSON, J. C. PARRISH-JOHNSON, G. L. KIRCHNER & D. C. MARTIN. 1986. Attention, distraction and reaction time at age 7 years and prenatal alcohol exposure. Neurobehav. Toxicol. Teratol. **8**(6): 717-725.

29. WEST, J. R., Ed. 1986. Alcohol and Brain Development. Oxford University Press. New York, NY.

30. MEYER, L. S. & E. P. RILEY. 1986. Behavioral teratology of alcohol. *In* Handbook of Behavioral Teratology. E. P. Riley & C. V. Vorhees, Eds. Plenum Press. New York, NY.

Alcohol-Related Birth Defects: Assessing the Risk[a]

CLAIRE B. ERNHART,[b,c] ROBERT J. SOKOL,[d] JOEL
W. AGER,[d] MARY MORROW-TLUCAK,[c] AND
SUSAN MARTIER[d]

[b] *Case Western Reserve University*
University Circle
Cleveland, Ohio 44106

[c] *Cleveland Metropolitan General Hospital*
Department of Psychiatry
3395 Scranton Road
Cleveland, Ohio 44109

[d] *Wayne State University*
Department of Obstetrics and Gynecology
4707 St. Antoine Boulevard
Detroit, Michigan 48201

The risk of adverse effects on the fetus of the pregnant woman who drinks has received systematic attention only in recent years.[1] Not surprisingly, early studies of alcohol-related neonatal status centered on the most dramatic manifestation of the problem, the pattern termed fetal alcohol syndrome (FAS) by Jones and Smith in their seminal report.[2]. FAS is diagnosed in the infants of some, but not all, women who consume large quantities of alcohol during pregnancy.

The diagnosis of FAS requires evidence of (a) growth retardation, (b) neuropsychological impairment, as mental retardation, and (c) the presence of craniofacial and other anomalies. Early failures to recognize FAS as a distinctive condition may have been due, in part, to the fact that growth retardation and mental retardation are not specific to FAS. Furthermore, the most important feature of FAS, mental retardation, is not readily diagnosed in the newborn, hence its association with maternal drinking has been difficult to assess.

The individual anomalies are seldom all present in a given case. Considered individually, these anomalies would not be considered as major or as having any notable functional sequelae. Single specific features are not unusual; in the cohort of 359 infants in the prospective portion of this study, only 26 were without any noted anomaly. Even an infant presenting a moderate number of anomalies might not be identified in a routine examination. Nevertheless, the pattern, when seen, is clearly related to fetal alcohol exposure.

[a] Supported in part by National Institute on Alcohol Abuse and Alcoholism (NIAAA) Grant AA06571, National Institute of Child Health and Human Development Grant HD 14883 to CBE, and NIAAA Grants AA03282 and AA06334 to RJS and by the Perinatal Clinical Research Center, United States Public Health Service Grant M01-RR00210.

These features of FAS, anomalies that may not be detected without expert examination, growth retardation that may be due to other conditions, and mental retardation that cannot be diagnosed in infancy, have complicated studies on FAS. Even in a high risk population, the number of neonates who present an easily diagnosed FAS pattern is small. Research on FAS is thus almost invariably retrospective. Studies of partial effects enable us to use prospective methodology to study critical issues. The identification of a threshold is one such issue.

In the period since the FAS was linked to heavy drinking, numerous warnings about the adverse effects of drinking on the fetus have been made in professional journals and in the media. These warnings can produce considerable anxiety for the woman who has engaged in social drinking prior to learning that she is pregnant. Determination of the threshold of effect, the dose at which risk of effect can be identified, is of considerable importance to these women and to those who counsel them.

In the present study, a tally of neonatal anomalies was used as a marker for fetal alcohol effects. It is generally recognized that the first trimester, particularly the period from two to eight conceptual weeks, is critical for the induction of anatomic abnormalities. In previous reports[3,4] we used the data from a prospective study cohort to relate several measures of average ounces of alcohol per day (AA/day) to these anomalies. While first trimester AA/day was related to craniofacial anomalies for a small sample, the strongest results were those relating an estimate of embryonic AA/day to a full tally, to a subgroup of craniofacial anomalies, and, to a lesser extent, to the remaining, or "other" anomalies. While plotted data were suggestive of a threshold of effect, the sample size was too small to be able to describe a break point in the function so that a "no effect" area could be specified with reasonable confidence.

The major aim of this study was to evaluate the threshold question in greater depth by using three different indicators of alcohol consumption and by using the data from the much larger sample from which the cohort was selected in order to provide replication of the threshold analyses and increase statistical power. A second aim was to use the threshold findings to describe the prevalence of risk in the population of disadvantaged mother-infant pairs studied in this program.

Since few women are available for study very early in pregnancy, information about drinking at this time is dependent on later self-report. Furthermore, self-report about alcohol use in pregnancy is subject to possible underreporting.[4-10] This and other methodological concerns will be reviewed with respect to the findings of the study.

METHOD OF STUDY

Selection of Subjects and Procedure

During a period of almost three years, 7764 women who registered in the antenatal clinics associated with Cleveland Metropolitan General Hospital were screened for alcoholism. These clinics serve primarily disadvantaged patients; almost all women were in Hollingshead Social Classes IV and V. The screening instrument was the Michigan Alcoholism Screening Test (MAST).[11] Demographic data and information about smoking and the use of other drugs were collected and each woman was interviewed regarding her use of alcohol in the preceding two-week period.[12]

Approximately 11% of the registrants were positive on the MAST (score of 5 or more). These women and an equal number of MAST— women matched on race, smoking, parity, date of recruitment, drug abuse, prepregnancy weight, and weeks gestation at registration formed the antenatal sample. The portion of the interview covering alcohol use during the previous two-week period was repeated at each antenatal visit.

In addition to the usual neonatal examination, 1284 offspring of the women followed through pregnancy were examined under protocol for FAS-linked anomalies. Examiners were blinded to antenatal data. (Some selected infants were not included because of illness, delivery at a different hospital, and delivery and discharge on unstaffed days.)

Of these infants, those born in a 15 month period were considered for a study relating fetal alcohol exposure and child development. After exclusions for preterm delivery and other health-related reasons, parental refusal, primary language other than English, adoption and plans to move from the area, 359 mother-infant pairs were recruited into a prospective child development cohort.

Postpartum maternal and neonatal behavioral examinations were conducted. Psychological examinations of the children and assessments of the caretaking environment were conducted in the home through the preschool years. Attrition in this period was slightly over 25%. Attrition was unbiased, *i.e.,* not related significantly to any variable measured in the perinatal period. At 4 years, 10 months, 239 mother-child pairs remained in the study. (Data from an additional 22 fostered children are available for analyses not discussed in this report.)

In order that the examiners of the children could be blind to the alcohol use data, no further queries were made about alcohol until the visit at 4 years, 10 months. Two staff members conducted this visit; one tested the child while the other interviewed the mother, in a different room, about the child's behavior and about her alcohol use.

The Anomalies Tallies

The primary marker of effect was the total tally of anomalies[3,4] that characterize FAS children. Since the most notable and specific feature of FAS is the presence of craniofacial anomalies, a subgroup of craniofacial items was also identified. This craniofacial tally included the FAS features related to the head, including eyes, nose, ears, maxilla, mandible, and lips. The total tally also included cardiac murmurs and cutaneous, renogenital, skeletal, and muscular anomalies. Because these other anomalies were less prevalent, threshold analyses, while consistent, were less definitive and are not included in this report.

Indices of Alcohol Exposure

As noted above, the critical period for the dysmorphology of alcohol-related birth effects is considered to be in the embryonic period, a period when women are generally not receiving professional care and are not readily accessible to research personnel. Measures of exposure are thus based on information obtained during or after pregnancy. We are reporting on three indices, each assumed to be related to drinking in the critical early portion of pregnancy.

First, we assume that if a woman drinks during pregnancy, a period when drinking is usually decreased, she was probably drinking at least as much in the embryonic period. The first index, then, is AA/day in pregnancy. Second, a retrospective report of drinking while pregnant can avoid the underreporting and denial involved in an in-pregnancy self-report and thus may be a more valid index of alcohol use. Third, an estimate of embryonic AA/day, based in large part on MAST scores, provides an estimate of the amount being drunk at or shortly after conception.

AA/day in Pregnancy

The interviews at screen and at ensuing visits during pregnancy covered alcohol use for the two weeks prior to the respective visit. The data for each visit consisted of the volumes of the specific beverages for each drinking day in the period. These data were converted into two indices, AA/day for the screening interview and the corresponding index for the entire pregnancy. The latter is the in-pregnancy index to be used in analyses to be reported.

Retrospective AA/Day

The interview conducted five years after the pregnancy included a questionnaire regarding both current alcohol use and recall of alcohol use during the index pregnancy. The MAST was also readministered. The collection and coding of these data resembled as closely as possible that used for the in-pregnancy data.[10] An effort was made to obtain a description of the typical in-pregnancy drinking pattern (usual days on which drinking occurred, beverage used and quantity of each beverage on each day). Binging and changes in amounts drunk during pregnancy were also reviewed. For most respondents, the retrospective reports were coded easily into AA/day data. In some instances, only partial or limited reports could be elicited. These reports were blindly coded to agreement by two coders.

Estimated Embryonic AA/Day

Neither the screen AA/day obtained from the first antenatal visit nor the full pregnancy index reflected alcohol use during the period at, or shortly after, conception, i.e., before a woman knew she was pregnant. Because this period is critical for alcohol-related dysmorphology, an additional method of estimating embryonic AA/day was sought. An equation was developed from the data of a later, independent, sample of antenatal registrants who were screened and interviewed following the same protocol but from whom self-report data were also obtained relative to drinking at or shortly after conception. The embryonic AA/day scores derived from this report were highly correlated with MAST scores. This embryonic AA/day was used as the criterion measure in devising a regression equation with the MAST score and the screening AA/day score as predictors. The resulting equation was then applied to the screening data of participants in the full study to yield estimated embryonic AA/day scores.

Exclusion of Data

Data obtained from one of the examiners who administered the MAST at screen and from another one who conducted neonatal examinations were found to be highly aberrant; it is clear that some of these data were incorrect. Data collected by both examiners were excluded from the analyses reported herein.

With the exclusion of questionable data, the sample sizes were 873, and 791, respectively, for the analyses of AA/day in pregnancy and estimated embryonic AA/day. These sample sizes differed because valid MAST scores were needed for the estimation of embryonic AA/day.

Embryonic AA/day was also calculated for the entire population of 7764 women screened during the study period. (This included those women not selected for in-pregnancy, neonatal and child development study and thus represents an essentially complete survey of this population of women using the services of these clinics.) After discarding the data of women to whom the MAST had been administered by the examiner whose work was questionable, this baseline dataset consisted of 7123 measures of estimated embryonic AA/day.

The tenure of the neonatal examiner whose work was questionable did not overlap recruitment of the developmental cohort, thus none of the 239 cases with the retrospective maternal interview were excluded from the analyses of retrospective AA/day. It was possible to identify and correct affected MAST scores for this cohort so no estimated embryonic AA/day data were discarded for this group.

ANALYTIC STRATEGY

The scales of the respective AA/day indices were divided into groups to provide easily interpreted units of alcohol consumption with adequate numbers in the extreme groups. The first grouping for each index was a baseline, or abstention, category. The distributions of the three AA/day indices differed appreciably and the choice of categories for each was adjusted accordingly. Because the range of the in-pregnancy AA/day index was limited with few cases at higher values, only three categories, aside from the abstaining group, were selected for this measure. With a larger range of values, four categories, in addition to the abstaining group, were specified for the retrospective and estimated embryonic indices.

For each index, the overall differences between the AA/day categories were tested by analysis of covariance (ANCOVA) in which the anomalies data were adjusted for relevant covariates. Since the adjustments represented within-group regressions, the list of plausible covariates was reduced to those that were significantly correlated with the anomalies tally. These were parity, smoking, race and year of study. In most analyses race, parity, and year of study were statistically significant; the effect of smoking was marginal.

The major function of the ANCOVA was the adjustment of the data for the planned comparisons between groups. The test between groups was not optimal for the assessment of the threshold issue, since it was hypothesized that there would be little effect among the abstaining and low AA/day groups, in which the frequencies were highest, but that there would be significant differences between these and the high AA/day groups. Planned tests among groups were made by one-tailed t-tests.

This use of pairwise one-tailed tests, as opposed to traditional post hoc tests reflected a concern with type II error, the possibility that we would fail to detect an important difference between the abstainers and those reporting drinking small amounts of alcohol. For these analyses power analyses were used to determine whether the sample sizes were adequate for the detection of small effects.

RESULTS

Descriptive Statistics, AA/Day Indices

The means, standard deviations and ranges of the indices are provided in TABLE 1. The relationship of the means to the respective standard deviations and maximum values reflect the marked positive skewness, with numerous 0.0 scores (abstainers) in the dataset. The categories chosen for the analyses using each index and the frequencies in each category are shown in TABLES 2-7.

TABLE 1. Descriptive Statistics for Indices of Alcohol Exposure

AA/Day Index	N	$\overline{X}$	SD	Range	Intercorrelations[a] Retrospective	Intercorrelations[a] Estimated Embryonic
In-pregnancy	873	0.12	0.39	0-5.79	0.67 (0.59)[b]	0.55 (0.76)[c]
Retrospective	239	0.61	1.71	0-13.47		0.43 (0.50)[b]
Estimated embryonic	791	0.90	1.09	0-9.33		

[a] The Pearson r correlations are followed by Spearman ρ correlations in parentheses.
[b] N = 239.
[c] N = 791.

The differences among the three indices are notable and highly significant. The in-pregnancy AA/day measures are much lower and more restricted in range than those from either the retrospective or the estimated embryonic index. The mean retrospective AA/day score was lower than that for the estimated embryonic index and the range and standard deviation were attenuated for the latter index because these values resulted from the application of an estimation equation.

In spite of these differences, both Pearson and Spearman correlations indicate a high degree of interrelatedness among the three indices. This is important since each is considered to be an indicator of alcohol exposure early in gestation.

TABLE 2. Adjusted Means and Probabilities for Differences among In-Pregnancy AA/Day Groups, Total Anomalies Tally

AA/Day Group	n	Mean	Probabilities[a] for Contrasts of AA/Day Groups		
			0.0	>0.0, ≤0.1	>0.1, ≤0.5
0.0	356	2.53			
>0.0, ≤0.1	325	2.60	0.28		
>0.1, ≤0.5	153	2.62	0.28	0.45	
>0.5	39	3.29	0.005	0.010	0.016

[a] Pairwise one-tailed *t*-tests.

TABLE 3. Adjusted Means and Probabilities for Differences among In-Pregnancy AA/Day Groups, Tally of Craniofacial Anomalies

AA/Day Group	n	Mean	Probabilities[a] for Contrasts of AA/Day Groups		
			0.0	>0.0, ≤0.1	>0.1, ≤0.5
0.0	356	1.85			
>0.0, ≤0.1	325	1.92	0.26		
>0.1, ≤0.5	153	2.03	0.10	0.22	
>0.5	39	2.47	0.005	0.01	0.04

[a] Pairwise one-tailed *t*-tests.

TABLE 4. Adjusted Means and Probabilities for Differences among Retrospective AA/Day Groups, Total Anomalies Tally

AA/Day Group	n	Mean	Probabilities[a] for Contrasts of AA/Day Groups			
			0.0	>0.0, ≤0.1	>0.1, ≤0.5	>0.5, ≤1.5
0.0	86	2.71				
>0.0, ≤0.1	63	2.81	0.37			
>0.1, ≤0.5	37	2.80	0.40	—		
>0.5, ≤1.5	24	3.48	0.03	0.06	0.08	
>1.5	29	4.31	0.000	0.000	0.000	0.049

[a] Pairwise one-tailed *t*-tests.

TABLE 5. Adjusted Means and Probabilities for Differences among Retrospective AA/Day Groups, Tally of Craniofacial Anomalies

AA/Day Group	n	Mean	0.0	> 0.0, ≤ 0.1	> 0.1, ≤ 0.5	> 0.5, ≤ 1.5
0.0	86	1.84				
> 0.0, ≤ 0.1	63	2.10	0.15			
> 0.1, ≤ 0.5	37	1.94	0.37	—		
> 0.5, ≤ 1.5	24	2.65	0.01	0.07	0.036	
> 1.5	27	3.15	0.000	0.001	0.001	0.12

Header spanning: Probabilities[a] for Contrasts of AA/Day Groups

[a] Pairwise one-tailed *t*-tests.

TABLE 6. Adjusted Means and Probabilities for Differences among Estimated Embryonic AA/Day Groups, Total Anomalies Tally

AA/Day Group	n	Mean	0.0	> 0.0, ≤ 1.0	> 1.0, ≤ 2.0	> 2.0, ≤ 3.0
0.0	233	2.18				
> 0.0, ≤ 1.0	300	2.41	0.06			
> 1.0, ≤ 2.0	166	2.45	0.06	0.40		
> 2.0, ≤ 3.0	55	3.15	0.000	0.002	0.045	
> 3.0	37	3.90	0.000	0.000	0.000	0.018

Header spanning: Probabilities[a] for Contrasts of AA/Day Groups

[a] Pairwise one-tailed *t*-tests.

TABLE 7. Adjusted Means and Probabilities for Differences among Estimated Embryonic AA/Day Groups, Tally of Craniofacial Anomalies

AA/Day Group	n	Mean	0.0	> 0.0, ≤ 1.0	> 1.0, ≤ 2.0	> 2.0, ≤ 3.0
0.0	233	1.60				
> 0.0, ≤ 1.0	300	1.81	0.042			
> 1.0, ≤ 2.0	166	1.91	0.14	0.22		
> 2.0, ≤ 3.0	55	2.37	0.000	0.003	0.18	
> 3.0	37	2.85	0.000	0.000	0.000	0.049

Header spanning: Probabilities[a] for Contrasts of AA/Day Groups

[a] Pairwise one-tailed *t*-tests.

Thresholds for Anomalies

In-Pregnancy AA/Day

In the ANCOVA tests, the between groups Fs with 3,865 df were 2.20, $p = 0.09$ and 2.40, $p = 0.07$ for the total anomalies tally and for the tally limited to craniofacial anomalies. The adjusted means for the total anomalies tally, shown in TABLE 2, increased with increasing alcohol exposure. One-tailed t-tests revealed no significant differences between the two lowest categories and the abstainer group. For power analysis a "small" effect size, or difference between means, was arbitrarily defined as one fifth of the standard deviation or approximately 1% of the variance.[13] For the contrast of the first group, (with n = 325) and the abstainers (n = 358), the power for alpha = 0.05, one-tailed, was 0.90; for the second group (n = 153), power = 0.77. The power for these two comparisons considered together provides strong support for the inference that there is little if any effect for the groups of women whose drinking was reported to be infrequent and small in quantity.

The heaviest drinking group, however, did differ significantly from the abstaining group and from the low AA/day groups. A closely parallel pattern of results, shown in TABLE 3, was obtained in analyses limited to craniofacial anomalies. The data support the hypothesis of a threshold of effect at about an average of 0.5 ounces of alcohol per day, or an average of about one drink per day.

Retrospective AA/Day

This index was available for the women interviewed five years later. Because recruitment to the prospective cohort was restricted in time and by exclusion criteria, and because of attrition, the sample size was smaller (n = 239). In contrast to the analyses of in-pregnancy AA/day, the categories for retrospective AA/day are not equal in interval sizes, but were selected to provide reasonable numbers of cases through the range of measurement.

Analyses of covariance among groups were statistically significant for the total anomalies tally and the craniofacial tally (with $df = 4,231$, $F = 4.87$, $p = 0.0009$ and 4.77, $p = 0.001$ respectively). The results of the t-tests provided in TABLES 3 and 4 contrasting the two low AA/day groups and the abstention group support an inference of no effect at these AA/day levels. With the smaller sample size, the power terms for these two contrasts for the detection of a small effect size were 0.47 and 0.39. Considered alone, these analyses are not sufficient for a strong statement on the issue.

Notable and significant increases in the total and the craniofacial anomalies tallies were obtained at the two highest drinking levels. The breakpoint or threshold for this index appears to be near 0.5 ounces of alcohol per day, or about one drink per day.

Estimated Embryonic AA/Day

This index is an estimate of the amount drunk very early in pregnancy and the categories listed in TABLES 5 and 6 to describe the range of values are appreciably higher than those for the other indices. The ANCOVAs for the total anomalies tally and for the subgroup of craniofacial anomalies, were statistically significant with $p <$ 0.0001. The Fs, each with 4,782 df were 9.97 and 8.33, respectively.

The pattern of adjusted group means, shown in TABLES 6 and 7, shows small increases in both the total and the craniofacial tallies in the contrast of the abstaining group and the low AA/day groups. The difference approached statistical significance for the total tally and was marginally significant for the craniofacial anomalies. In each case the observed effect size was less than 1% of the variance. The power for the contrast of the first group with the abstainers was 0.84; that for the second group was 0.75.

The effect sizes for these contrasts, however, are small when compared with the marked, and highly significant, differences between the two highest groups and both the abstaining and the low AA/day groups. With this index, as with the other two, a clear breakpoint, or threshold, is seen in the comparisons of the heavy-drinking groups with the abstainers and with the low AA/day groups. The estimated lower boundary of alcohol use for these groups was greater than AA/day = 2.0, or about an average of four drinks per day in the embryonic period.

TABLE 8. Summary of Results of Threshold Analysis

	Threshold Analysis		
	In-Pregnancy	Retrospective	Estimated Embryonic
Threshold (AA/day)	0.5	0.5	2.0
Per cent positive	4%	22%	12%

Integration of Threshold Information

While each of the analyses for threshold supports the inference that there is a non-effect or "safe" range of alcohol exposure and a threshold above which an effect is found, the three indices yielded different quantitative results. Threshold values, summarized in TABLE 8, can be expressed either in terms of amount of alcohol (AA/ day) or in terms of percent positive (above threshold). In the latter case, percentile data can be used to derive an estimated amount of drinking in the indicated period. The latter approach was chosen as a way of resolving the differences among the indices.

The rationale which guides this integration follows. The anomalies tally, which is the marker variable for the specification of the threshold, reflects exposure in the embryonic period. The intercorrelations among the indices used in this study and the fact that the threshold pattern was obtained with each indicates that each is a valid indicator of alcohol use very early in pregnancy. Nevertheless, the descriptive statistics for the three indices are not the same and should not be expected to be the same. The first difference, of course, is that both the in-pregnancy and the retrospective indices measured alcohol use during pregnancy when drinking is known to decrease.[14] The estimate of embryonic AA/day was based on a prediction of quantities drunk prior to knowledge of pregnancy.

The proportion of cases above the threshold identified with the in-pregnancy index is extremely low. Even though many women reduce drinking during pregnancy, underreporting was suggested by the fact that only 4% reported drinking an average of one or more drinks per day in a sample selected to include a high proportion of MAST+ women. In retrospective interviews, this figure was 22%, and for some women the amount reported was dramatically higher. Since it is unlikely that women would overreport in the later interview, the discrepancy is interpreted as in-pregnancy underreporting.[10] Although underreporting was related to MAST scores,[15] these data were too variable for simple analytic adjustment. Because of the amount of underreporting, the in-pregnancy data were not used to try to define threshold values.

The estimated embryonic index threshold, AA/day = 2.0, was not affected by pregnancy-induced reductions in drinking. If the MAST score, which contributes heavily to this index, was subject to denial or underreporting, this was not detected in the results of readministration in the later interview. The sample size on which the threshold analysis was conducted was ample. This threshold value is thus identified as a plausible candidate in setting a drinking level of concern. 12% of the 791 cases in the analysis were positive for risk by this criterion.

Another approach is to set the proportion of at-risk cases at a value determined by the analyses yielding the largest proportion of positive, *i.e.*, above threshold, cases. In the analyses of the retrospective index, 53 or 22% of the 239 cases were above threshold. Of these cases, only 25, or 10% were positive by the criterion of estimated embryonic AA/day = 2.0. By applying he 22% cut-off to the 791 women of the sample used in the analysis of the estimated embryonic index, the highest drinking 174 women would be selected. The estimated embryonic AA/day cut-off for these cases is about 1.5, or an average of about three drinks per day. This threshold, based on the information from the retrospective index and from the estimated embryonic index, provides a more conservative criterion for the range of risk than that based solely on the analysis of the estimated embryonic AA/day index.

The Prevalence of Risk-Level Drinking among Inner-City Indigent Women

One aim of the study was to use the threshold findings to describe the prevalence of risk among disadvantaged mother-infant pairs.

The women whose data entered the analyses we have reported were selected using a protocol planned to recruit 50% MAST+ women. This selection was made from the population of 7764 women screened at their first antenatal visits. Screening AA/day data and MAST scores, available for all screened women, were used to compute estimated embryonic AA/day scores for the population. Exclusion of the data of the aberrant screener reduced this data pool to 7123.

The estimated embryonic AA/day measures of 251 of these women were above the threshold value of AA/day = 1.5. Based on this index, the risk for alcohol-related neonatal anomalies was limited to the 3.5 per cent of women who drank three or more drinks per day, or 21 or more drinks per week at or during the period shortly after conception.

DISCUSSION

The offspring of women drinking small amounts of alcohol early in pregnancy did not differ notably from the offspring of abstaining women with respect to the marker variable, FAS-related neonatal anomalies. This was so for the full tally and for the subgroup of craniofacial anomalies. This result was obtained for two of the three different indices of alcohol use; for the third measure the effect, significant only for the craniofacial tally, was marginal and probably of no importance in the context of the full set of analyses. Large samples for two of the measures provided enough power for the detection of a small increase in risk. Considered altogether, the data support the assertion that there is little risk of an increase in alcohol-related anomalies associated with having had an occasional drink in the earliest part of pregnancy.

At the same time, the results do support an inference of a threshold with significant effects related to heavy drinking. Clearly, heavy drinking places the fetus at risk for increased neonatal anomalies, including those craniofacial anomalies that, as a group, characterize fetal alcohol syndrome.

What is striking about this set of analyses is the consistency with which the threshold of effect was seen with the three different indices. Although direct measures of drinking in early pregnancy were not available, the effect was strong enough to be replicated with the three instruments, each of which had limitations as an estimate of the exposure involved. Each was based on self-report. One index was subject to underreporting by a number of women, one was based on a five year retrospective recall, and one was an estimate based primarily on a history of alcohol-related problems rather than actual reported drinking.

While the three indices are sufficiently correlated for each to be considered as a reasonable measure of alcohol exposure, the differences among them are important in connection with two difficult, interrelated questions: what is the "safe" level of drinking? and how do we identify women whose drinking will increase the risk of alcohol-related anomalies?

Following the rationale described above, we arrived at a conservative threshold value of AA/day = 1.5, or an average of about three drinks per day during the period prior to knowledge of pregnancy. It should be mentioned that this average, for a number of the heavy-drinking women, resulted from weekend drinking. Thus many of the fetuses whose mothers averaged three drinks per day were often subject to much heavier doses.

The findings are limited to the estimate of a threshold for drinking effects in the earliest part of pregnancy; this is not a license for drinking later in pregnancy. The results reported are for neonatal anomalies, which is the feature associated with the period of embryogenesis. It is still prudent to advise pregnant women to stop or greatly limit drinking during pregnancy. The effects of drinking during pregnancy on size measures and on neuropsychological development remain to be analyzed.

Although the below-threshold results should be reassuring for the woman who drinks occasionally and finds herself pregnant, the above-threshold results do serve to remind us that the heavy drinking engaged in by 3.5 per cent of this population remains a public health concern. The problem is not, of course, limited to the population we studied; similar data for determining the prevalence for other groups are not available.

The identification of women whose drinking may place their fetuses at risk is not easy. We found strong evidence of underreporting in response to questions asked about drinking in pregnancy. The discrepancy between the in-pregnancy and retrospective reports we obtained is presumably due to denial associated with the stigma of drinking in pregnancy. This discrepancy was not seen in a similar five year follow-up of nonpregnant women.[16] It appears, then, that an in-pregnancy interview regarding one's current drinking has limited validity for research and is not sufficiently sensitive for clinical use.

In spite of the imprecision of recall over a five year period, the retrospective AA/day index was correlated as highly with the alcoholism measure (the MAST) as was the in-pregnancy AA/day index. Furthermore, the retrospective index was related more highly than the in-pregnancy index to the neonatal anomalies tally. Even though a retrospective report may help to overcome the denial seen with in-pregnancy interviewing, it is rather impractical for research and, of course, of no value for clinical use.

The validity of the estimated embryonic index appears to be due to the contribution of the MAST score. This provides an interesting clue for the identification of women whose infants are at risk of alcohol-related birth effects since questions about a history of alcohol-related problems do not usually elicit as much denial as does an interview about drinking in pregnancy. The MAST is a useful research tool, but it is unduly long for clinical application. Our experience with this study has contributed to the plans for several interrelated studies now ongoing to validate a short set of questions that can be used for the identification of the pregnant woman who is a problem drinker.

We are heartened by our ability to offer some reassurance to those women concerned about having had an occasional drink early in their pregnancies, but continue to be concerned about the offspring of women who are alcohol dependent. It is important that women who may become pregnant be informed that there is a risk associated with heavy drinking in the period shortly after conception.

REFERENCES

1. ABEL, E. L. 1984. Fetal Alcohol Syndrome and Fetal Alcohol Effects. Plenum Press. New York, NY.
2. JONES, K. L. & D. W. SMITH. 1973. Recognition of the fetal alcohol syndrome in early infancy. Lancet 2: 999-1000.
3. ERNHART, C. B., A. W. WOLF, P. L. LINN, R. J. SOKOL, M. J. KENNARD & H. F. FILIPOVICH. 1985. Alcohol-related birth defects: Syndromal anomalies, intrauterine growth retardation, and neonatal behavioral assessment. Alcohol. Clin. Exp. Res. 9: 447-453.
4. ERNHART, C. B., R. J. SOKOL, S. MARTIER, P. MORON, D. NADLER, J. W. AGER & A. W. WOLF. 1987. Alcohol teratogenicity in the human: A detailed assessment of specificity, critical period, and threshold. Am. J. Obstet. Gynecol. 156: 33-39.
5. RUSSELL, M. 1982. Screening for alcohol-related problems in obstetric and gynecologic patients. *In* Fetal Alcohol Syndrome. E. Abel, Ed. Vol 2: 1-20. CRC Press. Boca Raton, FL.

6. RUSSELL, M. 1982. The epidemiology of alcohol-related birth defects. *In* Fetal Alcohol Syndrome. E. Abel, Ed. Vol 2: 89-126. CRC Press, Boca Raton, FL.
7. ARMOR, D. J., J. M. POLICH & H. B. STAMBUL. 1976. Alcoholism and Treatment. Rand. Santa Monica, CA.
8. FULLER, R. K., K. K. LEE & E. GORDIS. 1988. Validity of self-report in alcoholism research: Results of a Veterans Administration cooperative study. Alcohol. Clin. Exp. Res. **12:** 201-205.
9. POLICH, J. M. 1982. The validity of self-reports in alcoholism research. Addictive Behav. **7:** 123-132.
10. ERNHART, C. B., M. MORROW-TLUCAK, R. J. SOKOL & S. MARTIER. 1988. Underreporting of alcohol use in pregnancy. Alcohol. Clin. Exp. Res. **12:** 506-511.
11. SELZER, M. L. 1971. The Michigan Alcoholism Screening Test: The quest for a new diagnostic instrument. Am. J. Psychiatry **127:** 1653-1658.
12. SOKOL, R. J., S. MARTIER & C. B. ERNHART. 1985. Identification of alcohol abuse in the prenatal clinic. *In* Early Identification of Alcohol Abuse. National Institute on Alcohol Abuse and Alcoholism, Research Monograph **17:** 209-227.
13. COHEN, J. 1977. Statistical Power Analysis for the Behavioral Sciences. Academic Press. New York, NY.
14. LITTLE, R. E. 1982. Maternal alcohol use during pregnancy: A review. *In* Fetal Alcohol Syndrome. E. Abel, Ed. Vol 2: 47-64. CRC Press. Boca Raton, FL.
15. MORROW-TLUCAK, M., C. B. ERNHART, R. J. SOKOL, S. MARTIER & J. AGER. 1988. Assessment of risk drinking during pregnancy. Alcohol. Clin. Exp. Res. **12:** 338.
16. CZARNECKI, D., M. RUSSELL & D. SALTER. 1987. Five year retrospective reliability of alcohol consumption in a gynecologic population (abstract). Alcohol. Clin. Exp. Res. **11:** 223.

The Behavioral and Neuroanatomical Effects of Prenatal Alcohol Exposure in Animals

EDWARD P. RILEY AND SUSAN BARRON

Department of Psychology
College of Sciences
San Diego State University
San Diego, California 92182

One of the most devastating and obvious long-term effects of prenatal alcohol exposure is its impact on the developing nervous system. In fact, one criterion for a diagnosis of fetal alcohol syndrome (FAS) is some evidence of a central nervous system (CNS) dysfunction such as microcephaly or mental retardation.[1] Even in the absence of the full FAS, learning and behavioral deficits such as shortened attention span and overactivity are frequently reported in children with heavy maternal alcohol histories.[2,3]

Rodent models have proved useful in the study of the behavioral effects and underlying mechanisms involved in alcohol's behavioral teratogenic effects. In this paper, we discuss some behavioral data collected following prenatal and neonatal alcohol exposure using rodent models concentrating on data gathered in our laboratory. We have tried to relate these results to clinical findings in children exposed to alcohol in utero and also in terms of potential brain areas that might be involved in these dysfunctions.

In our laboratory, alcohol is administered in a liquid diet with vitamin and mineral supplements. This diet is designed to provide 35% of the total caloric content as ethanol (35% ethanol-derived calories (EDC)). An isocaloric 0% EDC pair-fed liquid diet group and a nontreated ad libitum water and chow group are included in all of our studies in order to rule out possible nutritional effects.

Recently, we have also begun investigating neonatal alcohol exposure in rats. While the pattern of development of the CNS is relatively similar across species, the timing in which birth occurs in relation to CNS development differs greatly.[4,5] In rats, early postnatal life coincides with a period of rapid CNS growth and proliferation that occurs in humans during the third trimester of development.[4,5] Therefore, it has been argued that administration of alcohol to neonatal rats is a useful model to examine the effects of alcohol during the equivalent of the human third trimester "brain growth spurt."[6]

To deliver alcohol neonatally, we use the "pup-in-the-cup" technique, in which pups are surgically implanted with an intragastric cannula and artificially reared.[6,7] A milk formula containing alcohol or maltose/dextrin in an isocaloric concentration is delivered via an infusion pump at scheduled periods throughout the day. We also include a sham-surgery, suckled control that is kept with its dam to control for possible effects of the artificial rearing procedure.

RESPONSE INHIBITION DEFICITS

One of the more frequent general characteristics reported following prenatal alcohol exposure is a response inhibition deficit. For example, in clinical studies, infants with maternal alcohol histories took longer to habituate to a novel stimulus than controls,[8] preschool and school-age children performed more poorly in vigilance tasks,[2,3] and these children were frequently diagnosed as being hyperactive.[3] These deficits have been explained, in part, by an inability to inhibit responding to external stimuli.[3]

A number of the behavioral abnormalities reported in rats following prenatal alcohol exposure can also be attributed to response inhibition deficits. One of the most frequent and consistent findings following *in utero* alcohol exposure is overactivity as measured in open-fields,[9] running wheels,[10] and nose-poke and head-dip apparatus.[11] The overactivity observed in these paradigms has been explained as an inability to inhibit activity and/or exploration or as a deficit in habituation to a novel environment. This alcohol-related overactivity appears to be both dose and age related. Young, weanling-age subjects or animals tested in old age typically exhibit overactivity, while young or mature adult subjects do not.[12,13]

Other behavioral paradigms that require the subject to inhibit responding are also affected in rats following prenatal alcohol exposure. Passive avoidance learning requires the subject to learn to remain in one location to avoid shock. This response is usually learned quite rapidly by even fairly young animals. However, following prenatal alcohol exposure, subjects took longer to reach the learning criterion.[14] Again, this deficit appears to be age related. When tested in adulthood, subjects with a history of prenatal alcohol exposure showed no deficits relative to controls.[12] However, it may be that the task was so easy for the adult that the response inhibition deficit was masked by the simplicity of the task.

When tested in a T-maze without any extrinsic rewards, rats typically alternate between the two arms of the maze. This tendency to "spontaneously alternate" develops at about the same time that cholinergic inhibitory systems are maturing in the rat and therefore this alternation is thought to reflect inhibitory tendencies. Alcohol-exposed offspring (35% EDC and 17% EDC) perseverated more in their behavior than controls, *i.e.*, they required an increased number of trials prior to their first alternation.[15] Once again, the effects of alcohol exposure were age dependent. Prenatal alcohol exposure altered alternation in younger subjects but not in adults.[12]

Both activity and passive avoidance have also been studied in rodents following neonatal alcohol exposure. After such exposure, overactivity was reported in rats 16-20 or 90 days of age.[16] In passive avoidance, 23-day-old alcohol-exposed females took more trials to reach criterion than controls. However, alcohol-exposed males were unaffected (Barron *et al.*, in preparation). This sex difference is consistent with recent data reported by Kelly *et al.* in which alcohol-exposed females but not males, displayed deficits in a Morris-maze.[17]

The hippocampus has been implicated in these response inhibition deficits following prenatal alcohol exposure. Behavioral comparisons between rodents with prenatal alcohol histories and those with hippocampal damage show many similarities.[18] In agreement with this, prenatal alcohol exposure has been associated with a number of hippocampal anomalies including a decreased number of pyramidal cells in the CA1 region,[19] aberrant mossy fiber terminal fields,[20] and altered postlesion-induced sprouting.[21] Following neonatal alcohol exposure a reduction in hippocampal area,[22] decreased cell number,[23] and disruptions in mossy fiber development[24] have been reported. While alcohol altered the hippocampus following both exposure periods, the effects were not identical and may explain some of the behavioral variations observed in the two exposure models.

FEEDING AND SUCKLING BEHAVIOR

Human newborns with a history of maternal alcohol abuse frequently exhibit abnormalities in feeding. These infants are typically described as being "poor feeders," easily distracted when suckling, or easily fatigued and displaying a weak suck.[25,26] Experimentally, alcohol-exposed newborns displayed longer nipple attachment latencies and exerted less pressure on a nonnutritive nipple than control newborns.[26] These early feeding problems may contribute to the postnatal growth deficiencies that are typically reported in alcohol-exposed offspring.

Feeding abnormalities have also been reported in rodents following prenatal alcohol exposure. Until approximately 9 days of age, 35% EDC pups exhibited longer latencies to attach to the nipple of an anesthetized dam when compared to controls.[27] Since this increase in attachment latency was seen in pups with no prior suckling experience,[28] it suggests that the deficit observed was not due to some differential suckling experience in alcohol-exposed offspring. Suckling pressure has also been measured in rats following prenatal alcohol exposure by inserting an intraoral cannula in the pup and attaching this to a pressure transducer. At 6-10 days of age, the alcohol exposed-offspring exerted less pressure than controls and also had altered patterns of suckling.[29] These effects were not apparent at 15-16 days of age.[30]

BALANCE AND GAIT DISORDERS

Both balance and gait appear to be affected in FAS children. Clinical observations suggest that these children have problems with motor tasks, balance, and coordination.[31] Recently, Marcus reported on 5 children diagnosed with FAS and found a range of cerebellar-related disorders including axial ataxia and kinetic tremors as well as balance and gait abnormalities.[32]

Rodent studies also report deficits in tasks that require balance and motor coordination. Following prenatal alcohol exposure, developmental indices which require motor coordination such as the righting reflex[33] and negative geotaxis[34] are delayed. The walking pattern or gait of the animal also appears to be affected. The 35% EDC subjects exhibited significantly shorter stride lengths, had an increased angle of placement of the hind paws, and had less symmetry in their gait relative to controls. These types of gait anomalies suggest a form of "ataxia" in these animals.[35]

Neonatal alcohol exposure has also been associated with deficits in various tasks that require balance and motor abilities such as traversing parallel horizontal rods.[36] Examination of walking patterns revealed that at 45 and 65 days of age alcohol exposed subjects displayed shorter stride lengths and increased hindfoot step angle relative to controls.[37] These anomalies were not seen, however, at 21 days of age.

Damage to the cerebellum is frequently associated with deficits in motor skills and balance. In clinical studies, cerebellar dysgenesis has frequently been noted in autopsies of FAS children,[38] and it has been suggested that cerebellar hypoplasia is one of the most frequently observed anomalies.[39] In rodents, structural alterations in the cerebellum have also been reported following prenatal alcohol exposure,[40] although these effects appear more robust following neonatal alcohol administration.[41,42] This is not surprising since the cerebellum undergoes considerable growth in the early neonatal period.

EARLY LEARNING ABILITIES

In the clinical literature, there are very few studies examining learning in infants with a history of maternal alcohol abuse. However, it has been shown that prenatal alcohol exposure has been associated with deficits in habituation to a novel stimulus,[8] orienting[43] and operant performance.[44]

In our laboratory, we have assessed learning in neonatal rats in odor associative and taste aversion paradigms following prenatal alcohol exposure. In the taste aversion paradigm, a novel taste was paired with an injection of lithium chloride which made the animal mildly ill. At 15 days of age, the 35% EDC offspring did not form as strong a conditioned taste aversion as controls. At 10 days of age, there were no differences in the strength of the aversion between groups and at 5 days of age, no evidence of learning in any of the groups.[45] The absence of learning in the 5-day-old offspring may be due to the fact that taste is probably not the most salient cue for newborn pups. Rather than taste or any other sense, olfaction appears to be the most critical and functionally developed sense in infant rats.[46] When odor aversion learning was assessed by pairing a novel odor with LiCl-induced toxicosis at 10 days of age, the 35% EDC offspring demonstrated little evidence of learning an aversion as compared to controls. When appetitive odor associative learning was examined by pairing milk infusion with a novel odor in 3-day-old offspring, again, the 35% EDC offspring showed no evidence of learning any association between the milk and the odor. The control groups, in contrast, preferred the odor previously associated with milk reward.[47]

In this paper we have tried to review some of our data collected using rodent models of prenatal and neonatal alcohol exposure. We believe that the findings discussed coincide well with the clinical literature and provide strong evidence for the relevance of these animal models. We believe that these types of investigations may prove useful in delineating the mechanisms underlying some of the effects resulting from prenatal alcohol exposure. They may also be useful in determining risk factors that predispose an infant to fetal alcohol effects and in developing therapies useful in the treatment of behavioral dysfunctions resulting from prenatal alcohol exposure.

REFERENCES

1. CLARREN, S. K. & D. W. SMITH. 1978. N. Engl. J. Med. **298:** 1063-1067.
2. STREISSGUTH, A. P., D. C. MARTIN, H. M. BARR, B. M. SANDMAN, G. L. KIRCHNER & B. L. DARBY. 1984. Dev. Psychol. **20:** 533-541.
3. STREISSGUTH, A. P. 1986. The behavioral teratology of alcohol: Performance, behavioral, and intellectual deficits in prenatally exposed children. *In* Alcohol and Brain Development. J. R. West, Ed.: 3-44. Oxford University Press. New York, NY.
4. DOBBING, J. 1981. The later development of the brain and its vulnerability. *In* Scientific Foundations of Pediatrics. 2nd edit. J. A. Davis & J. Dobbing, Eds.: 744-759. Saunders. Philadelphia, PA.
5. DOBBING, J. & J. SANDS. 1979. Early Hum. Dev. **3:** 79-83.
6. SAMSON, H. H. & J. DIAZ. 1982. Effects of neonatal ethanol exposure on brain development in rodents. *In* Fetal Alcohol Syndrome, Vol. III. Animal Studies. E. L. Abel, Ed.: 131-150. CRC Press. Boca Raton, FL.
7. WEST, J. R., K. M. HAMRE & D. R. PIERCE. 1984. Alcohol **1:** 213-222.
8. STREISSGUTH, A. P., D. C. MARTIN & H. M. BARR. 1983. Child Dev. **54:** 1109-1118.
9. ABEL, E. L. 1984. Fetal Alcohol Syndrome and Fetal Alcohol Effects. Plenum Press. New York, NY.

10. MARTIN, D. C., J. C. MARTIN, G. SIGMAN & B. RADOW. 1978. Physiol. Psychol. **6:** 362-365.
11. RILEY, E. P., N. R. SHAPIRO & E. A. LOCHRY. 1979. Pharmacol. Biochem. Behav. **11:** 513-519.
12. ABEL, E. L. 1982. Alcohol. Clin. Exp. Res. **6:** 369-376.
13. ABEL, E. L. & B. A. DINTCHEFF. 1986. Drug Alcohol Depend. **16:** 321-330.
14. RILEY, E. P., E. A. LOCHRY & N. R. SHAPIRO. 1979. Psychopharmacology **62:** 47-52.
15. RILEY, E. P., E. A. LOCHRY, N. R. SHAPIRO & J. BALDWIN. 1979. Pharmacol. Biochem. Behav. **10:** 255-259.
16. KELLY, S. J., D. R. PIERCE & J. R. WEST. 1987. Exp. Neurol. **96:** 580-593.
17. KELLY, S. J., C. R. GOODLETT, S. A. HULSETHER & J. R. WEST. 1987. Behav. Brain Res. **27:** 247-257.
18. RILEY, E. P., S. BARRON & J. H. HANNIGAN. 1986. Response inhibition deficits following prenatal alcohol exposure: A comparison to the effects of hippocampal lesions in rats. *In* Alcohol and Brain Development. J. R. West, Ed.: 71-102. Oxford University Press. New York, NY.
19. BARNES, D. E. & D. W. WALKER. 1981. Dev. Brain Res. **1:** 333-340.
20. WEST, J. R., C. A. HODGES & A. C. BLACK, JR. 1981. Science **211:** 957-959.
21. PIERCE, D. R. & J. R. WEST. 1987. Neurotoxicol. Teratol. **9:** 129-141.
22. WEST, J. R., S. L. DEWEY & M. D. CASSELL. 1984. Dev. Brain Res. **12:** 83-95.
23. WEST, J. R., K. M. HAMRE & M. D. CASSELL. 1985. Alcohol. Clin. Exp. Res. **9:** 196.
24. WEST, J. R. & K. M. HAMRE. 1985. Dev. Brain Res. **17:** 280-284.
25. OULETTE, E. M., H. L. ROSETT, N. P. ROSMAN & L. WEINER. 1977. J. Pediatr. **297:** 528-530.
26. MARTIN, D. C., J. C. MARTIN, A. P. STREISSGUTH & C. A. LUND. 1977. Sucking frequency and amplitude in newborns as a function of maternal drinking and smoking. *In* Currents in Alcoholism. M. Galanter, Ed. Vol. 5: 359-366. Grune & Stratton, New York, NY.
27. CHEN, J. S., C. D. DRISCOLL & E. P. RILEY. 1982. Teratology **26:** 145-153.
28. RILEY, E. P., S. L. BUNIS & N. GREENFELD. 1984. Bull. Psychon. Soc. **22:** 239-240.
29. ROCKWOOD, G. A. & E. P. RILEY. 1986. Teratology **33:** 145-151.
30. RILEY, E. P. & G. A. ROCKWOOD. 1984. Nutr. Behav. **1:** 289-299.
31. CLARREN, S. K. 1981. J. Am. Med. Assoc. **245:** 2436-2439.
32. MARCUS, J. C. 1987. Neuropediatr. **18:** 158-160.
33. SHAYWITZ, B. A., G. G. GRIFFIETH & J. W. WARSHAW. 1979. Neurobehav. Toxicol. **1:** 113-122.
34. LEE, M. H., R. HADDAD & A. RABE. 1980. Neurobehav. Toxicol. **2:** 189-198.
35. HANNIGAN, J. H. & E. P. RILEY. Alcohol. In press.
36. MEYER, L. S., L. E. KOTCH & E. P. RILEY. Neurotoxicol. Teratol. In press.
37. MEYER, L. S., L. E. KOTCH & E. P. RILEY. Alcohol. Clin. Exp. Res. In press.
38. CLARREN, S. K. 1986. Neuropathology in fetal alcohol syndrome. *In* Alcohol and Brain Development. J. R. West, Ed.: 158-166. Oxford University Press. New York, NY.
39. CLARREN, S. K. 1981. J. Am. Med. Assoc. **246:** 2436-2439.
40. KORNGUTH, S. E., J. J. RUTLEDGE, E. SUNDERLAND, F. SIEGEL, I. CARLSON, J. SMOLLENS, U. JUHL & B. YOUNG. 1979. Exp. Brain Res. **37:** 299-308.
41. BAUER-MOFFETT, C. & J. ALTMAN. 1977. Brain Res. **119:** 249-268.
42. BORGES, S. & P. D. LEWIS. 1983. Brain Res. **271:** 388-391.
43. SMITH, I. E., C. D. COLES, J. LANCASTER, P. M. FERNHOFF & A. FALEK. 1986. Neurobehav. Toxicol. Teratol. **8:** 375-381.
44. MARTIN, J. C., D. C. MARTIN, A. P. STREISSGUTH & C. A. LUND. 1977. Alcoholism **1:** 243-247.
45. RILEY, E. P., S. BARRON, C. D. DRISCOLL & J. S. CHEN. Teratology **29:** 325-331.
46. ALBERTS, J. R. 1976. Olfactory contributions to behavioral development in rodents. *In* Mammalian Olfaction, Reproductive Processes and Behavior. R. L. Doty, Ed.: 67-94. Academic Press. New York, NY.
47. BARRON, S., W. A. GAGNON, S. N. MATTSON, L. E. KOTCH, L. S. MEYER & E. P. RILEY. 1988. Neurotoxicol. Teratol. **10:** 333-339.

Role of Prostaglandins in Alcohol Teratogenesis

CARRIE L. RANDALL, RAYMOND F. ANTON,
HOWARD C. BECKER, AND NANCY M. WHITE

Veterans Administration Medical Center
and
Department of Psychiatry and Behavioral Sciences
Medical University of South Carolina
109 Bee Street
Charleston, South Carolina 29403

Our laboratory has been working on animal models of fetal alcohol syndrome for a number of years. We, among others, have shown that mice are sensitive to alcohol-induced birth defects.[1,2] With confidence that we could produce birth defects reliably by administering high doses of alcohol to pregnant C57BL/6J mice, recently we chose to focus our attention on possible ways to reduce or prevent these birth anomalies.

A number of studies demonstrated that prostaglandin (PG) inhibitors such as aspirin and indomethacin were capable of reducing several alcohol-related behaviors in mice. For example, PG synthesis inhibitors injected prior to alcohol were shown to reduce alcohol-induced loss of righting reflex following narcotic doses of alcohol,[3,4] alcohol-induced hypothermia,[5] alcohol-induced hyperactivity,[6] and alcohol-induced mortality.[7] It was proposed that alcohol caused an increase in brain PG levels that was blocked by PG-inhibitor pretreatment. This speculation recently was confirmed by the same investigators.[8]

We considered the implications of this line of work for the teratogenic actions of alcohol. After all, PGs are known to play important roles in reproduction and pregnancy.[9] Moreover, exogenous administration of PGE and PGF have been shown to be teratogenic in mice.[10]

We reasoned that if 1) alcohol caused an increase in maternal PGE/PGF and 2) elevated levels of these PGs were teratogenic, then pretreatment with a PG inhibitor *prior* to alcohol administration should reduce birth defects. Treatment *after* alcohol should not have any effect.

As reported by Randall and Anton,[11] nulliparous C57BL/6J mice were time bred and injected s.c. on gestation day 10, 3 hours with either vehicle or 150 mg/kg aspirin (acetylsalicylic acid). This dose was selected because our unpublished work demonstrated that it reduced alcohol-induced sleep time in this strain of mice.

One hour later, the mice received either 5.8 g/kg alcohol or an isocaloric sucrose solution by gavage. This experimental design resulted in the following four treatment groups: vehicle-alcohol, vehicle-control, aspirin-alcohol, and aspirin-control. The alcohol dose and day of administration were selected based on a paper by Webster *et al.*,[12] demonstrating an increased incidence of limb defects.

The results on fetal weight are shown in FIGURE 1. As can be seen, the vehicle-alcohol group weighed less than all other groups ($p < 0.05$) and, while there was a

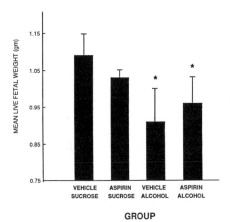

FIGURE 1. Effect of aspirin and alcohol on fetal weight. Mean ± SE fetal weight as a function of alcohol and aspirin treatment (N = 8-11 litters/group). *Significantly differs from sucrose-treated groups ($p < 0.001$).

tendency for the aspirin-pretreatment to increase body weight toward control levels, the data did not reach statistical significance.

FIGURE 2 shows the effect of aspirin pretreatment on alcohol-induced birth defects. As expected, the vehicle-alcohol group had more fetuses with birth defects than the other groups. The aspirin-control and vehicle-control groups were similar, indicating that aspirin, itself, was not teratogenic. Of major importance, however, was the significant decrease in birth defects in the aspirin-alcohol group. Thus, our hypothesis that pretreatment with a PG inhibitor would reduce alcohol-induced birth defects was supported.[11]

Our hypothesis also predicted that aspirin treatment following alcohol administration should be without any protective effect. PGs would already have been released in response to maternal alcohol administration.

In this study,[9] a similar methodology was followed to that described above except that aspirin or vehicle injections followed alcohol incubation by one hour instead of preceding it. The same drug doses and routes of administration were employed. The

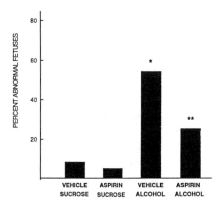

FIGURE 2. Effect of aspirin pretreatment on alcohol-induced fetal malformations. Mean percent abnormal fetuses as a function of alcohol and aspirin treatment (N = 8-11 litters/group). *Significantly differs from sucrose-treated groups ($p < 0.05$). **Significantly differs from vehicle-alcohol group ($p < 0.05$).

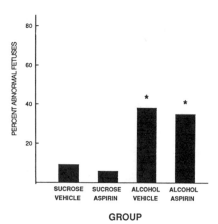

FIGURE 3. Effect of aspirin postalcohol treatment on fetal malformations. Mean percent abnormal fetuses as a function of alcohol and aspirin treatment (N = 11-16 litters/group). *Significantly differs from sucrose-treated groups ($p < 0.05$).

data are shown in FIGURE 3. It can be seen that although the frequency of birth defects was higher in the two alcohol-treated groups than the control groups, the percent of abnormal fetuses in the alcohol-aspirin group was not different from the alcohol-vehicle group. These data taken together with those from the previous study imply that PG inhibitors are only effective in reducing the teratogenic actions of alcohol if given *prior* to alcohol administration.

As mentioned in the beginning of this paper, aspirin is a prostaglandin synthesis inhibitor. It works by inhibiting the enzyme cyclooxygenase.[13] If inhibition of PG synthesis is, in fact, an important event in the protective effect of aspirin, then another cyclooxygenase inhibitor like indomethacin should also antagonize alcohol-induced birth defects.[14]

Briefly, various doses of indomethacin were injected s.c. on day 10 of gestation in C57BL/6J mice prior to administration of 5.8 g/kg alcohol by gavage. Aspirin was included in this experiment as a positive control. As can be seen in FIGURE 4, indomethacin protected in a dose-related manner against alcohol-induced birth defects, but only the highest dose was statistically different from the vehicle-alcohol group. As we had shown previously,[11] aspirin significantly reduced alcohol-induced birth

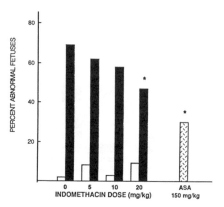

FIGURE 4. Effect of indomethacin on alcohol-induced fetal malformations. □ Sucrose; ■ alcohol. Mean percent abnormal fetuses as a function of alcohol treatment and indomethacin dose (N = 6-12 litters/group). Aspirin-treated alcohol group was included as a positive control. *Significantly differs from vehicle-alcohol group ($p < 0.05$).

defects even more than did the highest dose of indomethacin. We interpreted these data to indicate that cyclooxygenase inhibitors that cross the placenta easily are more likely to protect against alcohol-induced birth defects than those that do not.[15]

It will be noted that in all of the studies described above, the dose of aspirin employed was 150 mg/kg. We recently completed a study evaluating the effects of several doses of aspirin on alcohol teratogenesis. Our results indicate that aspirin dose-dependently reduced alcohol-induced birth defects. That is, while a dose of 18.75 mg/kg was not effective, 37.5 mg/kg was marginally effective, and doses of 75, 150, and 300 mg/kg were equally effective in reducing alcohol-induced birth defects (unpublished data). Interestingly, we were not able to completely "block" alcohol-induced birth defects even when the dose was doubled to 300 mg/kg. It is unlikely that higher doses can be used effectively without introducing some teratogenic potential of their own. Although these results strongly suggest aspirin is reducing PG levels elevated by alcohol, without direct measurement of PG levels in the mother and/or embryo, this hypothesis can never be directly proved.

Most recently, our laboratory has been working on developing a method to reliably measure prostaglandins in these critical tissues. Studies are in progress to measure not only PGE and PGF, but the vasoactive prostaglandins, thromboxane and prostacyclin, as well. It is likely that alterations in prostaglandins that regulate placental blood flow may play an important role in the etiology of alcohol-induced birth defects.

We do not mean to imply that PGs mediate all of the adverse effects of alcohol on fetal growth and development. It may be that only some of the teratogenic actions of alcohol are mediated via the PG system.[16] Even if our PG hypothesis turns out to be too simplistic or ultimately is rejected, our data clearly show that PG inhibitors reduce alcohol-induced birth defects in C57BL/6J mice. While this does not appear to be true for CD-1 mice,[17] this does not weaken the significance of our findings. The data with C57BL/6J mice are some of the first to demonstrate a reduction in alcohol-induced birth defects and, as such, may reveal potential mechanisms for the teratogenic actions of alcohol.

REFERENCES

1. RANDALL, C. L. & W. J. TAYLOR. 1979. Prenatal ethanol exposure in mice: Teratogenic effects. Teratology **19:** 305-311.
2. SULIK, K. K., M. C. JOHNSTON & M. A. WEBB. 1981. Fetal Alcohol Syndrome: Embryogenesis in a mouse model. Science **214:** 936-938.
3. GEORGE, F. R. & A. C. COLLINS. 1979. Prostaglandin synthetase inhibitors antagonize the depressant effects of ethanol. Pharmacol. Biochem. Behav. **10:** 865-869.
4. SEGARNICK, D. J., D. M. CORDASCO & J. ROTROSEN. 1982. Biochemical and behavioral interactions between prostaglandin E₁ and alcohol. *In* Clinical Uses of Essential Fatty Acids. pp. 175-189. Eden Press. Buffalo, NY.
5. GEORGE, F. R., S. J. JACKSON & A. C. COLLINS. 1981. Prostaglandin synthetase inhibitors antagonize hypothermia induced by sedative hypnotics. Psychopharmacology **74:** 241-244.
6. RITZ, M. C., F. R. GEORGE & A. C. COLLINS. 1981. Indomethacin antagonizes ethanol-induced but not pentobarbital-induced behavioral activation. Subst. Alcohol Actions Misuse **2:** 289-299.
7. GEORGE, F. R., G. I. ELMER & A. C. COLLINS. 1982. Indomethacin significantly reduces mortality due to acute ethanol overexposure. Subs. Alcohol Actions Misuse **3:** 267-274.
8. GEORGE, F. R. & A. C. COLLINS. 1985. Ethanol's behavioral effects may be partly due to increases in brain prostaglandin production. Alcohol. Clin. Exp. Res. **9:** 143-146.

9. RANDALL, C. L., R. F. ANTON & H. C. BECKER. 1987. Alcohol, pregnancy, and prostaglandins. Alcohol. Clin. Exp. Res. **11:** 32-36.
10. PERSAUD, T. V. N. 1978. Prostaglandins and organogenesis. *In* Advances in Prostaglandin
   and Thromboxane Research. Vol. 4 139-156. Raven Press. New York, NY.
11. RANDALL, C. L. & R. F. ANTON. 1984. Aspirin reduces alcohol-induced prenatal mortality
   and malformations in mice. Alcohol. Clin. Exp. Res. **8:** 513-515.
12. WEBSTER, W. S., D. A. WALSH, S. E. MCEWEN & A. H. LIPSON. 1983. Some teratogenic
   properties of ethanol and acetaldehyde in C57BL/6J mice: Implications for the study
   of the fetal alcohol syndrome. Teratology **27:** 231-243.
13. VANE, J. R. 1978. 1978. Inhibitors of prostaglandin, prostacyclin, and thromboxane synthesis. *In* Prostaglandins and Perinatal Medicine. Advances in Prostaglandin and Thromboxane Research. Vol. 4: 27-44. Raven Press. New York, NY.
14. RANDALL, C. L., R. F. ANTON & H. C. BECKER. 1987. Effect of indomethacin on alcohol-
   induced morphological anomalies in mice. Life Sci. **41:** 361-369.
15. KLEIN, K. L., W. J. SCOTT, K. E. CLARK & J. G. WILSON. 1981. Indomethacin-placental
   transfer, cytotoxicity, and teratology in the rat. Am. J. Obstet. Gynecol. **141**(4): 448-452.
16. RANDALL, C. L., R. F. ANTON, H. C. BECKER & C. K. WILLIAMS. 1987. Brain/body
   weight reduction after acute prenatal alcohol exposure in C57 mice: Effects of aspirin
   pretreatment. Soc. Neurosci. Abstr. **13**(1): 691.
17. GUY, J. F. & M. E. SUCHESTON. 1986. Teratogenic effects on the CD-1 mouse embyro
   exposed to concurrent doses of ethanol and aspirin. Teratology **34:** 249-261.

Clinical Studies of Infants and Children Exposed Prenatally to Heroin

GERALDINE S. WILSON

Department of Pediatrics
Baylor College of Medicine
and
Meyer Center for Developmental Pediatrics
Texas Children's Hospital
Clinical Care Center
6621 Fannin Street
Houston, Texas 77030

For almost a century, the newborn drug withdrawal syndrome has been a predictable consequence of opiate dependency in pregnant women.[1] Over the ensuing years this once life-threatening condition has been well described and effectively treated.[2,3]

In recent years, the increasing popularity of recreational drug use and abuse by all segments of society has led to an interest in possible long-term effects on children exposed prenatally to these drugs. Follow-up studies involving children exposed prenatally to heroin have been particularly difficult to interpret because of the variability inherent in the addicts' life style as well as limitations in study design. Samples have been small and poorly defined, and comparison groups were either absent or failed to match for important life-style characteristics. Data was often based solely on interview, and test batteries did not utilize well-standardized instruments.

Early studies were largely descriptive in nature. In the first such study, half of thirteen children of heroin-addicted mothers who were followed through at least one year of age showed difficulty in regulating their behavior, but were otherwise developmentally normal.[4] A sequel to this preliminary study compared the neurodevelopmental and behavioral function of twenty-two preschool heroin-exposed children with that of controls.[5] Controls were children at environmental risk (*i.e.,* raised by drug-dependent parent but not exposed in utero), children with other nondrug-related perinatal risk factors, and children of similar sociodemographic background without specific risk factors. By parental report heroin-exposed children had more adjustment problems than controls, but they did not differ on objective measures of attention, activity, or other observed behavior. Lower performance on tasks involving perception, organization and short-term memory suggested that heroin-exposed children might be at risk for later school problems.

Olofsson has reported the outcome at one to ten years of 72 children exposed in utero to a variety of drugs (heroin, methadone or tranquillizers).[6] Based on screening tests and interview data, he reported impaired psychomotor development in 21 percent of the sample and behavioral abnormalities (lack of concentration, hyperactivity, aggressiveness and lack of social inhibition) in 50 percent. He linked psychomotor deficits with deprivation.

Several studies reporting disturbed function in children of addicts have failed to separate those exposed to heroin in utero from unexposed children raised by addicted parents. Nichtern surveyed 95 children whose parents were addicted, and found a history of problems with physiologic patterning, behavioral concerns, developmental lags and learning problems.[7] Sowder focused on 34 children three to seven years old raised by addicted parent(s); 44 percent reported that their children were exposed to heroin and/or other drugs gestationally.[8] On the basis of screening tests, 42 percent of the children of addicts and 20 percent of neighborhood controls from drug-free homes were considered at high risk for early school problems and socioemotional development. Of interest is the finding of lower visual motor functioning in children of addicts.[8]

Herjanic et al. conducted a controlled study of 32 children ages six to 17 years raised in the household of their heroin-addicted fathers.[9] By history, they were unexposed to opiates in utero. Forty-four percent were considered slow in mental development on the basis of screening tests and school performance, as compared to ten percent of controls. Reports of behavioral concerns were comparable in the early elementary years, but by age twelve conduct disorders and school behavior problems were much more common in children of addicts.

Each of these studies has contributed to our understanding of the problems to be expected in children of addicted parents, yet none has been comprehensive enough to elucidate the specific factors related to poor outcome. Aylward has reviewed many methodological issues stultifying the study of direct sequelae of drug exposure in children of methadone-maintained mothers.[10] These same issues are magnified in the untreated addict because their contact with investigators during the period of pregnancy is so limited. Moreover, variance is introduced postnatally by a wide spectrum of child care experiences related to the mother's lack of involvement in parenting.

Controlled Longitudinal Study, Infancy to Preschool

Such methodologic issues were considered in designing a comprehensive follow-up study of children exposed to heroin during gestation.[11] Through Houston's city-county hospital, pregnant narcotic-dependent women were offered comprehensive medical care, social services, and referral for drug treatment at their first prenatal contact, which ranged from eight weeks gestation to delivery.

Drug-dependent women were divided into two groups based on their pattern of drug use during pregnancy.[11] The first was comprised of 29 untreated heroin-dependent women; the second consisted of 39 women enrolled in methadone maintenance programs for a period of at least two months during pregnancy. Drug groups did not differ on educational background, age, or obstetrical risk factors. The significantly greater number of white and married women in the methadone-treated group (versus single black untreated women) suggests a possible selection bias in the subgroup of addicts choosing to enter methadone treatment. The rate of prenatal care among methadone-treated women (95%) was significantly greater than that of the untreated (48%). All but three methadone-treated women (93%) used psychoactive drugs, either illicit or prescribed, in addition to methadone, as compared with only fifty-nine percent of untreated addicts.[11] Less frequent contact with untreated women may have affected the reliability of these reports.

In order to control for other risk factors associated with drug use, a drug-free comparison group of 57 women from the same obstetrical service was matched for age, race, socioeconomic level, and marital status. The protocol also matched for the duration of pregnancy at the onset of prenatal care, but too few drug-free women without prenatal care consented to participate. Maternal measures included duration of prenatal care, weight gain during pregnancy, prenatal risk score and a narcotic score derived from the reported use of methadone, heroin, and other psychoactive drugs during each trimester of pregnancy. Urine samples were tested at each prenatal visit for heroin, methadone, diazepam, amphetamines, and barbiturates. Reports of drug screening and methadone dosage were also provided by cooperating methadone maintenance programs.

The longitudinal study included medical and neurodevelopmental assessments of infants and interview of the mother or caretaker for social and behavioral information at six weeks and at three month intervals during the first year, at eighteen months, at two years, and annually thereafter. A research team composed of a developmental pediatrician, nurse, and social worker coordinated all aspects of medical care and provided social services.

Infancy

As reported in previous studies, drug-exposed infants were significantly smaller at birth and had a higher incidence of intrauterine growth regardation than infants born to drug-free controls.[12] However, a multifactorial analysis adjusting for infant sex, race, prenatal care, maternal weight gain, prenatal risk score, maternal education, and smoking eliminated the differences related to drug use.[13]

While the incidence of severe neonatal abstinence syndrome was comparable for both drug groups (69% in infants of untreated women, 87% in those of methadone-treated), the methadone-exposed infants required a longer course of pharmacologic treatment. Following hospital discharge, signs of continuing physiologic disruption (excessive crying, feeding difficulties, and sleep disturbances) were reported more frequently in infants of untreated mothers, but the difference was statistically not significant. Transient hypertonia, significantly increased in infants of untreated mothers in comparison with methadone-treated and drug-free groups, subsided by six to nine months.[11]

Static neurologic deficits identified in four infants during the first year included hypotonic cerebral palsy in a drug-free control. The other impaired children were born to untreated heroin-dependent women who had no prenatal care. One child had spastic diplegia, one had spastic quadriparesis in association with hydrocephalus, optic atrophy, and global delay, and the third was hypotonic, mildly retarded, and had features consistent with fetal alcohol syndrome.

Parenting and Home Environment

Untreated heroin-dependent women were more likely to relinquish the role of parent than were methadone-treated mothers.[14] By their first birthday 48 percent of infants of untreated women were living with substitute parents, and by the preschool years only two children (9%) remained with their biologic mother. In contrast, almost half of the methadone-treated women continued to care for their preschool children. Characteristics of the child's primary caretaker and of his home environment were evaluated when subjects were three years of age by structured interview and use of the HOME instrument.[15] The three groups did not differ on educational or occupational classification of the head of the household, on HOME scores, or on a measure of family stability reflecting factors such as regularity of income and involvement in illegal activities.

Compliance

Ninety-four percent of subjects remained in the study through the first year, and 73 percent through three years. Heroin-exposed children had a remarkably high follow-up rate, with 97 percent compliance at one year, 93 percent at the two year visit, and 87 percent evaluated at three years or older. Subjects lost to study prior to the three year visit did not differ from those remaining on the following measures: socioeconomic status, race, sex, gestational age, birth measurements, severity of newborn withdrawal symptoms, neurologic status, or developmental performance at age nine months.

Cognitive Performance

During the first two years of life, cognitive function was measured by the Bayley Scales of Infant Development.[16] The McCarthy Scales of Children's Abilities, which includes a general cognitive index (GCI) and five additional scales, was administered at ages three, four, and five years.[17] Sequential mean values for cognitive performance are shown in TABLE 1. Values reported exclude scores for a heroin-exposed child who was institutionalized in infancy because of profound retardation and quadriparesis secondary to hydrocephaly and for those children whose tests could not be scored because of inadequate cooperation. McCarthy evaluations were not obtained for all subjects at three years of age because of a lapse in funding; thus the McCarthy scores reflect testing done at ages ranging from three to five years.

With the exception of lower performance by the heroin-exposed group at 18 months (see TABLE 1), there were no significant differences in cognitive function between drug-exposed and drug-free children. The pattern of gradual decline over time is consistent with the performance of a disadvantaged population.[18,19]

The comparability of group means, however, obscures atypical patterns of development within the drug-exposed population. Particularly among the heroin-exposed children, developmental performance fluctuated widely over time; uneven performance was found most often in children living in unstable or disadvantaged homes. This variance and lack of predictability suggests that cross-sectional studies of this population may be of limited value, since environmental changes appear to influence cognitive function dramatically.

Case Reports

TR was hypertonic but showed average developmental function at age nine months (Bayley MDI 86), when brought for evaluation by her mother. Her retarded performance at 18 months (MDI < 50) was felt in part to reflect the absence of nurturing and stimulation in the group foster home where she had lived since one year. Following adoption, developmental quotients rose to borderline at two and three years, and by age five she was again performing in the low average range (McCarthy GCI 86).

JV was raised primarily by drug-dependent natural parents. His mother was an intelligent but highly emotional woman whose life was in constant turmoil. JV had intermittent exposure to a preschool program during extended stays with his grandmother, but no consistent enrichment until kindergarten entry. At nine and eighteen months JV appeared to have good potential (MDI 93 and 98 respectively), but tested in the retarded range (MDI 62) at age two. His GCI was 80 at three years, but fell to 60 by four years, with deficits on quantitative and verbal scales. Toward completion of the first grade, full scale IQ as measured by the WISC-R was 94, well within the average range.

TABLE 1. Sequential Measures of Cognitive Performance (Mean ± SD)

Developmental Performance	Untreated Heroin-Exposed	Methadone-Exposed	Drug-free Controls
Bayley MDI			
9 months	100.6 ± 17.8 (n = 27)	98.4 ± 13.9 (n = 33)	105.5 ± 15.6 (n = 54)
18 months	86.5 ± 10.7[a] (n = 27)	92.0 ± 14.5 (n = 29)	97.4 ± 14.4 (n = 42)
24 months	84.4 ± 16.4 (n = 27)	88.8 ± 15.5 (n = 32)	90.2 ± 14.6 (n = 48)
McCarthy GCI			
3 to 5 years	85.3 ± 15.7 (n = 25)	90.4 ± 13.0 (n = 26)	89.4 ± 10.8 (n = 41)

[a] Heroin/control, $p < 0.01$.

Lifschitz analyzed the relationship of intellectual function to maternal drug use, perinatal factors, and environmental factors in the 92 subjects who completed the McCarthy at three to five years.[20] Multivariate analysis failed to demonstrate a relationship between the GCI and maternal narcotic score, birth size, or the severity of neonatal abstinence. Predictive factors included the obstetric prenatal risk score, amount of prenatal care, and quality of the home environment.

Despite comparable group means on the McCarthy GCI and on each of the five McCarthy scales, retardation was most common in heroin-exposed children.[21] Five heroin-exposed children and one control performed in the mildly retarded range, with GCI scores ranging from 56 to 68. In addition, the institutionalized heroin-exposed child was profoundly retarded. These figures are not statistically significant. While the small sample may obscure statistical significance, a 24 percent rate of mental retardation is certainly clinically important.

Preschool Behavior

Behavioral measures included parental interviews and ratings of behavior during psychometric and neurologic assessment with a modification of the Behavioral Record of the Bayley Scales.[16] Behavioral patterns observed during preschool evaluation did not differentiate between drug-exposed children and the comparison group. Attention and activity level were rated independently by a psychologist and pediatrician unaware of the child's background. Disturbances in attention and activity level were considered clinically significant in six controls, six methadone subjects, and in two heroin-exposed children. The mean values on a 5-point rating of activity-attention did not differ significantly between groups. However, regression analysis indicated that the only independent variable related significantly to the activity-attention rating was the maternal narcotic score (coefficient = 0.073, SD = 0.036, p <0.05).

Preschool Neurologic Function

The only subject with persistent signs of static encephalopathy on the preschool evaluation was the heroin-exposed child with congenital hydrocephalus and profound retardation. Sporadic neurologic abnormalities included strabismus in one methadone-exposed child and tremors with dysmetria in three heroin-exposed, one methadone-exposed and two drug-free children. Articulation disorders were found in 15 percent of heroin-exposed and methadone-exposed children, and in five percent of drug-free controls. From 30 to 40 percent of subjects in each of the three groups demonstrated motor incoordination, as shown by immature motor patterns, weakness in gross or fine motor performance or weak visual-motor skills. Multiple logistic regression found a significant association between motor incoordination and the severity of newborn withdrawal. Calculation of an odds ratio indicated that after adjustment for possible confounding variables, the likelihood for motor incoordination was 2.9 times greater in children who were treated for newborn narcotic withdrawal than in those who were either asymptomatic or had mild withdrawal symptoms and required no medication.

Heroin-Exposed Children in School

Grant support permitted follow-up of the study population only through the preschool years. However, reports of school performance were obtained for subjects who responded to contact by mail or telephone. Sixty-eight percent of the original heroin-exposed subjects responded but only 30 percent of the methadone-exposed and 36 percent of the drug-free controls. The low rate of response among the methadone and drug-free groups raises concern about bias, so data are interpreted with caution. For this reason the ensuing description is limited to the school performance of heroin-exposed children, and data from the longitudinal cohort is provided in TABLE 2 for comparative purposes only.

Descriptive Study, School Performance of Heroin-Exposed Subjects

Reports of school performance have been obtained for 40 children whose mothers were heroin-dependent during the pregnancy; methadone-exposed subjects are not included. Twenty of the school-aged children participated in our longitudinal study, and 20 had been assessed by the investigator during infancy and at least once in the preschool years as participants in earlier studies.[4,5]

Subjects ranged in age from six to eleven years at the time of survey. Nineteen (48%) were male. Eighteen subjects (45%) were black, nine (23%) were Hispanic

TABLE 2. The Incidence of School-Related Problems in Children of Addicts and Longitudinal Study Subjects

	Combined Heroin-Exposed Subjects (n = 40)	Longitudinal Study Subjects		
		Heroin-Exposed (n = 20)	Methadone-Exposed (n = 12)	Drug-Free Controls (n = 12)
		n (%)		
IQ 1-2 SD below norm	11 (27)	4 (20)	1 (8)	1 (5)
IQ >2 SD below norm	5 (13)	4 (20)	—	—
LLD[a]	5 (13)	2 (10)	1 (8)	1 (5)
Repeated 1 or more grades	12 (30)	5 (25)	3 (25)	6 (29)
Special education	20 (50)	8 (40)	2 (16)	4 (19)
Mental retardation	2	1	—	—
LLD class	4	2	—	—
Emotionally disturbed	1	1	—	—
Other	14	4	2	4
Expulsion	2 (5)	—	—	—
Behavioral problems	26 (65)	15 (75)	9 (75)	10 (48)
Psychiatric referral	7 (17)	5 (25)	2 (16)	1 (5)

[a] Language learning disabled.

and 13 (32%) were white. Five of the children (12%) lived with their biologic mother. Twenty-four subjects lived with extended family or friends, ten had been legally adopted, and a profoundly retarded child was institutionalized.

Families provided written consent for release of reports from the child's school. School reported the child's present grade level, record of past or present grade repetition or special educational services, and results of intelligence or achievement tests done by the school. The teacher was asked to rate the child's competence in Reading, Spelling and Math, and report rate of absences. They also rated behavioral/interpersonal characteristics.

Ideally, psychometric and academic testing should be done after the first grade to identify children with language learning disabilities. Since financial constraints prohibited such evaluation, test measures reflect each subject's most recent formal assessment. Twenty-nine children who were six years old or older when tested completed the WISC-R, a standardized test of intellectual potential. Ten children, ages three to six years at their last evaluation, completed the McCarthy Scales of Children's Abilities. The institutionalized child was not tested. The Wide Range Achievement Test (WRAT), a measure of academic ability, was completed by 19 of the subjects seen at age six or older. The Bender Gestalt Test of visual-motor performance had been completed by 27 children aged six or above.

Grade Placement

At the time school reports were obtained, 70 percent of these heroin-exposed subjects were in the first or second grade, and 30 percent in grades three through five. School reports identified no academic problems or need for special educational services in 14 subjects (35%). The remainder of the population repeated one or more grades and/or required special educational services, as outlined in TABLE 2.

Learning Profile

The mean intellectual quotient (IQ) for the 40 subjects was 87.5 ± 16.8 with IQ ranging from below 50 to 124. Sixteen subjects (40%) scored greater than one standard deviation below the norm, with three of the 16 in the mentally retarded range (below 2 SD). A significant discrepancy between Verbal and Performance scales was recorded in almost one-third of the 29 subjects who completed the WISC. The Verbal IQ was lower in two subjects, while low Performance IQ indicated relative deficits in visual-perceptual-motor function in seven.

Five children met the criteria for a specific language-learning disability (LLD). Two boys from disadvantaged homes did not receive remediation for LLD, and both were ultimately expelled from elementary school for disciplinary reasons. Seven children (26% of the 27 tested) had standard scores greater than 2 SD below the mean on the Bender Gestalt test of visual-motor performance.

Behavior

Behavioral reports were taken from the most current information on each child; school and parental reports were supplemented by the psychologist and pediatrician's observations for those children tested at six or older. Twenty-six children, two-thirds of the sample, were felt to have problematic behavior by the family, school and/or the evaluation team. Seven children were referred for psychiatric evaluation and treatment because of overtly deviant behavior and/or significant concerns based on responses to projective testing.

The school completed forms rating work habits and factors affecting classroom performance for 31 children. As shown in TABLE 3 lack of self-discipline and inattention were reported for half, while low self-confidence and peer relations were also common. Characterization of behavior by the school report and observations of the research team defined two separate patterns of inattention. Half of the inattentive children were described as fidgety, impulsive, and disruptive in class, while the other half were rated as passive, withdrawn, nervous daydreamers. Two subjects, boys aged six to seven years at time of observation, were diagnosed as Attention Deficit Disorder. From school reports we suspect that several additional children might have met diagnostic criteria had they been tested at school age.

Within this school-aged sample, relationships between demographic and environmental variables, measures of maternal drug use, severity of newborn withdrawal syndrome, IQ score, Bender visual-motor score, behavioral problems and school performance were studied by correlational analyses. The intellectual quotient was most strongly associated with the quality of the home environment ($r = 0.4$, $p < 0.05$), and did not relate to prenatal or perinatal variables. The IQ also related to special educational placement ($r = 0.36$, $p < 0.05$), but not to grade repetition. The Bender score was negatively related to the severity of maternal drug abuse ($r = 0.37$) and to the quality of the home ($r = 0.40$), but neither correlation was significant. No direct relationship was seen between behavior and perinatal variables or school performance, and behavioral problems were only weakly associated with environmental variables.

TABLE 3. Behavioral Attributes of 31 Heroin-Exposed Elementary School Children

	n (%)
Inattention	15 (48)
Poor self-discipline	16 (52)
Low self-confidence	12 (39)
Poor peer relations	10 (32)
Fails to participate	10 (32)
Excessive absence	3 (10)

COMMENTS

While the statistical strength of this study is impaired by the fact that it encompasses more variables and outcome measures than subjects, nevertheless patterns of clinical import emerge from the data.

Early separation from their biologic mothers is perhaps the most obvious factor distinguishing children of untreated heroin addicts from those of methadone-treated women and drug-free control mothers. Conventional wisdom is divided between the extremes of advantage and disadvantage of this to the separated child. Neither seems relevant to this population, since the spectrum of determinant factors influencing child behavior and development expands exponentially beyond the simple "with or without mother" condition. Important factors such as the child's age and developmental stage at the time of separation, the number of times the primary caretaker has changed, and the quality of life afforded by the substitute parent(s) have been difficult to assess. The comparable ratings of parental and environmental factors in our untreated and comparison groups obscure very broad ranges of socioeconomic condition and parenting practice among the substitute homes.

Contrary to our expectations, we found the similarities between children of untreated addicts and those of the controls more impressive than their differences. Behaviorally, addicts' children were not unique following completion of subacute withdrawal, a period during which physiologic patterns were disrupted. Although the extent of maternal narcotic use was shown to relate directly to measures of activity and inattention in the preschool child, the absence of clinically significant attentional deficit disorder was reassuring. Preliminary reports of high activity level, impulsivity, and inattention in toddlers gave rise to our concerns that attentional deficits might persist.[4] This survey of school-aged children of addicts indicates that, while poor attention is a common concern of teachers, inattention was as frequently associated with passivity, nervousness, and preoccupation as it was with the impulsive and disruptive profile common to children with an organic attentional deficit.

Our longitudinal study suggests also that heroin-exposed children do not differ from controls in the area of school performance. However, the possibility that bias may have been introduced by the selective responses of both methadone-maintained and drug-free control groups cannot be ignored, and conclusions concerning incidence of school problems cannot be drawn from this limited sample.

In the larger combined sample of school-aged heroin-exposed children, the incidence of grade repetition was 30 percent, and an additional 35 percent received special educational services. No single factor appeared to be responsible for this high incidence of school problems. The combination of limited cognitive potential, weak visual-motor-perceptual skills, disadvantaged environment, and lack of preschool enrichment is compounded by behavioral attributes of the children. As a group they have poor work habits and little self-confidence. The 13 percent incidence of language learning disabilities identified may be an underestimate, since LLD cannot be excluded in children not fully tested (IQ and academic achievement) at school age.

While it has been pointed out that heroin-exposed children do not have distinctive neurologic findings, we find a continuing thread of weakness in the area of motor coordination and visual-motor-perceptual function. This is particularly intriguing because of the apparent relationship to the extent of maternal drug use and severity of newborn withdrawal symptoms.

A concern raised by this study is that of impaired cognitive potential in children of heroin-addicted mothers. While most prior controlled studies have looked at sequelae of maternal methadone use, the general concensus has been that cognitive function of drug-exposed children, while lower than the norm, is comparable to that of socioeconomic controls.[22] In our study, the rate of mental handicap in the heroin-exposed group was alarmingly high—six of 25 children evaluated in the preschool years functioned within the retarded range. This 24 percent rate is eight times greater than the expected incidence and suggests the need for incidence studies in a much larger sample.

The retarded subjects in this study were all born to untreated addicts who had limited prenatal care and limited involvement in infant care after delivery. In two infants retardation was associated with malformations (hydrocephalus and fetal alcohol syndrome), but no etiology could be identified in the other three babies. We speculate that episodes of maternal drug withdrawal or overdose and the unreported abuse of a variety of noxious substances may combine with maternal malnutrition, infection and untreated obstetrical complications to compromise the developing fetus, and that a poor environment during childhood may further compound prenatal influences. Methadone-treated women, while reporting more extensive polydrug use than the untreated addicts, did not produce mentally retarded infants.[11]

In conclusion, the overwhelming number of confounding prenatal and environmental influences and the small number of drug-exposed subjects who have been carefully evaluated in a prospective fashion preclude the statistically meaningful analysis of long-term effects of intrauterine narcotic exposure. Investigators concur that children of addicts have a high incidence of behavioral and school-related problems, whether they were exposed to drugs prenatally or merely raised within a drug milieu.[7-9]

IMPLICATIONS

It is unlikely that more definitive studies of long-term effects of intrauterine heroin exposure will be forthcoming. Thus we must glean what we can from available data in an effort to improve the outlook for addicted women and their children. Improved utilization of prenatal care and drug treatment programs by addicted women during pregnancy must be a primary goal, since lack of prenatal care appears to be a common factor to all severely impaired children. This may entail modification of both obstetric and drug programs to accommodate the special needs of the pregnant addict.

Of perhaps greater importance will be efforts directed toward improving the child's postnatal environment. This might be accomplished by improving the resources and parenting skills of drug dependent women, and by facilitating adoptive placement when their children are unwanted. A nurturing environment might be expected to prevent some of the behavioral and school problems observed in our study population. However, adoptive parents should be made aware of the possible increased risk of intellectual impairment and visual motor problems in the offspring of addicts.

Although the studies reviewed do not address the issue of drug abuse in the children of drug abusers, children who show evidence of poor adjustment and failure in the elementary school may be at risk for later behavioral deviance. Thus comprehensive programs for drug dependent women and their children may prove vital weapons in our war to prevent drug abuse.

REFERENCES

1. HAPPEL, T. J. 1900. Morphinism from the standpoint of the general practitioner. J. Am. Med. Assoc. **35:** 407-409.
2. HILL, R. M. & M. M. DESMOND. 1963. Management of the narcotic withdrawal syndrome in the neonate. Pediatr. Clin. of North Am. **10:** 67-85.
3. VOLPE, J. J. 1987. Teratogenic effects of drugs and passive addiction. *In* Neurology of the Newborn. J. J. Volpe, Ed. W. B. Saunders. Philadelphia, PA.
4. WILSON, G. S., M. M. DESMOND & W. W. VERNIAUD. 1973. Early development of infants of heroin-addicted mothers. Am. J. Dis. Child. **126:** 457-462.
5. WILSON, G. S., R. MCCREARY, J. KEAN & J. C. BAXTER. 1979. The development of preschool children of heroin-addicted mothers: A controlled study. Pediatrics **63:** 135-141.
6. OLOFSSON, M., W. BUCKLEY, G. E. ANDERSEN & B. FRIIS-HANSEN. 1983. Investigation of 89 children born by drug-dependent mothers. Acta Paediatr. Scand. **72:** 407-410.
7. NICHTERN, S. 1973. The children of drug users. J. Am. Acad. Child Psychiatry. **12**(1): 24-31.

8. SOWDER, B. J. & M. R. BURT. 1980. Children of Heroin Addicts. J. A. Inciardi, Ed. Praeger. New York, NY.
9. HERJANIC, B. M., V. H. BARREDO, M. HERJANIC & C. J. TOMELLERI. 1979. Children of heroin addicts. Int. J. Addictions 14(7): 919-931.
10. AYLWARD, G. P. 1982. Methadone outcome studies: Is it more than the methadone? J. Pediatr. 101(2): 214-215.
11. WILSON, G. S., M. M. DESMOND & R. B. WAIT. 1981. Followup of methadone-treated and untreated narcotic-dependent women and their infants: Health, developmental and social implications. J. Pediatr. 98: 716-722.
12. ZELSON, C., E. RUBIO & E. WASSERMAN. 1971. Neonatal narcotic addiction: Ten-year observation. Pediatr. 48: 178-189.
13. LIFSCHITZ, M. H., G. W. WILSON, E. O. SMITH & M. M. DESMOND. 1983. Fetal and postnatal growth of children born to narcotic-dependent women. J. Pediatr. 102: 686-691.
14. LAWSON, M. S. & G. S. WILSON. 1980. Parenting among women addicted to narcotics. Child Welfare 59: 67-79.
15. CALDWELL, B. M. 1978. Manual for the Home Observation for Measurement of the Environment. University of Arkansas. Little Rock, AR.
16. Bayley Scales of Infant Development. 1972. The Psychological Corp. New York, NY.
17. McCarthy Scales of Children's Abilities. 1972. The Psychological Corp. New York, NY.
18. McCALL, R. B. 1979. The development of intellectual functioning in infancy and the prediction of later IQ. In Handbook of Infant Development. J. D. Osofsky, Ed. Wiley. New York, NY.
19. EGBUONO, L. & B. STARFIELD. 1982. Child health and social status. J. Pediatr. 69: 350-357.
20. LIFSCHITZ, M. H., G. S. WILSON, E. O. SMITH & M. M. DESMOND. 1985. Factors affecting head growth and intellectual function in children of drug addicts. Pediatrics 75: 269-274.
21. SONDEREGGER, T., A. ZIMMERMAN & G. WILSON. Heroin/morphine in perinatal substance abuse: Research findings and clinical implications. In Perinatal Substance Abuse: Research Findings and Clinical Implications. T. Sonderegger, Ed. John Hopkins Univ. Press. Baltimore, MD. In Press.
22. KALTENBACH, K. & L. FINNEGAN. 1984. Developmental outcome of children born to methadone maintained women: A Review of longitudinal studies. Neurobehav. Toxicol. Teratol. 6: 271-275.

Developmental Consequences of Prenatal Exposure to Methadone[a]

SYDNEY L. HANS

Department of Psychiatry, Box 411
The University of Chicago
5841 South Maryland Avenue
Chicago, Illinois 60637

Use of opioid drugs is a major and long-standing social problem in the United States[1] and one that has endured throughout changing fashions in drug use, including the current popularity of cocaine. Illicit heroin is currently the most widely used opioid. For over twenty years, the treatment of choice in the United States for heroin abuse has been methadone maintenance—administration of daily, medically-supervised doses of methadone, a synthetic opioid drug, as a substitute for heroin.[2]

The opioid-drug-using population includes an increasing proportion of women. In the early 1980s, the proportion of women admitted to drug treatment programs funded by the National Institute on Drug Abuse had reached a record level of thirty percent.[3] The vast majority of women entering drug treatment programs are of childbearing age. While there are few statistics available on the numbers of children born in the United States to women using opioid drugs—primarily heroin and methadone, the numbers may be as high as 10,000 per year.

Opioid drugs cross the placental barrier,[5] and their effects on the health of the pregnant woman and developing fetus are great. Pregnancies of opioid-dependent women are often complicated by problems such as toxemia, maternal syphilis and hepatitis, placental problems, and abnormal presentation;[6-8] opioid-exposed infants are especially likely to show signs of fetal distress and to be born at low birthweight even when receiving adequate prenatal care.[9-13] The effects of prenatal opioid exposure on the behavior of newborn infants are also dramatic. During the first week after birth, most opioid-exposed infants show a well-documented neonatal abstinence syndrome that includes a variety of behaviors associated with central and automatic nervous system hyperarousal such as tremors, hypertonus, hyperactive reflexes, high-pitched crying, poor sleeping and feeding, fever, and rapid respiration.[14-19] These signs attenuate dramatically during the first month of life, and by one month of age only subtle differences can be observed between exposed and unexposed infants.[18-19]

Because opioid-drug-using women are a difficult population to involve and maintain in longitudinal research, there are relatively few data about the development of their infants after the neonatal period. However, these few longitudinal studies of opioid-exposed infants present a rather consistent pattern of results across samples. As a group, opioid-exposed infants show normal motor and cognitive development during the first two years of life,[18,20,21-23] but they generally lag slightly behind unexposed infants of the same race and socioeconomic background. Yet despite the consistency

[a] Supported by National Institute on Drug Abuse Grant PHS 5 R18 DA-01884.

195

of these findings, there remain questions about whether long-term differences between opioid-exposed and unexposed infants are due to the toxic effects of the drugs.

Human teratology research employs quasi-experimental designs with nonrandom assignment of individuals to groups, and there are many factors that distinguish opioid-exposed infants from other infants besides their opioid exposure. Several of these could plausibly cause or accentuate differences between opioid-exposed and comparison infants.[1,24–27]

> 1. *Exposure to other teratogens.* Women who use opioid drugs, including those in methadone maintenance, generally continue to use and abuse other licit and illicit drugs, some of which have been shown to have teratogenic effects.
> 2. *Pregnancy and birth complications.* Opioid-drug use during pregnancy is associated with various perinatal complications some of which have directly damaging effects to the fetus outside of any toxic effect of the opioid drug.
> 3. *Impoverished social environment.* Opioid-drug-using women may provide their infants with a less optimal rearing environment than women not using drugs.
> 4. *Genetic factors.* Drug-using women (and their spouses) may have genetically determined neurobehavioral impairment that may have predisposed them to drug abuse and that could be passed on to their offspring.

This paper will present data on the neurobehavioral development of a cohort of two-year-old children who were exposed prenatally to methadone and who have been followed since before birth. These data will be analyzed to look at the behavior of methadone-exposed toddlers and a comparison group, but also to examine how other nonteratogenic risk factors may be related to the behavior of drug-exposed children.

METHODS

Sample

Between the years of 1978 and 1982, 36 women who used opioid drugs throughout pregnancy were recruited during pregnancy at the prenatal clinics of Chicago Lying-In Hospital. During the four-year recruitment period, these women delivered 42 infants, including one pair of twins. These opioid-using women were all involved in low-dose methadone-maintenance programs for the treatment of chronic heroin addiction; their dosages during pregnancy ranged from 3 to 40 mg per 24-hour period with a mean of less than 20 mg. Most had been involved in methadone-maintenance throughout pregnancy, some had sought treatment during pregnancy. Most of the women occasionally used other drugs in addition to methadone, most commonly alcohol, marijuana, heroin, cocaine, Valium, or Talwin. Drug-using mothers were excluded from the sample who had chronic medical problems such as diabetes, obvious mental illness, or who were not between the ages of 18 and 35.

A comparison group of 43 pregnant women who used no opioid drugs was recruited from the same prenatal clinics. The comparison-group mothers delivered 47 infants during the duration of the recruitment, including one pair of twins. In addition to the age and illness exclusion criteria used for the methadone group, women were excluded from the comparison group who had any reported history of opioid use or abuse or who consumed more than one drink a day of alcohol.

All women from methadone and comparison groups were black and from low-income inner-city neighborhoods. All women received good quality prenatal care. All infants remained with their mothers' or fathers' families after birth.

Mothers' drug use status was determined both through their self report on the University of Washington Pregnancy and Health Questionnaire[28] and by repeated urine toxicology screening during pregnancy. During pregnancy, mothers were assessed through a lengthy battery of interviews and tests that have been described elsewhere.[29] Among these assessments were the Wechsler Adult Intelligence Scale[30] and the Schedule for Affective Disorders and Schizophrenia-Life Version (SADS-L.[31] Socioeconomic status was scored using the Hollingshead three-factor Index of Social Position.[32] DSM-III[33] Axis I through V diagnoses were made for each mother.

The behavior of the infants was assessed using the Neonatal Behavioral Assessment Scale with Kansas supplements[34,35] twice during the neonatal period, at one day and at four weeks of age. The pattern of behavior observed in this sample was typical of other reports of narcotics abstinence syndrome. Children were hypertonic, jerky, tremulous, hyperactive, and generally irritable. These signs attenuated considerably between the one-day and one-month period, although the children remained somewhat hypertonic.[19]

TABLE 1. Sources of Attrition between Birth and Two-Year Assessment

	Methadone	Comparison
Birth sample	42	47
Neonatal death	2	0
Postneonatal death	2	0
Stroke	1	0
Cerebral palsy	0	1
Unavailable at 2-year assessment	2	0
Withdrawal from study	5	2
Failure to locate	0	0
Two-year sample	30	44

The behavior of the infants was followed longitudinally to the age of two years. At that time, the sample included 74 toddlers each within two weeks of their second birthday. Several of the methadone-group toddlers who were born at less than 37 weeks gestational age were assessed two years after their estimated 40-week gestational date. TABLE 1 indicates the sources of attrition between birth and twenty-four months of age. Attrition was greater for the methadone group (30%) than the comparison group (6%), although almost half of the attrition from the methadone group was due to death or disablement of the infants.

TABLE 2 shows the characteristics of the mothers and infants remaining in the twenty-four-month sample. At the twenty-four-month assessment, as at the time of recruitment, the two groups were well matched on sociodemographic characteristics and maternal intelligence. Mothers in both groups were black, from the lowest socioeconomic levels, had completed an average of eleven years of formal education, and typically were unmarried. Both groups had mean IQ scores of about 90. There were strong differences between the comparison and methadone mothers in psychiatric functioning. On DSM-III ratings of severity of psychosocial stressors (Axis IV) and highest level of adaptive functioning (Axis V), methadone mothers showed much poorer functioning than comparison women. Methadone-using women also experienced more pregnancy and birth complications as assessed by the Rochester Research Obstetrical Scale[36] (with methadone use not tallied as a complication).

Two-Year Assessment Procedures

Two-year-olds and their mothers were transported to a laboratory at the University of Chicago for assessment on the Bayley Scales of Infant Development.[37] Carefully

TABLE 2. Demographic Characteristics of 24-Month Follow-up Sample: Means and Standard Deviations by Drug Group

	Methadone n = 30	Comparison n = 44	X^2	$t(72)$
Maternal Demographic				
Race (black)	100%	100%		
Years education	11.1 (1.5)	11.3 (1.3)		0.35
Hollingshead SES	4.5 (0.7)	4.4 (0.8)		0.66
Parity	3.2 (1.2)	2.9 (1.0)		1.14
Mother's age	27.3 (3.7)	25.4 (4.1)		2.06*
Married	20%	32%	1.26	
Maternal Functioning				
WAIS full-scale IQ	89.1 (9.4)	89.7 (12.0)		0.23
Adaptive functioning	4.8 (0.8)	3.3 (0.8)		8.05***
Stressors	4.7 (0.7)	4.2 (0.4)		3.61**
Birth outcome				
Sex (male)	50%	57%	0.33	
Birthweight	2862 (605)	3236 (395)		3.15**
Apgar 1	8.0 (1.7)	8.4 (1.2)		1.22
Research Obstetric Scale	5.3 (2.9)	3.6 (2.4)		2.81**

    * $p < 0.05$.
   ** $p < 0.01$.
  *** $p < 0.001$.

trained female examiners who were blind to any information about the mothers' drug use or infants' medical history administered the examination.

The Bayley Scales of Infant Development consist of three parts. The Psychomotor Developmental Index (PDI) and the Mental Development Index (MDI) assess acquisition of milestones in motor and mental functioning and are scored on an IQ-type scale. The Infant Behavior Record (IBR) is a series of 9- and 5-point items rating qualitative aspects of the infant's behavior. They are completed by the examiner at the end of the testing session and are based on clinical impressions made throughout the session. Included in the IBR are several items reflecting aspects of neurobehavioral functioning that could plausibly be affected by teratogenic action: attention span, activity level, tension, gross motor coordination, and fine motor coordination.

After administration of the Bayley scales, children's height, weight, and head circumference were measured.

RESULTS

Eleven dependent variables were selected for study representing aspects of physical growth, motor behavior, and mental behavior: height, weight, head circumference; Bayley PDI, IBR activity level, IBR tension, IBR gross motor coordination, IBR fine motor coordination; Bayley MDI, IBR attention span. Analyses of variance were computed on each of these variables using drug exposure and child's sex as independent variables. There were no significant drug by sex interactions. Compared to female infants, male infants were taller ($F(1,70) = 3.89$) and had larger head circumferences ($F(1,70) = 19.12$). Compared to unexposed infants, drug-exposed infants were shorter ($F(1,70) = 4.54$), had smaller head circumferences ($F(1,70) = 6.97$), had poorer Psychomotor Development Indexes ($F(1,70) = 5.19$), were more tense ($F(1,70) = 5.54$), had poorer gross motor coordination ($F(1,70) = 6.08$), and had poorer fine motor coordination ($F(1,70) = 4.29$). Means for both the methadone-exposed and comparison groups were well within the range of normal development for all the outcome variables. TABLE 3 presents group means for methadone and comparison groups and summary statistics by drug and sex.

Three variables selected for further analysis that represent nonteratological aspects of risk: socioeconomic status (Hollingshead), maternal intelligence (WAIS full-scale), and pregnancy and birth complications (Research Obstetrical Scale). Two of these—SES and IQ—were independent of maternal drug use in this sample; ROS scores were greater in the methadone group (TABLE 2). SES and maternal IQ were correlated with each other ($r = 0.31$), but not with ROS. Because preliminary analyses with these risk factors and maternal drug use showed a number of risk factors by drug interaction effects, it was decided to look more closely for drug effects within levels of risk factors. The following analytic model was used. For each of the risk factors, the sample was dichotomized into high and lower risk groups, and drug-use effects were examined within these risk groups using analysis of variance. In all analyses, sex was entered into the model as an independent variable. Results will be reported in terms of *eta* coefficients to allow for direct comparison of effect sizes between analyses based on differing sample sizes.

The sample was first dichotomized according to socioeconomic status: lowest SES families were those at Hollingshead level 5; higher SES families were those at Hollingshead level 4 or 3. Typically, the Level 5 mothers were on Public Aid, lived in public housing or in the worst slums of the city, and perhaps had completed some high school. The best of the Level 4 and 3 mothers had finished high school, had some work skills or lived with men who had some skills, and lived in poor but not the worst neighborhoods of the city. Analyses of variance computed within the higher

TABLE 3. Differences between Methadone-Exposed and Comparison Infants: Group Means, Standard Deviations, and Summary Statistics

	Methadone n = 30	Comparison n = 44	Sex $F(1,70)$	eta	Drug $F(1,70)$	eta
Physical						
Height (cm)	85.1 (4.3)	87.3 (2.9)	3.89*	.24	4.54*	.26
Weight (kg)	12.3 (1.8)	12.7 (1.3)	3.13*	.22	0.45	.08
Head circumference (cm)	48.4 (1.4)	49.5 (1.5)	19.12***	.47	6.97*	.28
Motor						
Psychomotor Development Index	100.8 (12.6)	108.5 (14.6)	0.04	.02	5.19*	.26
IBR activity level	5.8 (0.9)	5.4 (1.1)	1.82	.16	2.81	.19
IBR tension	4.3 (0.8)	4.0 (0.6)	3.42	.20	5.54*	.26
IBR gross motor coordination (high = poor)	2.6 (0.8)	2.2 (0.7)	3.62	.21	6.08*	.28
IBR fine motor coordination (high = poor)	2.8 (0.6)	2.5 (0.7)	0.87	.11	4.29*	.24
Mental						
Mental Development Index	92.0 (13.1)	95.8 (12.4)	0.82	.11	1.62	.15
IBR attention span	5.4 (1.2)	5.8 (0.9)	0.04	.02	2.77	.19

* $p < 0.05$.
** $p < 0.01$.
*** $p < 0.001$.

SES group (with sex as a covariate), showed that methadone-exposed infants lagged behind comparison infants in physical growth (height, weight, and head circumference) and motoric functioning (PDI, gross and fine motor coordination). Within the very low SES group, methadone-exposed infants lagged behind comparison infants in physical growth (height and head circumference), motoric functioning (PDI, activity level, tension, gross and fine motor coordination), as well as cognitive development (MDI and attention span). TABLE 4 presents eta coefficients for the differences between methadone-exposed and comparison infants by SES level. For all comparisons, differences were in favor of the comparison group; eta coefficients lower than 0.20 were deleted from the table to improve readability. TABLE 5 also presents mean scores on three of the dependent variables (head circumference, PDI, MDI) by level of socioeconomic risk.

Next, the sample was dichotomized according to maternal IQ: the low IQ group mothers were those with IQs less than 90 (mean = 81); the higher IQ group mothers were those with IQs greater than or equal to 90 (mean = 99). For the higher IQ group, methadone-exposed infants were poorer than comparison-group infants in their physical growth (height, weight, and head circumference) and on their motoric functioning (fine motor coordination). For the low IQ group, methadone-exposed infants were poorer than the comparison group in physical growth (head circumference), motoric functioning (PDI, tension, gross and fine motor coordination), and cognitive development (MDI, attention span). TABLES 4 and 5 summarize these data.

Similarly, the sample was dichotomized by pregnancy and birth complications: the many-complications group included those with ROS scores greater than 4 (mean = 7.0); the few-complications group included those with ROS scores of four or less (mean = 2.6). In the few-complications group, most of the complications were also minor, such as use of anesthesia or analgesia during delivery; in the many-complications group most infants showed some signs of fetal distress. Analyses of variance on the infants with few pregnancy and birth complications indicated that methadone-exposed infants lagged behind comparison infants in one measure of physical growth (height), and in motoric functioning (PDI, gross and fine motor coordination). For the infants in the group with many pregnancy and birth complications, methadone-exposed infants lagged behind comparison infants in physical growth (height, weight, and head circumference), and motoric functioning (activity level, tension, fine motor coordination). TABLES 4 and 5 summarize these data.

Because of the particularly strong difference between the head circumferences of methadone and comparison infants among those with pregnancy and birth complications (eta = 0.55), it was decided to explore further the relationships among these

TABLE 4. Differences between Methadone-Exposed and Comparison Infants at Different Levels of Risk, Controlling for Sex of Child (Pearson eta Coefficients[a])

	Socioeconomic Status		Maternal IQ		Pregnancy & Birth Complications	
	Very Low	Higher	Low	Higher	Many	Few
n (comparison)	23	21	25	19	14	30
n (methadone)	18	12	16	14	15	15
Physical						
Height (cm)	0.31	0.29		0.42	0.36	0.21
Weight (kg)		0.29		0.26	0.25	
Head circumference (cm)	0.27	0.34	0.29	0.36	0.55	
Motor						
Psychomotor Development Index	0.21	0.31	0.52			0.29
IBR activity level	0.28				0.40	
IBR tension	0.39		0.47		0.44	
IBR gross motor coordination (high = poor)	0.29	0.22	0.44			0.38
IBR fine motor coordination (high = poor)	0.22	0.26	0.25	0.32	0.22	0.28
Mental						
Mental Development Index	0.41		0.29			
IBR attention span	0.23		0.38			

[a] Coefficients < 0.20 omitted from table; all differences involved greater physical growth, better developmental quotients, lower tension and activity for comparison children.

variables. Since methadone infants tended to be smaller at birth than comparison infants, it might have been possible that the differences between the groups at two years was related to differing birthweights. Analyses were recomputed examining drug effects in the many-birth-complications groups, controlling for the effects of birth weight and sex. There remained a sizable methadone effect for two-year head circumference ($eta = 0.48$). Analyses were also computed looking at the relation of pregnancy and birth complications to two-year growth within the methadone group. Partial correlations between ROS scores and two-year growth controlling for sex were negligible for height and weight, and 0.44 for head circumference. Partial correlations between ROS scores and two-year growth controlling for the effects of birthweight as well as sex were also negligible for height and weight, and 0.46 for head circumference.

TABLE 5. Mean Scores on Selected Outcome Variables by Drug and Other Risk Factors

	Socioeconomic Status		Maternal IQ		Pregnancy & Birth Complications	
	Very Low	Higher	Low	Higher	Many	Few
Head circumference (cm)						
Methadone	48.6	48.1	48.6	48.1	48.3	48.7
Comparison	49.2	49.7	49.3	49.7	49.8	49.3
Psychomotor Development Index (PDI)						
Methadone	98	104	97	105	99	102
Comparison	104	113	112	104	104	111
Mental Development Index (MDI)						
Methadone	86	101	90	94	91	93
Comparison	97	95	98	93	94	97

DISCUSSION

The present study produced evidence that the effects of prenatal exposure to methadone can be observed in the physical, motor, and mental development of human infants at two years of age. The data also suggest that such effects, particularly in cognitive development, may be mediated by other nonteratological risk factors. These findings are reviewed below.

Physical Growth

Methadone-exposed infants showed poorer physical growth than unexposed infants, particularly head circumferences on average 1 centimeter smaller than those of comparison infants and linear height on average 2 centimeters shorter than that of comparison infants. The means for both methadone and comparison infants were within the normal range for physical growth.

While there is a large literature suggesting *in utero* growth disturbance in human newborns exposed to opioid drugs. There are fewer reports of growth disturbances in opioid-exposed toddlers and preschool children. Wilson, McCreary, Kean, and Baxter[38] found an increased incidence of subnormal stature and head circumference in preschool children of heroin addicts when compared to high-risk controls. Ting, Keller, Berman, and Finnegan[39] found a disproportionate number of head circumference measures below the third percentile in methadone-exposed toddlers and preschoolers. Johnson, Diano and Rosen[20] observed no differences in growth parameters of methadone-exposed infants at 24 months except a higher incidence of head circumferences below the third percentile. However, not all researchers have found growth differences between methadone-exposed and unexposed infants[40] or have reported growth catch-up by the second year of life.[41]

Animal research has confirmed the prenatal growth retarding effects of methadone,[42] although it has generated little data on long-term physical growth. Such research has suggested that methadone has direct effects on growth that are independent of nutritional status, possibly related to a disturbance of the ornithine decarboxylase/polyamine system that regulates nucleic acid, protein synthesis, and tissue growth during development.

In the present sample, head circumference differences showed a moderate association with prenatal and perinatal complications within the methadone-exposed group. Methadone-exposed infants with high numbers of pregnancy and birth complications had slightly smaller heads than methadone-exposed infants with few complications or than comparison infants with many complications. These relationships were unrelated to sex of child or birthweight. One can only speculate whether this relationship between complications and later outcome in methadone children is because pregnancy and birth complications cause later growth retardation in opioid-exposed children or because a subgroup of opioid-exposed fetuses are most affected by drug exposure and that the effect of the drug is manifested both by problems in utero and postnatally.

Motoric Development

In the present study methadone-exposed infants lagged behind unexposed infants in their motor development. They showed poorer fine and gross motor coordination assessed by clinical ratings and greater body tension. Much weaker evidence suggested elevated activity levels in the methadone-exposed infants. Methadone-exposed infants also scored approximately 8 points lower on a standardized measure of motor milestones—a difference that translates into a lag behind comparison infants of about 2 months of developmental age. For all motoric measures, the mean scores for both methadone and comparison groups were well within the normal range. Differences in motoric functioning were independent of other risk factors.

These results are similar to those in other follow-up studies in the clinical and animal literatures. Johnson, Diano, and Rosen[20] reported poorer performance on the Bayley Psychomotor Developmental Index in methadone-exposed two-year-olds (mean methadone = 99.1, mean comparison = 108.4) that produced group means almost identical to those in the present study (mean methadone = 108.5, mean comparison = 100.8). In this same sample, Rosen and colleagues reported that methadone-exposed infants also showed poorer performance on a neurological examination that evaluated tone, reflexes, and coordination as well as developmental milestones. Strauss, Lessen-Firestone, Chavez and Stryker[43] reported that at age five, children exposed to methadone in utero were more active and energetic during testing, showed more task-irrelevant activity, and tended to show poorer fine-motor coordination than comparison children.

Animal research provides clear evidence of disturbances in motoric functioning soon after birth in rodents exposed prenatally to methadone,[1] but only provides hints of long-term motoric dysfunctioning, specifically elevated bar press rates in conditioning tasks.[44,45]

Cognitive Development

There are conflicting reports in the literature about whether prenatal opioid-exposure is related to problems in cognitive development in toddlers and preschoolers. Johnson, Diano, and Rosen[20] reported poorer Bayley Mental Development Index scores in methadone-exposed two-year-olds than in comparison two-year-olds. On the other hand, Kaltenbach, Graziani, and Finnegan[46] found no differences between methadone and comparison two-year-olds, but among four-year-olds found an 8-point performance differential in intelligence.[47] Strauss, Lessen-Firestone, Chavez and Stryker[43] found no methadone effects on cognitive functioning at age five. Wilson and her colleagues[38] reported that three- to six-year-old children whose mothers were addicted to heroin had poorer performance on several perceptual and memory tasks.

In the present study, when looked at as a group, the methadone-exposed infants differed little from comparison infants in their cognitive development—either in attention span or in acquisition of developmental milestones. When examining only those infants being raised in families at the lowest socioeconomic levels, there were clear differences between methadone-exposed and unexposed infants on the Bayley Mental Development Index. The combination of prenatal methadone exposure and very low SES appears to be particularly devastating to infants by the age of two years. Methadone exposure may increase the vulnerability of children to the effects of impoverished environments. More work is needed to clarify the nature of the rearing environments experienced by children in drug-using families.

SUMMARY

This paper has presented evidence of growth and behavioral effects related to prenatal methadone exposure. The data suggest that methadone may have a small direct teratological effect reflected in reduced head circumference, poorer motor coordination, increased body tension, and delayed acquisition of motor milestones in methadone-exposed toddlers. In the sample as a whole, there are no direct effects of methadone exposure on mental development. However, methadone-exposed infants reared in extremely poor environmental circumstances show very delayed mental development. They function more poorly than nonexposed infants reared in such environments and more poorly than methadone-exposed infants reared in more adequate (although still economically poor) environments. This finding is important because it suggests that in the cognitive domain, methadone may not cause a behavioral deficit, but instead create a vulnerability in these children that then makes them more susceptible to impoverished environments.

The results from this study indicate that a large subgroup of methadone-exposed children are clearly at risk for poor early intellectual development and that the source of the risk is to a large degree related to environmental factors. These findings suggest that preventive interventions—focused both on enriching the early experiences of such children (*e.g.*, high-quality infant day care) and improving the quality of caregiving provided in the homes—might be particularly effective.

ACKNOWLEDGMENTS

The author acknowledges the major roles of Joseph Marcus, Rita J. Jeremy, Carrie B. Patterson, Victor J. Bernstein, and Linda Henson in the careful design and execution of this study. Susan Lutgendorf, Wendy Rabinowitz, Karen Freel, and Ora Aviezer were responsible for examining the infants.

REFERENCES

1. ZAGON, I. S. & P. J. MCLAUGHLIN. 1984. An overview of the neurobehavioral sequelae of perinatal opioid exposure. *In* Neurobehavioral Teratology, J. Yanai, Ed.: 197-234. Elsevier. Amsterdam.
2. SENAY, E. C. 1985. Methadone maintenance treatment. Int. J. Addictions. **20:** 803-821.
3. NIDA STATISTICAL SERIES. 1982. Annual Data 1981. Data from CODAP, Series E, Number 25, United States Department of Health and Human Services. U.S. Government Printing Office. Washington, DC.
4. BUSHORE, R. A., J. S. KETCHUM, K. J. STAISCH, C. T. BARRETT & E. G. ZIMMERMAN. 1981. Heroin addiction and pregnancy. West. J. Med. **134:** 506-514.
5. BLINICK, G., C. E. INTURRISI, E. JEREZ & R. C. WALLACH. 1975. Methadone assays in pregnant women and progeny. Am. J. Obstet. Gynecol. **121:** 617-621.
6. FINNEGAN, L. P. 1975. Narcotics dependence in pregnancy. J. Psychedelic Drugs **7:** 299-311.
7. PERLMUTTER, J. F. 1974. Heroin addiction and pregnancy. Obstet. Gynecol. Surv. **29:** 439-446.
8. REMENTERIA J. L. & K. LOTONGKHUM. 1977. The fetus of the drug-addicted woman: Conception, fetal wastage and complications. *In* Drug Abuse in Pregnancy and Neonatal Effects. J. L. Rementeria, Ed.: 1-18. Moseley. Saint Louis, MO.
9. CONNAUGHTON, J. F., L. P. FINNEGAN, J. SCHUR, & J. P. EMICH. 1973. Current concepts in the management of the pregnant opiate addict. Addictive Dis. **2:** 21-36.
10. NAEYE, K. L., W. BLANC, W. LEBLANK, & M. A. KHATAMEE. 1973. Fetal complications of maternal heroin addiction: Abnormal growth, infections, and episodes of distress. J. Pediatr. **83:** 1055-1061.
11. ZELSON, C. 1973. Infant of the addicted mother. N. Engl. J. Med. **288:** 1393-1395.
12. STRAUSS, M. E., M. ANDRESKO, J. C. STRYKER, J. N. WARDELL & L. D. DUNKELL. 1974. Methadone maintenance during pregnancy: Pregnancy, birth and neonate characteristics. Am. J. Obstet. Gynecol. **120:** 895-900.
13. KANDALL, S. R., S. ALBUM, E. DREYER, M. COMSTOCK, & J. LOWINSON. 1975. Differential effects of heroin and methadone on birth weights. Addictive Dis. **2:** 347-355.

14. DESMOND, M. M. & G. S. WILSON. 1975. Neonate abstinence syndrome: Recognition and diagnosis. Addictive Dis. **2:** 113-121.

15. FINNEGAN, L. P., J. F. CONNAUGHTON, R. E. KRON, & J. P. EMICH. 1975. Neonatal abstinence syndrome: Assessment and management. Addictive Dis. **2: 141-158.**

16. Zelson, C. 1976. Neonatal narcotic addiction. *In* The Neonate: Clinical Biochemistry, Physiology and Pathology. D. S. Young & J. M. Hicks, Eds. Wiley. New York, NY.

17. KRON, R. E., S. L. KAPLAN, L. P. FINNEGAN, M. LITT & M. D. PHOENIX. 1975. The assessment of behavioral change in infants undergoing narcotic withdrawal: Comparative data from clinical and objective methods. Addictive Dis. **2:** 257-275.

18. STRAUSS, M. E., R. H. STARR, E. M. OSTREA, JR., C. J. CHAVEZ & J. C. STRYKER. 1976. Behavioral concomitants of prenatal addiction to narcotics. J. Pediatr. **89:** 842-846.

19. JEREMY, R. J. & S. L. HANS. 1985. Behavior of neonates exposed *in utero* to methadone as assessed on the Brazelton scale. Infant Behav. Dev. **8:** 323-336.

20. JOHNSON, H. L., A. DIANO & T. S. ROSEN. 1984. 24-month neurobehavioral follow-up of children of methadone-maintained mothers. Infant Behav. Dev. **7:** 115-123.

21. KALTENBACH, K., L. J. GRAZIANI & L. P. FINNEGAN. 1979. Methadone exposure *in utero:* Effects upon developmental status at 1 and 2 years of age. Pediatr. Res. **13:** 332.

22. WILSON, G. S., M. M. DESMOND & R. B. WAIT. 1981. Follow-up of methadone-treated and untreated narcotic-dependent women and their infants: Health, developmental, and social implications. J. Pediatr. **98:** 716-722.

23. HANS, S. L., J. MARCUS, R. J. JEREMY & J. G. AUERBACH. 1984. Neurobehavioral development of children exposed *in utero* to opioid drugs. *In* J. Yanai, Ed. Neurobehav. Teratol. Elsevier. Amsterdam.

24. AYLWARD, G. P. 1982. Methadone outcome studies: Is it more than the methadone? J. Pediatr. **10:** 214-215.

25. MARCUS, J. & S. L. HANS. 1982. A methodological model to study the effects of toxins on child development. Neurobehav. Toxicol. Teratol. **4:** 483-487.

26. GREENSPAN, S. I. 1982. Developmental morbidity in infants in multi-risk factor families: Clinical perspectives. Public Health Rep. **97:** 16-23.

27. HUTCHINGS, D. E. & W. P. FIFER. 1986. Neurobehavioral effects in human and animal offspring following prenatal exposure to methadone. *In* Handbook of Behavioral Teratology. E. P. Riley & Charles V. Vorhees, Eds.: 141-160. Plenum. New York.

28. University of Washington Pregnancy and Health Study. 1974. Pregnancy and Health Interview (adapted with permission of A. P. Streissguth). Department of Psychiatry and Behavioral Sciences, University of Washington. Seattle, WA.

29. MARCUS, J., S. L. HANS, C. B. PATTERSON & A. J. MORRIS. 1984. A longitudinal study of offspring born to methadone-maintained women. I. Design, methodology, and description of women's resources for functioning. Am. J. Drug Alcohol Abuse **10:** 135-160.

30. WECHSLER, D. 1955. Wechsler Adult Intelligence Scale. The Psychological Corporation. New York, NY.

31. ENDICOTT, J. & R. L. SPITZER. 1978. A diagnostic interview: The schedule for affective disorders and schizophrenia. Arch. Gen. Psychiatry **35:** 837-844.

32. HOLLINGSHEAD, A. B. & F. C. RIDLICK. 1958. Social class and mental illness: A community study. Wiley. New York.

33. American Psychiatric Association. 1980. Diagnostic and Statistical Manual of Mental Disorders. 3rd edit. American Psychiatric Association. Washington, DC.

34. BRAZELTON, T. B. 1973. Neonatal Behavioral Assessment Scale. Clinics in Developmental Medicine. No. 50. Lippincott. Philadelphia, PA.

35. HOROWITZ, F. D., J. W. SULLIVAN, & P. LINN. 1978. Stability and instability in the newborn infant: The quest for elusive threads. *In* Organization and Stability of Newborn Behavior: A Commentary on the Brazelton Neonatal Behavioral Assessment Scale. Monographs of the Society for Research in Child Development, 43. A. J. Sameroff, Ed.: 29-45. University of Chicago Press. Chicago, IL.

36. ZAX, M., A. J. SAMEROFF & H. M. BABIGIAN. 1977. Birth outcomes in the offspring of mentally disordered women. Am. J. Orthopsychiatry **47:** 218-230.

37. BAYLEY, N. 1969. Bayley Scales of Infant Development. The Psychological Corporation. New York, NY.

38. WILSON, G. S., R. MCCREARY, J. KEAN, & J. C. BAXTER. 1979. The development of preschool children of heroin-addicted mothers: A controlled study. Pediatrics **63:** 135-141.
39. TING, R., A. KELLER, P. BERMAN & L. FINNEGAN. 1974. Follow-up studies of infants born to methadone-addicted mothers. Pediatr. Res. **8:** 346.
40. LIFSHITZ, M. H., G. S. WILSON, E. O'B. SMITH & M. M. DESMOND. 1983. Fetal and postnatal growth of children born to narcotic dependent women. J. Pediatr. **102:** 686-691.
41. CHASNOFF, I. J., K. A. BURNS, W. J. BURNS & S. H. SCHNOLL. 1986. Prenatal drug exposure: Effects on neonatal and infant growth and development. Neurobehav. Toxicol. Teratol. **8:** 357-362.
42. SLOTKIN, T. A. 1983. A critique. *In Research on the treatment of narcotic addiction: State of the art.* J. R. Cooper, F. Altman, B. S. Brown & D. Czechowicz, Eds. National Institute on Drug Abuse. Rockville, MD.
43. STRAUSS, M. E., J. K. LESSEN-FIRESTONE, C. J. CHAVEZ & J. C. STRYKER. 1979. Children of methadone-treated women at five years of age. Pharmacol. Biochem. Behav. **11:** 3-6.
44. HUTCHINGS, D. E., J. P. TOWEY, H. S. GERINSON & H. F. HUNT. 1979. Methadone during pregnancy: Assessment of behavioral effects in rat offspring. J. Pharmacol. Exp. Ther. **208:** 106-112.
45. MIDDAUGH, L. D. & L. W. SIMPSON. 1980. Prenatal maternal methadone effects on pregnant C57BL/6 mice and their offspring. Neurobehav. Toxicol. **2:** 307-313.
46. KALTENBACH, K., L. J. GRAZIANI & L. P. FINNEGAN. 1979. Methadone exposure *in utero:* Effects upon developmental status at 1 and 2 years of age. Pediatr. Res. **13:** 332.
47. KALTENBACH, K., L. J. GRAZIANI & L. P. FINNEGAN. 1978. Development of children born to women who received methadone during pregnancy. Pediatr. Res. **12:** 372.

Drug Use and Women: Establishing a Standard of Care

IRA J. CHASNOFF

*Perinatal Center for Chemical Dependence
and
Departments of Pediatrics and Psychiatry
Northwestern University Medical School
215 East Chicago Avenue, Suite 501
Chicago, Illinois 60611*

The societal issues which impinge on the care and treatment of the substance-exposed newborn are multiple, not the least of which are the legal and ethical guidelines in place in this country to protect the rights of both mother and infant. Progress in this area has been hampered by the lack of accurate information as to the epidemiology of substance abuse in pregnancy and its impact on the future of health care in the United States. In order to develop preliminary data as to the incidence of perinatal exposure to illicit substances of abuse, a hospital survey was conducted.

Forty hospitals were selected, representing different geographic areas across the country. The Chairman of Obstetrics, Pediatrics, Neonatology or Maternal-Fetal Medicine was contacted at each of these hospitals and informed as to the purpose of the study. A detailed questionnaire was administered, and any questions left unanswered were readministered one to two weeks later after the individual was able to obtain the information for his or her hospital. Of the initial 40 hospitals, 4 hospitals were unable to obtain the requested data, usually due to lack of a computerized discharge review system for the hospital. The survey thus included the remaining 36 hospitals, which represented a total annual delivery rate of 154,856. Substances included in the survey were heroin, methadone, cocaine, amphetamines, phencyclidine (PCP), and marijuana. For the purpose of this study, alcohol was not included.

Of the 36 hospitals, 35 described themselves as teaching hospitals and 21 defined themselves as private hospitals. The proportion of public aid (welfare) patients in the obstetric populations of the 36 hospitals varied widely with 3 of the hospitals having less than 25% of their population on public aid, 9 hospitals having between 25% and 50% of their population on public aid, and the remaining 24 hospitals having more than 50% of their obstetric population on public aid.

The overall incidence of substance abuse in pregnancy based on discharge diagnosis of the mother or infant in the 36 hospitals was 11% with a range from 0.4% to 27%. In order to account for this wide variability in the incidence of substance abuse in pregnancy among the study hospitals, the incidence was examined in relation to the proportion of public aid population in each hospital. As shown in TABLE 1, hospitals with a small or moderate number of public aid patients had an incidence of substance aubse in pregnancy similar to hospitals with greater than half their population on public aid. Thus, the incidence of substance abuse in pregnancy was not related to the proportion of public aid patients delivering at the particular hospital.

TABLE 1. Incidence of Substance Abuse in Pregnancy by Proportion of Public Aid Population

Public Aid Population	N	Incidence of Diagnosis
<25%	3	11.0%
≥25% <50%	9	10.8%
≥50%	24	11.3%

Each of the 36 hospitals was then categorized as to the thoroughness of the substance aubse assessment conducted in the prenatal or perinatal period (TABLE 2). Level I hospitals were those hospitals at which no substance abuse assessment by history or urine toxicology was performed by physicians or staff during or after pregnancy. Infants were evaluated with urine toxicology only if a severe complication occurred at the time of labor and delivery. Level II hospitals were those hospitals that had a policy, either written or unwritten, that all pregnant women were to be questioned regarding substance use and abuse, but no established protocol was in place and there was no monitoring of staff compliance. Neonates automatically had a urine toxicology performed if the mother had admitted to drug use or if complications occurred at labor and delivery or in the newborn period. Level III hospitals were those hospitals that had a protocol through which every pregnant women and/or neonate was assessed through history or urine toxicology for substance abuse or exposure.

As can be seen in TABLE 2, the reported incidence of substance abuse in pregnancy rose with the increased thoroughness of the assessment utilized by the hospital staff and physicians. Level I and II hospitals had an incidence similar to one another, while Level III hospitals had an incidence of diagnosis 3 to 5 times greater than the other two categories. Thus, the incidence of the diagnosis of substance abuse in pregnancy being made was a variable dependent on the thoroughness of assessment of pregnant women by medical professionals and support staff.

Among the 36 hospitals, 9 hospitals had conducted formal studies of the incidence of illicit drug use in pregnancy. These studies, listed by principal investigator's name and hospital, have been summarized in TABLE 3. It can be seen in this table that the incidence of substance abuse in pregnancy, particularly for cocaine, was consistent, regardless of the location of the hospital or the size of the population studied.

From these data, it is clear that substance abuse in pregnancy may be the most frequently missed diagnosis in all of obstetric and pediatric medicine. With this realization, the health care community must now move to establish a standard of care for pregnant women across the country. This standard of care would not involve urine toxicologies or other laboratory evaluations, but would bring physicians back to the basic practice of medicine; i.e., taking a complete history and performing a thorough physical exam. This approach would establish the necessity of evaluating lifestyle as a part of medical care and of instructing the patient as to the impact that that lifestyle

TABLE 2. Incidence of Substance Abuse in Pregnancy by Hospital Assessment

Assessment Level	N	Incidence of Diagnosis
I (none)	4	3.0%
II (history or clinical)	17	5.1%
III (protocol)	15	15.7%

TABLE 3. Substance Abuse Studies

Name/Hospital	Methodology	N	Rate
Little/Parkland	history: intake in prenatal clinic	3000	9.8% cocaine 3.0% amphetamines
Rogers/Shands	urine: all newborns	100	10.0% cocaine
Wong/San Francisco	urine: all newborns in 1 month	170	10.0% illicit drugs
Burkett and Bandstra/ Jackson Memorial	urine: all women at labor/delivery	300	12.5% cocaine
Bateman/Harlem	urine: all newborns	3000	15.0% cocaine
Rahman/Chicago Osteopathic	urine: all newborns in 2 months	158	16.0% cocaine
Zuckerman/Boston City	urine/history: all study participants	1600	17.0% cocaine 27.0% marijuana
Colmorgen/Christiana	urine: all women at first prenatal visit	1500	24.0% illicit drugs
Evans/University of California at Davis	urine: all women at labor/delivery	800	25.0% cocaine, amphetamines, heroin

may have on her unborn child. Training of medical students, residents and practicing physicians in substance abuse and its impact on health should emphasize the art of taking a substance abuse history. The overall goal must be to develop a sense of responsibility on the part of the health care community to ensure that every pregnant woman receives appropriate information and intervention in lifestyle issues which can affect future generations.

Neuroendocrine Consequences of Alcohol Abuse in Women[a]

NANCY K. MELLO, JACK H. MENDELSON, AND
SIEW KOON TEOH

Alcohol and Drug Abuse Research Center
Harvard Medical School—McLean Hospital
115 Mill Street
Belmont, Massachusetts 02178

INTRODUCTION

There is accumulating evidence that alcohol and other drugs adversely affect fetal growth and development, but the pathophysiological mechanisms underlying the fetal alcohol syndrome are unknown.[1–8] The relative influence of alcohol's direct toxic effects on the developing fetus through the placenta and/or alcohol's adverse effects on the mother are unclear.[9–11] Isolation of the effects of any toxins on a single component of the maternal-placental-fetal unit is difficult. Although it is possible that alcohol's disruptive effects on maternal reproductive hormones contribute to fetal dysmorphologies and behavioral impairments, there is little direct evidence to support or refute this hypothesis.[10]

The importance of these questions is illustrated by recent estimates that in the general population 1 to 3 of every 1,000 live births is afflicted with some variant of alcohol-related impairment.[12,13] Among alcoholic women, the prevalence of the fetal alcohol syndrome has been estimated at 21 to 29 per 1,000 births.[12] There is also an increased awareness that many women of reproductive age have alcohol-related problems. For example, alcoholism and alcohol abuse were the fourth most frequent of all psychiatric disorders among young women aged 18 to 24 according to a survey of major metropolitan areas sponsored by the National Institute on Mental Health.[14] Women accounted for 24% of 10,000 first admissions to a proprietary hospital system for alcoholism treatment.[15]

Until very recently there has been relatively little research on alcohol's effects on reproductive function in women.[16–19] The lack of research on women is especially surprising since it has long been known that alcohol is a gonadal toxin in men. Alcoholism is associated with testicular atrophy, low testosterone levels, gynecomastia, impotence and diminished sexual interest in men.[16,20–22] It now appears that alcohol inhibits testosterone biosynthesis by direct toxic effects on the testes,[19,23–25] but the

[a] Preparation of this review was supported in part by Grants DA 00101 and DA 00064 from the National Institute on Drug Abuse and Grants AA 04368 and AA06252 from the National Institute on Alcohol Abuse and Alcoholism, of the Alcohol, Drug Abuse and Mental Health Administration.

211

extent to which hypothalamic and pituitary factors contribute to alcohol-induced male reproductive system pathology remains controversial.[19,24]

This paper focuses on recent studies of alcohol's effects on reproductive hormones in women. Alcohol's effects in women who are alcohol dependent, alcohol abusers or social drinkers are examined. Experimental studies of the acute effects of alcohol on the hypothalamic-pituitary-gonadal-adrenal axis in normal women following stimulation with opioid antagonists and synthetic LHRH are described. Some possible implications of alcohol's disruptive effects on pituitary, gonadal and adrenal hormones for understanding the pathogenesis of fetal dysmorphologies and developmental impairments are discussed. Finally, the impact of polydrug abuse on the analysis of alcohol's effects on fetal growth and development is considered.

ALCOHOLISM AND REPRODUCTIVE SYSTEM DYSFUNCTION IN ALCOHOL-DEPENDENT WOMEN

Clinical studies have shown that alcoholic women may have several menstrual cycle-related disorders including amenorrhea,[26–29] anovulation and/or luteal phase dysfunction[26,27] and, in some instances, early menopause.[30,31] This information has been derived primarily from clinical history and endocrine evaluations made during sobriety at the time of admission for treatment of alcohol-related problems. Alcoholic women often have a number of medical disorders such as liver disease or pancreatitis, sometimes complicated by malnutrition or infectious disease.[15] Since these medical disorders can also contribute to reproductive dysfunction, it is not possible to attribute abnormal menstrual cycles in alcoholic women to alcohol alone. But, recent replications of these reproductive disorders in animal models under controlled conditions[32–38] and in healthy social drinkers[39] indicate the generality of observations on alcoholic women with other medical complications.[18]

Amenorrhea

Amenorrhea, or the complete cessation of menses, has been reported consistently by alcoholic women.[26–29] Twenty-two women admitted for the treatment of liver disease or pancreatitis were studied in Finland and in Paris.[26,29] Fourteen women showed a similar endocrine profile characterized by low levels of estrogens and high levels of LH and FSH in comparison to normal controls. Eight alcoholic amenorrheic women had normal estrogen levels and a positive estradiol response to stimulation with clomiphene or human chorionic gonadotropin (hCG).[26] Hyperprolactinemia was not observed in these amenorrheic alcoholic women and the prolactin response to TRH stimulation was normal.[29] Pituitary function was evaluated with synthetic luteinizing-hormone-releasing hormone (LHRH) (100mcg). The amenorrheic women showed no significant difference in the LH and FSH response to synthetic LHRH stimulation in comparison to normal controls.[26,29] The normal gonadotropin response to synthetic LHRH stimulation suggested that the pituitary may not be the primary site of alcohol's toxic effects in amenorrheic alcoholic women. The relative contribution of ovarian and hypothalamic factors remains undetermined. Ovarian pathology has been reported in postmortem studies of alcoholic women, alcohol-dependent rhesus monkeys and rats.[32,37,40] But low estrogen levels could reflect either impairment of ovarian function or disruption of gonadotropin secretory activity or both.

Hypothalamic amenorrhea as well as several other disorders of reproductive function in nonalcoholic women are associated with abnormal patterns of LH secretory activity.[41,42] Hypothalamic amenorrhea was often associated with a low frequency of LH pulses or an apulsatile pattern of LH secretion.[41,42] Treatment with pulsatile administration of synthetic LHRH restored normal ovulatory menstrual cycles in women with hypothalamic amenorrhea.[41–45] It is possible that alcohol-induced amenorrhea also reflects aberrant gonadotropin secretory patterns, but no systematic pulse frequency analyses of gonadotropin secretory activity of alcoholic women are as yet available to confirm or refute this hypothesis.

Anovulation and Luteal Phase Dysfunction

Alcoholic women who continue to menstruate may have anovulatory cycles or luteal phase dysfunction.[18,26,27] Luteal phase dysfunction is defined either as a *short luteal phase defect* (eight days or less from ovulation to menses) or an *inadequate luteal phase* when progesterone levels are abnormally low, but the interval from ovulation to menstruation is of normal length.[46–48]

Only one endocrine evaluation of alcoholic women with anovulatory cycles or luteal phase dysfunction has been reported.[26] Four women with *anovulatory* cycles had severe oligomenorrhea (scanty menses) and intermittent amenorrhea. Clomiphene administration induced a significant rise in LH and estradiol. Three of these alcoholic women had pancreatitis and one had cirrhosis.[26]

Six women with *luteal phase inadequacy* had mild oligomenorrhea and low plasma progesterone levels during the luteal phase. Menstrual cycles were of normal length and gonadotropin and estradiol levels during the late follicular phase were normal. hCG stimulation during the luteal phase increased progesterone levels above 10ng/ml in three of six women. Two women also had cirrhosis and four had pancreatitis.[26]

ALCOHOL EFFECTS ON REPRODUCTIVE FUNCTION IN SOCIAL DRINKERS

Alcohol related *luteal phase dysfunction* and *anovulation* have also been observed in healthy, well-nourished women who lived on a clinical research ward for 35 days.[39] After a seven day alcohol-free baseline, these social drinkers could self-administer alcohol for 21 consecutive days and were observed during a postalcohol period of seven days. Women could earn alcohol (beer, wine or distilled spirits) or money ($0.50) for 30 minutes of performance on a simple operant task, a second-order fixed-ratio 300 fixed-interval one-second schedule of reinforcement (FR 300 FI 1 sec:S). Points earned for alcohol and for money were not interchangeable.[39]

Women were classified as heavy, social or occasional alcohol users on the basis of the actual number of drinks consumed during three consecutive weeks of alcohol availability. Five women who consumed an average of 7.8 (± 0.69) drinks per day were classified as heavy drinkers. Twelve women who consumed an average of 3.84

(±0.19) drinks per day were classified as social drinkers and nine women who consumed an average of 1.22 (±0.21) drinks per day were classified as occasional drinkers. These drinking patterns were consistent with subjects' self reports of alcohol use before admission to the clinical research ward. The heavy, social and occasional alcohol users reported that they had used alcohol for an average of 7.5, 6.6. and 6.9 years respectively. Average peak blood alcohol levels measured in the social and heavy drinkers ranged from 109 (±16) to 199 (±13) mg/dl. Peak blood alcohol levels measured in the occasional drinkers averaged between 48 (±10) and 87 (±22) mg/ dl. Peak blood alcohol levels for *individual* heavy alcohol users ranged between 69 and 196 mg/dl. Peak blood alcohol levels for individual social alcohol users ranged between 27 and 233 mg/dl. Individual peak blood alcohol levels for the occasional alcohol users ranged between 5 and 159 mg/dl.[39]

Sixty percent of the heavy drinkers and fifty percent of the social drinkers who consumed more than three drinks per day had significant derangements of the menstrual cycle.[39] Three moderate (social) drinkers who consumed between 3.48 and 4.05 drinks per day had anovulatory cycles. An example of a prolonged follicular phase with delayed ovulation in a woman who drank an average of 4.10 (±0.77) drinks per day is shown in FIGURE 1. This subject did not ovulate until the 28th day of her menstrual cycle. Three heavy drinkers and one social drinker who consumed between 4.24 and 8.24 drinks per day had persistent hyperprolactinemia defined as elevations in plasma prolactin levels above 25 ng/ml during at least 7 of the 21 days of alcohol consumption. Illustrative data showing hyperprolactinemia in a heavy drinker who consumed an average of 8.24 drinks per day is shown in FIGURE 2. Plasma prolactin levels were significantly elevated within five days after initiation of drinking and peaked coincidentally with a normal LH surge on study day 16. This woman's prolactin levels remained elevated (above 25 ng/ml) throughout the luteal phase and after cessation of drinking.

These alcohol-related disorders appear to be alcohol dose dependent. There was no evidence of menstrual cycle dysfunction or abnormal reproductive hormone levels in the occasional drinkers or in two of the social drinkers who consumed less than an average of three drinks per day. Whereas five of the ten social drinkers who drank more than three drinks per day and three of the five heavy drinkers had significant derangements of the menstrual cycle and reproductive hormone function. The contrast between the occasional and heavy social drinkers suggests that the abnormalities observed can be attributed to alcohol and not to living conditions on the research ward per se. Since these women were otherwise healthy and well-nourished, it appears that alcohol and not extraneous factors accounted for the menstrual cycle derangements observed.[39]

It is important to emphasize that alcohol did not invariably cause menstrual cycle abnormalities. The woman who consumed the most alcohol (10 [±0.69] drinks per day) did not have abnormal menstrual cycles or hyperprolactinemia. It is possible that this heavy drinker had developed tolerance for alcohol.[39] The existence of repro-

FIGURE 1. Chronic alcohol effects on pituitary and gonadal hormones in a moderate social drinker. LH (ng/ml), prolactin (ng/ml), estradiol (pg/ml) and progesterone (ng/ml) levels were measured before, during and after 21 days of alcohol self-administration (*top and middle panel*). The number of drinks consumed ($\bar{x}$ = 4.10 [±0.77] drinks per day) and peak blood alcohol levels (mg/dl) during operant response-contingent alcohol self-administration on a clinical research ward is shown in the *lower panel*. This woman did not ovulate until day 28 of this menstrual cycle. (From Mendelson and Mello.[39] Reprinted by permission from the *Journal of Pharmacology and Experimental Therapeutics.*)

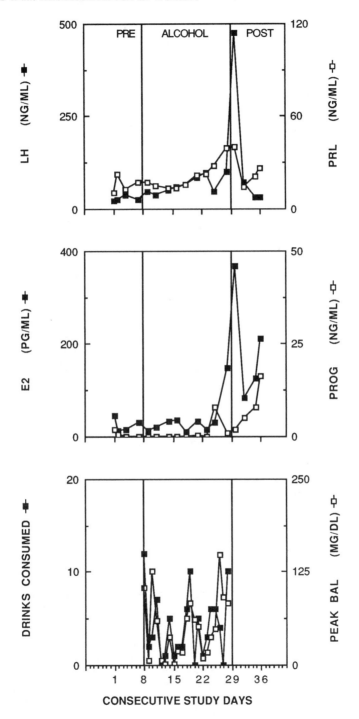

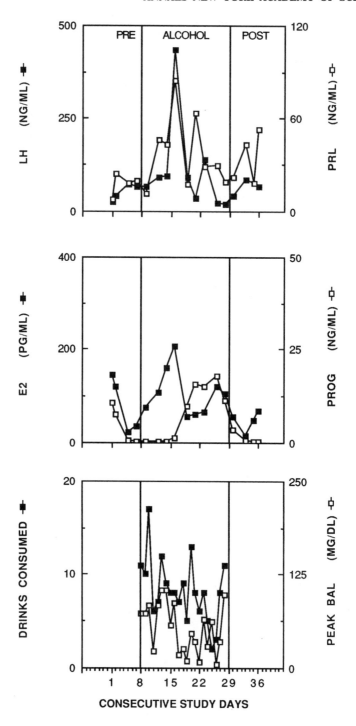

ductive system tolerance for alcohol can be inferred from the fact that many alcohol abusers and alcohol-dependent women have normal pregnancies.[49]

One implication of these data on the adverse effects of chronic alcohol intake on anterior pituitary and ovarian hormones in healthy women is that alcohol-related menstrual cycle and reproductive hormone dysfunctions may be more prevalent among social and heavy drinkers than had been assumed previously. This conclusion is concordant with survey evidence that drinking and reproductive dysfunction are related in the general, nonclinical population.[50] A stratified household sample of 917 women showed a strong association between alcohol consumption and several menstrual disorders, including dysmenorrhea, heavy menstrual flow and premenstrual discomfort. The incidence of these disorders increased as a concomitant of reported drinking levels. Women who consumed six or more drinks each day at least five times a week had elevated rates of gynecological surgery (other than hysterectomy) and obstetrical disorders.[50]

PATHOGENESIS OF ALCOHOL-RELATED REPRODUCTIVE SYSTEM DYSFUNCTIONS

Although there is increasing evidence that a wide spectrum of disorders of reproductive function are associated with alcohol dependence, alcohol abuse and moderate social drinking, very little is known about the mechanisms of alcohol's effects on the neuroendocrine regulation of the menstrual cycle.[18] Since data from alcohol abusers are often confounded by medical problems and/or polydrug abuse, animal models of alcoholism are essential for a systematic analysis of alcohol's effects on the hypothalamic-pituitary-gonadal-adrenal axis. Alcohol's effects can be studied in animal models under controlled conditions where other substance abuse, malnutrition and/or intercurrent illness cannot contribute to results obtained. Confirmation of pathology observed in women under controlled experimental conditions attests to the generality of these findings as well as the role of alcohol in the development of these disorders.

For example, persistent amenorrhea is usually reported in alcohol-dependent women who also have cirrhosis and/or pancreatitis.[26,27,29] Chronic alcohol self-administration also results in amenorrhea, atrophy of the uterus and decreased ovarian mass in otherwise healthy female macaque monkeys.[32] Daily self-administration of high doses of alcohol (2.9 to 4.4 g/kg/day) was accompanied by amenorrhea that persisted for 84 to over 200 days.[33] Amenorrheic monkeys developed postalcohol session blood alcohol levels ranging from 266 to 438 mg/dl,[32] *i.e.,* levels comparable to those observed in alcoholic men during intoxication.[51] In contrast, monkeys that self-administered relatively low doses of alcohol (1.3 and 1.6 g/kg/day) for 119 and 173 days respectively, continued to have stable ovulatory menstrual cycles.[32] Ano-

FIGURE 2. Chronic alcohol effects on pituitary and gonadal hormones in a heavy social drinker. LH (ng/ml), prolactin (ng/ml), estradiol (pg/ml) and progesterone (ng/ml) levels measured before, during and after 21 days of alcohol self-administration (*top and middle panel*). The number of drinks consumed ($\bar{x}$ = 8.24 [±0.75] drinks per day) and peak blood alcohol levels (mg/dl) during operant response-contingent alcohol self-administration on a clinical research ward is shown in the *lower panel*. This woman had recurrent hyperprolactinemia during daily alcohol consumption. (From Mendelson and Mello.[39] Reprinted by permission from the *Journal of Pharmacology and Experimental Therapeutics.*)

vulation and luteal phase dysfunction have been reported in alcohol-dependent women and in moderate social drinkers.[18] Our ongoing studies with the primate alcohol self-administration model have shown that chronic alcohol administration also suppresses ovulation and results in luteal phase dysfunction in otherwise healthy animals.

Examination of alcohol's effects on pituitary, hypothalamic, ovarian and adrenal function has been greatly facilitated by the availability of provocative tests commonly used in clinical endocrinology.[52-57] Each component of the hypothalamic-pituitary-gonadal-adrenal axis can be selectively stimulated to evaluate the primary site or sites of alcohol's toxic effects. Provocative tests provide a tool for analysis of alcohol's effects on the various facets of this complex, interrelated system. For example, synthetic LHRH can be used to directly stimulate pituitary release of LH and FSH,[52,58] and the effects of alcohol on LHRH stimulated gonadotropins can be examined.[18,59-61] Opioid antagonist drugs also stimulate release of pituitary gonadotropins, presumably by antagonism of endogenous opioid peptides which mediate the inhibitory regulation of endogenous LHRH in the hypothalamus.[53,62-65] Two opioid antagonists, naloxone and naltrexone, are used to stimulate hypothalamic release of endogenous LHRH followed by pituitary release of LH, FSH and prolactin.[53] Naltrexone also stimulates release of ACTH and cortisol in women.[65] One disadvantage of the short-acting narcotic antagonist naloxone is that it is only effective during the late follicular and luteal phases of the menstrual cycle.[53] In contrast, naltrexone, a long-acting opioid antagonist, significantly stimulates FSH and LH during the early follicular phase in women.[65] In the remainder of this section, some current hypotheses concerning the pathogenesis of amenorrhea, anovulation and luteal phase dysfunction will be reviewed and data from studies of alcohol's effects on synthetic LHRH or opioid antagonist-stimulated hormones will be described.

Possible Mechanisms Underlying Amenorrhea

The endocrine pathology underlying amenorrhea is poorly understood. A number of conditions other than alcohol abuse can contribute to the development of amenorrhea. Clinical disorders involving severe weight loss such as anorexia nervosa are often associated with persistent amenorrhea,[66] but obesity may also lead to amenorrhea.[67] In otherwise healthy, normal women, amenorrhea may be associated with weight reduction, jogging or professional athletic pursuits.[66-69] It is unlikely that a single endocrine disruption accounts for amenorrhea of such disparate origins. A number of medical disorders (e.g., liver, kidney, thyroid disease, polycystic ovaries and pituitary adenoma) can result in persistent amenorrhea.[66] A discussion of all of these conditions is beyond the scope of this review.

Amenorrhea and Gonadotropin Secretory Activity

It is possible that alcohol may suppress hypothalamic release of endogenous luteinizing-hormone-releasing-hormone (LHRH) with concomitant suppression of gonadotropin secretory activity. Contemporary understanding of the neuroendocrine regulation of the menstrual cycle is based upon the fundamental discovery of the importance of pulsatile gonadotropin secretion for normal reproductive function.[70-72]

When hypothalamic release of endogenous LHRH was disrupted in ovariectomized rhesus monkeys by lesions of the arcuate nucleus and the median eminence in the hypothalamus, LH and FSH secretory activity was abolished. Pulsatile administration of synthetic LHRH restored LH and FSH secretory patterns whereas continuous administration of LHRH did not.[70–72] Recent clinical data suggest that hypothalamic amenorrhea is associated with suppression of gonadotropin secretory activity.[41,42,73] A low frequency of LH pulses was most commonly associated with secondary hypothalamic amenorrhea, but pulses of low amplitude were also observed.[41,42,73] The most severe abnormalities were associated with a complete absence of LH pulses and low LH levels.[41,42] Normal ovulatory function was restored in amenorrheic patients by pulsatile infusion of synthetic LHRH.[41–43,45,74] In the female macaque monkey alcohol self-administration model, average LH levels were significantly lower during amenorrheic cycles (16.9 [± 1.2] to 24 [± 1.4] ng/ml) than during nonalcoholic control cycles (28 [± 1.2] to 30 [± 2.2] ng/ml) (p < 0.001).[33] These data in primates are consistent with the hypothesis that amenorrhea may be related to suppression of gonadotropin levels. However, there have been no systematic studies to confirm or refute the hypothesis that alcohol-induced amenorrhea reflects abnormal gonadotropin secretion. At present, it is not known if alcohol suppresses gonadotropin secretory activity by a direct effect on hypothalamic LHRH release or by stimulation of prolactin or corticotropin-releasing factor (CRF).

Hyperprolactinemia and Alcohol-Related Amenorrhea

Hyperprolactinemia associated with normal postpartum lactation or with pituitary adenomas may cause amenorrhea and other disruptions of menstrual cycle function.[55,75–77] Hyperprolactinemia developed in four healthy social drinkers during daily consumption of between 4.24 and 8.24 drinks per day.[39] However, hyperprolactinemia is not invariably associated with amenorrhea.[75,78,79] Amenorrhea with normal prolactin levels was observed in alcoholic women with liver disease.[29] These alcoholic women (ages 23–40) reported amenorrhea of 3 to 12 months duration and their basal prolactin levels averaged 10.6 (± 1.1) ng/ml.[29]

In one amenorrheic alcohol-dependent macaque monkey, prolactin levels increased from 16.5 to 63 ng/ml during chronic high-dose alcohol self-administration (3.4 g/kg/day) and immunocytochemical examination of the anterior pituitary showed apparent hyperplasia of the lactotrophs.[32] These data suggested that hyperprolactinemia might contribute to alcohol-induced amenorrhea in this model, but this hypothesis was not confirmed in subsequent studies.[33] Examination of four other amenorrheic cycles (85–194 days) indicated that although prolactin levels were intermittently elevated above 20 ng/ml, average prolactin levels during the amenorrheic cycles (14.7 [± 1.8] to 19.6 [± 1.5] ng/ml) did not differ significantly from prolactin levels during normal ovulatory menstrual cycles when no alcohol was available (19.7 [± 0.63] ng/ml).[33]

One monkey developed galactorrhea during a 97-day amenorrheic cycle when alcohol self-administration averaged 3.35 g/kg/day. But prolactin values averaged 19.6(± 1.5) ng/ml and ranged between 5.7 and 29.5 ng/ml. These data are shown in FIGURE 3. Galactorrhea and breast enlargement were first observed on cycle day 25 and persisted through cycle day 74. Days 27-45 were associated with unusually high levels of alcohol self-administration ranging between 4.68 and 9.24 g/kg/day.

Prolactin values ranged between 5.7 and 24 ng/ml during this period. LH levels averaged 19 [±2] ng/ml during this amenorrheic cycle.[33] Clinical studies indicate that galactorrhea does not invariably accompany hyperprolactinemia.[75,80,81] Galactorrhea with normal prolactin levels may reflect induction of prolactin receptors. These data suggest that hyperprolactinemia probably is not the primary mechanism underlying alcohol-induced amenorrhea in the female macaque monkey model.[33]

Studies of the effects of *acute* alcohol intoxication on prolactin in normal human subjects have yielded conflicting findings. Acute alcohol administration to normal women during the mid-luteal phase of the menstrual cycle significantly decreased prolactin levels over the first four hours of observation,[82] whereas a comparable alcohol dose given during the mid-follicular phase had no effect on prolactin except in women who complained of nausea and vomiting.[83] Acute alcohol administration to normal men has been shown to induce a small but statistically significant increase in prolactin levels, but the biological significance of these prolactin elevations is unclear.[84,85]

FIGURE 3. Plasma prolactin levels (ng/ml) (*closed squares*) during a 97-day amenorrheic cycle in an alcohol-dependent female rhesus monkey with no known pathology of the anterior pituitary. Alcohol self-administration (g/kg) during the 24 hours immediately preceding collection of the prolactin sample is shown as *open squares*. Galactorrhea was observed from day 25 through 74. (From Mello et al.[33] Reprinted by permission from the *Journal of Studies on Alcohol*.)

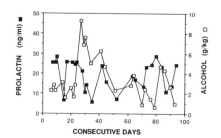

Corticotropin-Releasing Factor and Amenorrhea

A second possibility is that alcohol may stimulate corticotropin-releasing factor (CRF), ACTH and adrenal hormones which in turn suppress gonadotropin secretory activity and lead to amenorrhea. Alcohol, as well as stress, can stimulate CRF, ACTH and cortisol.[86–88] Administration of synthetic CRF inhibits pulsatile release of LH and FSH in ovariectomized rhesus females[89] but administration of ACTH and cortisol does not.[90] Synthetic CRF administration also suppressed endogenous LHRH measured in rat portal blood.[91] These data suggest that CRF induced suppression of LH and FSH is a central effect mediated through the hypothalamic/pituitary axis rather than through adrenal activation.[90] The role of alcohol-related increases in CRF to amenorrhea in alcohol-dependent females remains to be determined.

Alcohol-Induced Anovulation and Luteal Phase Dysfunction

The factors which account for anovulation and luteal phase dysfunction are also poorly understood. The relative contribution of hypothalamic-pituitary and ovarian factors to alcohol-induced anovulation is unclear. FSH is essential for normal follicular development and maturation during the follicular phase.[47,92] It is well established that suppression of FSH during the follicular phase could delay follicle maturation and ovulation or result in luteal phase dysfunction after timely ovulation.[46,47,93,94] Comprehensive studies of folliculogenesis in the primate ovarian cycle suggest that recruitment of the dominant follicle occurs during menstrual cycle days 1-4; a single follicle is selected during days 5-7; and that follicle achieves dominance during cycle days 8-12.[46,47,95] Although the determinants of the selection and dominance of a single ovulatory follicle are unclear, Goodman and Hodgen[47] postulate that nonsteroidal ovarian peptides, inhibins, critically affect this process through titration of FSH levels during folliculogenesis. If alcohol directly suppresses FSH or stimulates inhibin to down regulate FSH secretory activity, this could produce aberrations in folliculogenesis culminating in anovulation or luteal phase dysfunction.[18]

There is recent evidence that alcohol prevents synthetic LHRH stimulation of FSH during the follicular phase of the menstrual cycle in normal female rhesus monkeys.[59] In contrast, LH increased significantly within 15 minutes after synthetic LHRH stimulation when blood alcohol levels averaged 184 and 276 ng/dl. When an isocaloric sucrose solution was substituted for alcohol, both FSH and LH increased significantly after LHRH stimulation.[59] An alcohol-related inhibition of FSH responsivity to *endogenous* LHRH stimulation during the follicular phase could result in menstrual cycle irregularities commonly seen in alcohol-dependent females.

Inferential evidence for the importance of *ovarian factors* in modulating alcohol's effects on pituitary FSH is inferred from the fact that alcohol did not suppress LHRH-stimulated FSH in *ovariectomized* rhesus females.[60] LHRH-stimulated LH and FSH increased significantly in ovariectomized females when blood alcohol levels averaged 242 and 296 mg/dl.[60] The nonsteroidal ovarian peptide, inhibin, has been shown to suppress FSH without affecting LH.[96] In the human menstrual cycle, inhibin is inversely related to FSH during the mid- to late-follicular phase.[97] These data suggest that alcohol may suppress LHRH-stimulated FSH by stimulating ovarian inhibin, but data on alcohol's effects on inhibin are not yet available.

A second possibility is that alcohol may increase *estradiol* levels which in turn suppress FSH during the follicular phase and impair or delay follicle maturation and ovulation. There is considerable evidence that an increase in estradiol levels during the early follicular phase suppresses FSH and pre-ovulatory follicular growth and prolongs the follicular phase.[98–100] Luteal phase defects were consistently observed after 6 hours of exposure to 38.7 (±7.9) pg/ml estradiol on day 6 or 7 of the menstrual cycle.[98] An increase in estradiol levels of about 30 pg/ml significantly reduced FSH concentrations and prolonged the follicular phase.[100] Significant increases in estradiol levels during alcohol intoxication following naloxone and naltrexone stimulation of gonadotropins has been reported recently in normal women.[101,102] The alcohol-related augmentation of opioid antagonist-stimulated estradiol was 45 to 50 pg/ml; estradiol levels which are equivalent to those shown to selectively suppress FSH secretion in clinical studies (40 to 50 pg/ml.)[103]

Acute alcohol administration (0.695 g/kg) also induced a significant increase of 19.5 (±4.1) pg/ml in estradiol levels under basal (nonstimulated) conditions.[104] Plasma estradiol levels reached peak values within 25 minutes after initiation of drinking when blood alcohol levels averaged 34 mg/dl. These data are shown in FIGURE 4. Collection of plasma samples every five minutes permitted detection of an alcohol-related increase in plasma E_2 levels during the ascending phase of the blood alcohol curve. Previous studies of acute alcohol effects on estradiol levels used 20-minute integrated sample collection procedures,[83] and no significant changes in plasma estradiol levels were detected during the ascending, peak or descending phases of the blood alcohol curve. Alcohol (2.5 g/kg) also significantly increased estradiol within

150 to 210 minutes under basal (nonstimulated) conditions in mid-luteal phase rhesus females.[105]

These data converge to suggest that an alcohol-induced increase in estradiol could contribute to suppression of folliculogenesis with resulting anovulation and luteal phase dysfunction. Further research will be required to determine the relative contribution of alcohol-induced stimulation of ovarian steroid hormones and/or ovarian inhibins to anovulation and luteal phase dysfunction.

Alcohol-Induced Stimulation of Pituitary and Gonadal Hormones

Traditionally, disorders of reproductive function that are associated with alcoholism have been attributed to alcohol's suppressive effects on pituitary and gonadal hormones in both women and men. Alcohol-induced amenorrhea is usually attributed to a decreased frequency and/or amplitude of gonadotropin pulsatile secretory activity and/or suppression of ovarian hormones (estradiol, progesterone) essential for normal menstrual cycle function.[18] In alcoholic men, impotence, testicular atrophy and gynecomastia are associated with low testosterone levels reflecting inhibition of testosterone biosynthesis in the testes.[16,19,21–25,106,107] However, with the availability of provocative tests for evaluation of pituitary, hypothalamic and ovarian function and improved techniques for rapid plasma sample collection, a more complex picture of alcohol's effects has emerged. There now appears to be a disparity between *acute* and *chronic* effects of alcohol on the hypothalamic-pituitary-gonadal axis and the hypothalamic-pituitary-adrenal axis. Acute alcohol intoxication has been shown recently to *stimulate* rather than suppress gonadotropins and ovarian hormones under a variety of experimental conditions.[18] Recent data illustrating alcohol's stimulatory effects on pituitary, gonadal and adrenal hormones will be reviewed in this section and are summarized in TABLE 1.

Luteinizing Hormone

Alcohol did not attenuate synthetic LHRH or naloxone stimulation of luteinizing hormone in follicular phase rhesus macaque females and in rhesus males even though peak blood alcohol levels ranged between 200 and above 300 ng/dl.[59,108] These findings were subsequently replicated in mid-luteal phase women under conditions of naloxone stimulation.[101] Not only did alcohol fail to attenuate LH after exogenous stimulation of the hypothalamus or pituitary, but, under some conditions, alcohol augmented the LH response in comparison to placebo. Follicular phase women given the opioid antagonist, naltrexone[102] and ovariectomized rhesus females given synthetic LHRH[60] both showed a significant enhancement of LH after alcohol in comparison to placebo control conditions.[60,102] Illustrative data in LHRH-stimulated ovariectomized rhesus females are shown in FIGURE 5.

TABLE 1. Alcohol-Induced Stimulation of Pituitary, Gonadal and Adrenal Hormones

Subjects	Experimental Conditions	Alcohol Dose	BAL Peak	Pituitary Hormones				Gonadal Hormones			Adrenal Hormones	Sample Frequency	Reference
				LH	FSH	ACTH	PRL	E2	Prog	Test	Cortisol		
Women (n = 9) mid-luteal	Naloxone 5 mg i.v.	1 ml/kg	100 ±13 mg/dl	↑			↑↑ $p < .001$	↑↑ $p < .004$	≠			5–15 min	Mendelson et al., 1987 (101)
Women (n = 14) follicular	Naltrexone 50 mg P.O.	2.2 ml/kg	123 ±4.3 mg/dl	↑↑ $p < 0.05$			↑	↑↑ $p < 0.001$	↓ $p < 0.001$		↑	5–30 min	Teoh et al. 1988 (102)
Women (n = 12) follicular	Basal	350 ml	70–75 mg/dl					↑↑ $p < 0.01$				5 min	Mendelson et al., 1988 (104)
Rhesus females (n = 8) follicular	LHRH 100 mcg i.v.	2.5–3.5 g/kg	204 ± 11.45– 338 ± 21.9 mg/dl	↑	≠							15–20 min	Mello et al., 1986 (59)
Rhesus females (n = 5) OVX	LHRH 100 mcg i.v.	2.5–3.5 g/kg	245 ± 26– 296 ± 20 mg/dl	↑↑	↑							15–20 min	Mello et al., 1986 (60)
Rhesus males (n = 5)	Naloxone 0.5 mg/kg i.v.	2.5–3.5 g/kg	283 ± 9– 373 ± 17 mg/dl	↑						↑		30 min	Mello et al., 1985 (108)
Human males (n = 6)	LHRH 500 mcg	0.695 g/kg	83.1 ± 5.5 mg/dl	↑			↑↑ $p < 0.03$			↑↑ $p < 0.001$		5 min	Phipps et al., 1987 (61)

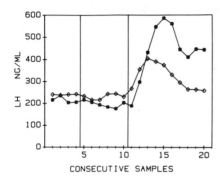

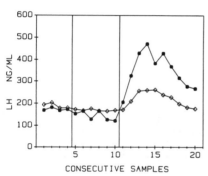

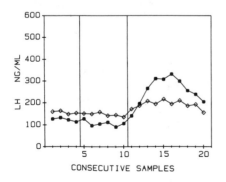

FIGURE 5. The effects of alcohol and sucrose on LHRH-stimulated LH in ovariectomized female rhesus monkeys. These data illustrate an alcohol enhancement of LHRH-stimulated LH in comparison to placebo control administration. Each data point represents a single integrated plasma sample for an individual monkey before and after sucrose control (*open diamond*) or 3.5 g/kg alcohol administration (*closed circle*). Alcohol or sucrose was administered after sample four via nasogastric intubation. Synthetic LHRH (100 mcg/iv) was administered after sample 10. Integrated plasma samples were collected at 20-minute intervals throughout the study except for the first hour after LHRH administration. Samples 11-14 were collected at 15-minute intervals. (From Mello *et al.*[60] Reprinted by permission from the *Journal of Pharmacology and Experimental Therapeutics.*)

Follicle-Stimulating Hormone

Alcohol also failed to attenuate an LHRH-stimulated increase in FSH in human males and ovariectomized rhesus females.[60,61] In follicular phase rhesus females, alcohol prevented an LHRH stimulation of FSH,[59] a finding which could reflect an alcohol-induced increase in ovarian inhibin as discussed earlier in the section on possible mechanisms of luteal phase dysfunction.

Prolactin

Alcohol significantly enhanced naloxone stimulation of prolactin in mid-luteal phase women and LHRH stimulation of prolactin in human males.[61,101] In follicular-phase women, alcohol did not block a naltrexone-stimulated increase in prolactin, but prolactin levels were not significantly higher after alcohol than after alcohol placebo administration.[102]

Gonadal Steroid Hormones

Gonadal steroid hormones in both males and females have shown a similar pattern of alcohol-related augmentation in comparison to placebo control conditions (TABLE 1). Opioid antagonist stimulation with naloxone or naltrexone significantly increased *estradiol* levels after alcohol in comparison to placebo control conditions.[101,102] Estradiol also increased significantly following alcohol administration, in comparison to placebo control, in follicular-phase women studied under basal (nonperturbated) conditions.[104] In human males, alcohol significantly increased testosterone levels in comparison to placebo control conditions after LHRH stimulation (500 mcg).[61] In rhesus males, alcohol failed to block a naloxone-stimulated increase in testosterone even though blood alcohol levels ranged between 283 and 373 mg/dl.[108]

These data indicating that alcohol may have either stimulatory or suppressive effects on pituitary and gonadal hormones depending on the duration of alcohol administration (acute or chronic) and conditions of gonadotropin stimulation (TABLE 1) greatly complicate analysis of the mechanisms by which alcohol intoxication induces derangements of the menstrual cycle.[18] It is increasingly apparent that the complex interrelationships between the hypothalamic-pituitary-ovarian axis and the hypotha-lamic-pituitary-adrenal axis precludes any simplistic conclusion that alcohol acts primarily at one specific target site. It remains to be determined how alcohol may affect the integration and regulation of these systems and how this may be related to alcohol-induced disorders of reproductive function.

Mechanisms of Alcohol-Related Pituitary and Gonadal Hormone Stimulation

The physiological basis for the alcohol-induced augmentation of LH, prolactin, estradiol and testosterone shown in TABLE 1 is unclear. It is possible that increased pituitary sensitivity to LHRH stimulation after alcohol administration may reflect a direct alcohol effect on endogenous LHRH or on other hormones, such as estradiol, which are known to modulate pituitary sensitivity to LHRH. Increased estradiol levels after alcohol administration could enhance the LH response to LHRH stimulation, just as the mid-cycle LH surge in normally cycling rhesus females is dependent upon the periovulatory increase in estradiol.[109] The sustained significant elevation in LHRH-stimulated LH after alcohol (165 minutes) in comparison to placebo control (105 minutes)[60] is consistent with earlier studies of estradiol pretreatment in ovariectomized monkeys.[110] There is also evidence that estradiol pretreatment increases pituitary sensitivity to LHRH stimulation in both normal and hypogonadal women[79,111] and in the intact diestrous rat.[112] Consequently, if alcohol administration did increase estradiol levels in ovariectomized monkeys,[60] this could have sensitized the pituitary to produce an augmented LH response to LHRH stimulation. Although ovariectomy reduces circulating estradiol by approximately 60 percent, estrogens are produced in the adrenal and peripheral conversion of androgens to estrogens.[30,31,92] Unfortunately, estradiol was not measured in the ovariectomized females in which alcohol-enhanced LHRH stimulated LH.[60]

The alcohol-related increase in plasma estradiol levels after naloxone and naltrexone stimulation[65,102] could be accounted for by several mechanisms. It is possible that alcohol may increase estradiol production or decrease estradiol metabolism. We have suggested elsewhere that since intrahepatic ethanol metabolism decreases NAD availability for other coupled oxidative reactions,[113–116] this in turn might reduce the rate of oxidation of estradiol to estrone and result in elevated estradiol levels.[65] Hepatic oxidative metabolism of steroids may become rate limiting during alcohol metabolism when relatively low blood alcohol concentrations (45 mg/dl or 10 mmol/1) may saturate human alcohol dehydrogenase isoenzymes and decrease the NAD to NADH ratio. This in turn could decrease the rate of oxidation of E_2 to estrone and result in increased E_2 levels.[102]

A similar hypothesis can be advanced to account for the alcohol-induced enhancement of LHRH-stimulated testosterone levels in males.[61] Acute alcohol administration may increase hepatic blood flow,[117–119] and ethanol catabolism causes a prompt and dramatic increase in the hepatic NADH to NAD ratio.[120,121] Increased testosterone levels after alcohol and concomitant gonadotropin stimulation may be due in part to increased hepatic conversion of precursor steroids such as androstenedione to testosterone as a consequence of increased NADH to NAD ratios during intrahepatic ethanol catabolism.

An alternative hypothesis is that since the LHRH-stimulated increase in LH preceded the increase in T both in human and macaque males,[61,108] it is possible that this elevation in LH levels was sufficient to stimulate testosterone during alcohol intoxication. We have interpreted these data to suggest that *acute* alcohol intoxication has minimal effects on hypothalamic-pituitary function.[108]

IMPLICATIONS OF ALCOHOL-INDUCED CHANGES IN MATERNAL REPRODUCTIVE HORMONES FOR PREGNANCY AND FETAL GROWTH AND DEVELOPMENT

The pathogenesis of fetal dysmorphologies and behavioral impairments associated with alcohol abuse, or the fetal alcohol syndrome, is unclear. Although it is reasonable to assume that alcohol's effects on maternal reproductive hormones may influence pregnancy outcome and affect fetal growth and development, very little is known about these critical interactions.[1,3,5,6,10,122] A comprehensive review of alcohol's effects on endocrine homeostasis and the possible implications for fetal development concludes that little information now exists on alcohol's effects on the endocrine system during pregnancy.[10]

We are aware of only one evaluation of pituitary and gonadal hormone levels during pregnancy in alcoholic mothers who gave birth to fetal alcohol syndrome infants.[49] Hormone levels were measured during pregnancy weeks 16 to 24 and increased levels of prolactin and low levels of estradiol and progesterone were reported.[49] Prolactin levels averaged 70 ng/ml by gestational week 24 and were significantly higher ($p < 0.025$) in alcoholic women than in abstinent control women at the same stage of pregnancy. However, prolactin levels in alcoholic women who gave birth to normal infants were not significantly different from prolactin levels in alcoholic women who had fetal alcohol syndrome infants.[49] The implications of elevated prolactin levels in all alcoholic women for fetal growth and development are unclear. But these findings are consistent with the alcohol-related enhancement of prolactin under basal conditions[39] and after naloxone and LHRH stimulation discussed earlier.[61,101]

Ovarian Steroid Hormones and Teratogenesis

There have been no comparable studies of alcohol's effects on maternal hormones during *early* pregnancy. Yet in the first trimester, the developing fetus is especially vulnerable to drug-induced malformations since this is the period of organogenesis.[7] During the second and third trimester, maternal drug use may impair fetal growth and functional development. The central nervous system continues to develop throughout pregnancy and consequently remains vulnerable to drug toxicity.[7]

Although a number of factors can contribute to adverse outcomes during the first trimester of pregnancy, it is well established that administration of exogenous estrogens such as diethylstilbesterol and progestogens (alone or in combination with estrogens) can result in spontaneous abortion and in fetal malformations.[123–125] Our recent findings that a single episode of alcohol intoxication can increase estradiol levels significantly in normal women under both basal (nonperturbated) and gonadotropin-stimulation conditions[101,102,104] suggests one possible factor that might contribute to alcohol-related abortion and the fetal alcohol syndrome. If alcohol stimulates a significant increase in estradiol during the first trimester of pregnancy when chorionic gonadotropin levels are high, this could be analogous to giving exogenous estrogen. Under basal conditions, alcohol stimulated an increase in estradiol of 19.5 (± 4.1) pg/ml.[104] The usual dosage regimen for diethylstilbesterol treatment was a gradual increase from 5 mg at week 6-7 to 25 mg between the 8th and 16th week of pregnancy,[126] although doses of 50 mg to 200 mg were sometimes prescribed.[127] Estradiol is approximately 100 times more potent than diethylstilbesterol, *i.e.*, 50 micrograms of estradiol is equivalent to 5,000 micrograms of diethylstilbesterol after parenteral administration.[57] But interpretation of the possible significance of these apparent differences in potency requires consideration of the dose-duration effects of the two estrogens. The greater initial potency of estradiol must be balanced against the longer duration of action of diethylstilbesterol. Although alcohol-induced increases in plasma E_2 occur rapidly when blood alcohol levels exceed 20-30 mg/dl and substrate saturation of hepatic alcohol dehydrogenase isoenzymes occurs,[104] the stability of such estradiol changes as a function of frequency of drinking is unknown. Under conditions of gonadotropin stimulation, plasma estradiol levels increased by about 45 pg/ml during the luteal phase of the menstrual cycle.[101] This may be analogous to hormonal conditions during the first trimester of pregnancy when levels of chorionic gonadotropin (a potent gonadotropin stimulator) are elevated. If so, an alcohol-induced stimulation of estradiol might be maximal during the first trimester when chorionic gonadotropin levels are high. However, the biologic significance of an alcohol-related increase in plasma estradiol levels during basal or naloxone-induced gonadotropin stimulation remains to be determined.

Hypothalamic-Pituitary-Adrenal Factors in Teratogenesis

There is considerable evidence that alcohol-induced changes in *hypothalamic-pituitary-adrenal* as well as hypothalamic-pituitary-gonadal function may be a significant factor in the pathogenesis of the fetal alcohol syndrome.[10,86] Alcohol-related stimulation of adrenocortical activity with concomitant increases in corticosteroid secretion could produce several adverse effects on the fetus. Corticosteroid administration during pregnancy has been associated with an increased frequency of abortions, fetal death, fetal growth retardation and congenital anomalies.[10] Studies with rat have revealed that alcohol stimulated an increase in basal corticosterone levels, stress-induced corticosterone and adrenal weight in pregnant animals as early as the eleventh day of gestation.[128] This may, in part, explain the observations of persistent increases in responsivity of the hypothalamic-pituitary-adrenal axis following an ethanol challenge in rats that were exposed to ethanol in utero.[129-131]

Both alcohol and stress stimulate corticotropin-releasing factor (CRF) release which in turn may inhibit gonadotropin secretion from the pituitary.[86-90] Administration of CRF antagonists reverse the inhibitory action of stress on pulsatile luteinizing hormone (LH) release in rat.[88] Recent studies have shown that CRF administration inhibits LH release in ovariectomized monkeys, whereas ACTH and cortisol do not affect LH secretory activity.[90] Consequently, a direct central effect of alcohol on CRF secretion may impair gonadotropin function essential for maintenance of normal pregnancy and fetal health.

Alcohol stimulation of the hypothalamic-pituitary-adrenal axis may also affect gonadal function. Cortisol directly suppresses plasma testosterone levels without concomitant changes in luteinizing hormone or prolactin in normal men,[132] and alcohol-induced increases in cortisol may be one factor which causes suppression of testosterone synthesis in alcoholic men. High levels of cortisol during pregnancy are associated with increased risk for premature births and fetal death.[10] To date, there have been no reports of controlled clinical studies of alcohol effects on the interaction of the hypothalamic-pituitary-adrenal and the hypothalamic-pituitary-gonadal axis in women.

Alcohol and Abortion

The adverse effects of moderate alcohol use on pregnancy also are indicated by accumulating data on abortion. A prospective survey of 32,019 women at their first antenatal visit to a Kaiser Hospital Clinic was conducted between 1974 and 1977.[133]

A total of 1,503 spontaneous abortions occurred during this period. During the first trimester (5-14 weeks), 714 abortions occurred and during the second trimester (15-27 weeks) 789 abortions occurred. The overall rate of abortion was 14.4% and 2.6% of these occurred during the second trimester.

Self-reports of drinking history indicated that women who had one or more drinks each day had more spontaneous abortions, primarily during the second trimester, than women who were abstinent or only occasional drinkers. The *second* trimester risk factor for spontaneous abortion was 1.03 for occasional drinkers, 1.98 for regular drinkers who consumed one to two drinks per day and 3.53 for women who had more than three drinks per day.

Alcohol did not significantly affect *first* trimester miscarriages. The relative risk of first trimester miscarriage was 1.12 in occasional drinkers, 1.15 in regular drinkers (one to two drinks per day) and 1.16 in women who had three drinks or more daily. These effects of alcohol appeared to be independent of the effects of cigarette smoking and alcohol influenced risk for abortion more than cigarette smoking.[133]

Similar conclusions concerning an association between spontaneous abortion and moderate drinking have been reached by other investigators.[134] Drinking frequency was compared in 616 women who had spontaneous abortions and 632 women who had normal deliveries. It was estimated that 25% of women who drank twice a week were likely to abort and about 14% of women who drank less frequently were likely to abort. One ounce of absolute alcohol was estimated to be the minimum harmful dose.

THE FETAL ALCOHOL SYNDROME AND POLYDRUG ABUSE

Despite the adverse effects of alcohol on menstrual cycle function, chronic alcoholic women do become pregnant and their children may be afflicted with physical, congenital anomalies, abnormal brain function, and pre- and postnatal retardation of growth and development. Behavioral disorders range from hyperactivity to mental retardation. Since alcohol diffuses freely across the placental barrier, the fetus is exposed to the same effective dose of alcohol as the mother. One important unresolved question is the range of alcohol doses that are likely to produce adverse consequences for the fetus. This information is important because most women (60%) of child bearing age use some alcohol[13] and confirmation of pregnancy often does not occur until midway into the first trimester, *i.e.*, the period of organogenesis. A second unresolved question is the effect of duration of alcohol abuse on risk for fetal abnormalities. Although tolerance for alcohol develops in many systems, there are provocative data suggesting that later pregnancies are more likely to be associated with severe fetal alcohol symptoms than early pregnancies.[9]

Historically, warnings against drinking during pregnancy have been traced to Aristotle, repeated in the Bible and reaffirmed in clinical observations in the early 19th and 20th centuries.[3,135] Yet, the 1973 report of the Fetal Alcohol Syndrome (FAS),[136] defined as a specific pattern of dysmorphologies and growth retardation in the children of alcoholic women, was met with considerable skepticism. Controversy over the extent to which alcohol is a specific teratogen was based on the fact that FAS mothers often used other drugs,[137] were malnourished and had inadequate medical care during pregnancy. Any of these factors alone, or in combination with alcohol, could lead to birth defects, and similar patterns of malformation could occur independently of alcohol abuse.[7] A specific attribution of birth defects to alcohol required conditions in which malnutrition and polydrug use could be controlled, a condition impossible to achieve in pregnant women.

Animal Models of FAS

Within the last decade, a number of animal models of alcoholism have been developed to address these issues.[3,4] Current evidence suggests that alcohol is a teratogen in several species studied under controlled laboratory conditions. In one primate model, administration of alcohol only once a week led to fetal malformation and behavioral retardation.[1,5,6] In the first series of studies, alcohol (2.5 to 4.1 g/kg) was administered by gavage once a week from 40 days postconception to delivery to four pregnant females. Within two hours after alcohol administration, average blood alcohol levels ranged between 240 to 256 ng/dl and 338 to 415 ng/dl respectively.[1] Under this alcohol regimen, there was one spontaneous abortion and three live births. Infants were followed for six months and compared with age and sex-matched controls. Prenatal exposure to the high alcohol dose (4.1 g/kg) resulted in neurologic, developmental and facial anomalies similar to those seen in human FAS infants. This infant showed profound retardation and neuropathological examination revealed cerebral asyetry, minimal cortical organization, and hydrocephalus exvacuo. The other two surviving infants exposed to 2.5 g/kg of alcohol prenatally showed no abnormalities in the female but hyperkinesis, developmental retardation and brain abnormality in the male.[1]

These alcohol-exposed macaque infants differed from human FAS infants in two respects: (1) all were abnormally large at birth whereas low birth weight is common in humans; (2) none showed malformations of heart, kidney or other organs often seen in human FAS infants. The absence of organ malformation is probably related to the fact that alcohol administration to the mother did not begin until the end of the organogenic period. The size of the macaque infants probably reflects the adequate nutritional status of the macaque mothers and the fact that they were exposed to alcohol once a week whereas alcoholic women usually drink daily.[1]

Further evidence for alcohol's teratogenic effects after weekly intoxication was obtained in a second series of studies. Fifty-four pregnant macaque monkeys (Macaca nemestrina) were given weekly doses of alcohol (or isocaric and isovolemic sucrose control solution) from the first or the fifth week of gestation until term.[6] Abortion was induced by alcohol doses of 2.5 gm/kg or more administered from the first week of gestation. Consequently, the final dose regimens were 1.8 g/kg from week 1 of gestation (Group 1) or 2.5 gm/kg from days 33 to 46 days postconception (Group 2). Sixteen of 28 infants had facial dysmorphia, growth deficiency and CNS dysfunction. Group 1 infants had more severe and consistent cognitive abnormalities than Group 2 infants despite exposure to higher alcohol doses in Group 2. At 6 months of age, Group 2 infants were more cognitively intact and showed less evidence of delayed development than Group 1 infants. Facial dysmorphia occurred in only one Group 1 infant, suggesting that behavioral teratogenic effects may occur independently of facial dysmorphia. Maternal blood alcohol levels of 240 mg/dl and above were associated with developmental retardation in 10 of 12 animals. Microcephaly occurred in the single surviving infant in the 4.1 gm/kg group.[6] These data indicate that alcohol-induced fetal impairments are related both to the dose and time of first exposure during pregnancy.

Evidence from well-controlled animal studies should further confirm (or refute) the hypothesis that alcohol is a specific teratogen. Although it seems likely that alcohol, in sufficient doses, is teratogenic, the extent to which the fetal alcohol syndrome is specific to alcohol remains unclear. As described throughout this volume, a number of other drugs are also fetotoxic and drug abuse during pregnancy can result in a profile of low birth weight, delayed development and brain malformations similar to those reported for alcohol abuse in human infants.[138]

Polydrug Abuse and Reproductive Function

The adverse consequences of maternal drug abuse for the developing fetus have been documented repeatedly throughout this conference. Although the relationship between drug effects on maternal reproductive hormones and consequent developmental anomalies in the fetus remains undetermined,[10] it is known that abused drugs have very similar effects on the neuroendocrine system. Marijuana,[139] opiate[16,140] and cocaine abuse[104,141–143] may lead to derangements of reproductive function similar to those reported for alcohol abuse. Illustrative data are summarized in TABLE 2.

TABLE 2. Derangements of Reproductive Function Reported in Alcohol, Cocaine, Marijuana, and Opiate Abusers[a]

	Alcohol	Cocaine	Marijuana	Opiate
Amenorrhea	X	X	X	X
Anovulation	X	X	X	X
Luteal phase dysfunction	X		X	X
Hyperprolactinemia	X	X		X
Spontaneous abortion	X	X	X	X

[a] References 11, 16, 18, 39, 104, 139-143.

Interpretation of these data is qualified by the fact that many subjects do not use only one drug, but rather may use several drugs in various combinations. Opiate addicts may also abuse alcohol, cocaine, marijuana and other available drugs. Cocaine abusers often use alcohol[142,144] as well as opiates and marijuana to modulate the cocaine high and crash. Alcohol abusers may also use marijuana, tobacco, opiates and cocaine. The prevalence and medical consequences of polydrug abuse has been recently reviewed by Kreek.[145,146] It appears that the combined effects of multiple drugs have more severe medical consequences than use of a single drug alone especially in instances when both drugs have similar effects. For example, both alcohol and cocaine are hepatotoxic and combined use may increase risk for liver disease.[145,146] It is likely that polydrug abuse also increases risk for derangements of reproductive system function, and a high incidence of sexual dysfunction (62%) has been reported in men who abuse both cocaine and alcohol.[142]

Polydrug abuse appears to be an increasingly prevalent drug use pattern, thereby defying efforts to categorize women by use or abuse of a single drug. The attribution of teratogenic properties to any one drug in a multiple drug user is obviously hazardous. For example, maternal tobacco smoking, like alcohol abuse, is associated with low birth weight.[147,148] There is evidence that marijuana use during pregnancy can induce behavioral impairments in infants, decreased length of gestation and increased risk of abortion.[11,149,150] Unraveling the relative contributions of poor prenatal care, marginal medical status and chronic drug abuse to fetal developmental anomalies and behavioral impairments presents a formidable challenge. From a public health perspective, drug avoidance may be extremely important for a successful pregnancy and a healthy baby.[7] From a scientific perspective, understanding how drugs compromise fetal development through direct toxic effects or through impairment of maternal health and disruption of maternal hormonal balance remains an important and increasingly timely question.

SUMMARY

Alcohol abuse and alcoholism are associated with a broad spectrum of reproductive system disorders. Amenorrhea, anovulation, luteal phase dysfunction, and ovarian pathology may occur in alcohol-dependent women and alcohol abusers. Luteal phase dysfunction, anovulation and persistent hyperprolactinemia have also been observed in social drinkers studied under clinical research ward conditions. The mechanisms underlying alcohol-related disruptions of the hypothalamic-pituitary-ovarian-adrenal axis are unknown. The reproductive consequences of alcohol abuse and alcoholism range from infertility and increased risk for spontaneous abortion to impaired fetal growth and development. Recent studies of alcohol's effects on pituitary gonadotropins and on gonadal, steroid and adrenal hormones in women are reviewed. Research on the acute effects of alcohol on opioid antagonist and synthetic LHRH-stimulated pituitary gonadotropins is summarized. The implications of alcohol's effects on reproductive hormones for impairment of fetal growth and development are discussed.

REFERENCES

1. BOWDEN, D. M., P. S. WEATHERSBEE, S. K. CLARREN, C. E. FAHRENBRUCH, B. L. GOODLIN & S. A. CAFFERY. 1983. A periodic dosing model of fetal alcohol syndrome in the pig-tailed macaque (Macaca nemestrina). Am. J. Primatol. **4:** 143-157.
2. Food and Drug Administration. 1981. Surgeon General's advisory on alcohol and pregnancy. FDA Drug Bull. **11:** 9-10.
3. STREISSGUTH, A. F., S. LANDESMAN-DWYER, J. C. MARTIN & D. W. SMITH. 1980. Teratogenic effects of alcohol in humans and laboratory animals. Science **209:** 353-361.
4. RANDALL, C. L. & E. NOBLE. 1980. Alcohol abuse and fetal growth and development. *In* Advances in Substance Abuse, Behavioral and Biological Research. N. K. Mello, Ed. Vol. 1: 327-367. JAI Press. Greenwich, CT.
5. CLARREN, S. K. & D. M. BOWDEN. 1982. Fetal alcohol syndrome: A new primate model for binge drinking and its relevance to human ethanol teratogenesis. J. Pediatr. **101:** 819-824.
6. CLARREN, S. K., S. J. ASTLEY & D. M. BOWDEN. 1988. Physical anomalies and developmental delays in nonhuman primate infants exposed to weekly doses of ethanol during gestation. Teratology **37**(6): 561-569.
7. BEELEY, L. 1986. Adverse effects of drugs in the first trimester of pregnancy. Clinics Obstet. Gynecol. **13**(2): 177-195.
8. HUTCHINGS, D. E. *et al.* 1989. This volume.

9. ABEL, E. L. 1984. Prenatal effects of alcohol. Drug Alcohol Depend. **14:** 1-10.
10. ANDERSON, R. A. 1981. Endocrine balance as a factor in the etiology of the fetal alcohol syndrome. Neurobehav. Toxicol. Teratol. **3:** 89-104.
11. SMITH, C. G. & R. H. ASCH. 1987. Drug abuse and reproduction. Fertil. Steril. **48**(3): 355-373.
12. ABEL, E. L. & R. J. SOKOL. 1987. Incidence of fetal alcohol syndrome and economic impact of FAS-related anomalies. Drug Alcohol Depend. **19:** 51-70.
13. Alcohol & Health. Fifth Special Report to the U. S. Congress on Alcohol and Health from the Secretary of Health and Human Services, 1984. DHHS Publ. No. (ADM) 84-1291. U.S. Government Printing Office. Washington, DC.
14. MYERS, J. K., M. M. WEISSMAN, G. L. TISCHLER, C. E. HOLZER, P. J. LEAF, H. ORVASCHEL, J. C. ANTHONY, J. H. BOYD, J. D. BURKE, M. KRAMMER & R. STOLTZMAN. 1984. Six month prevalence of psychiatric disorders in three communities. Arch. Gen. Psychiatry **41:** 959-967.
15. MENDELSON, J. H., T. F. BABOR, N. K. MELLO & H. PRATT. 1986. Alcoholism and prevalence of medical and psychiatric disorders. J. Stud. Alcohol. **47:** 361-366.
16. CICERO, T. J. 1980. Common mechanisms underlying the effects of ethanol and the narcotics on neuroendocrine function. *In* Advances in Substance Abuse, Behavioral and Biological Research. N. K. Mello, Ed. Vol. 1: 201-254. JAI Press. Greenwich, CT.
17. MELLO, N. K. 1980. Some behavioral and biological aspects of alcohol problems in women. *In* Alcohol and Drug Problems in Women: Research Advances in Alcohol and Drug Problems. O. J. Kalant, Ed. Vol 5: 263-298. Plenum Press. New York, NY.
18. MELLO, N. K. 1988. Effects of alcohol abuse on reproductive function in women. *In* Recent Developments in Alcoholism. M. Galanter, Ed. Vol. 6: 253-276. Plenum Press. New York, NY.
19. VAN THIEL, D. H. & J. S. GAVALER. 1982. The adverse effects of ethanol upon hypothalamic-pituitary gonadal function in males and females compared and contrasted. Alcohol. Clin. Exp. Res. **6:** 179-185.
20. MENDELSON, J. H. & N. K. MELLO. 1979. Biologic concomitants of alcoholism. N. Engl. J. Med. **301:** 912-921.
21. BOYDEN, T. W. & R. W. PAMENTER. 1983. Effects of ethanol on the male hypothalamic-pituitary-gonadal axis. Endocr. Rev. **4:** 389-395.
22. NOTH, R. H. & R. M. WALTER, JR. 1984. The effects of alcohol on the endocrine system. Med. Clin. North Am. **68:** 133-146.
23. ELLINGBOE, J. & C. C. VARANELLI. 1979. Ethanol inhibits testosterone biosynthesis by direct action on Leydig cells. Res. Commun. Chem. Pathol. Pharmacol. **24:** 87-102.
24. CICERO, T. J. 1982. Alcohol-induced deficits in the hypothalamic-pituitary-luteinizing hormone axis in the male. Alcohol. Clin. Exp. Res. **6**(2): 207-215.
25. CHIAO, Y.-B. & D. H. VAN THIEL. 1983. Biochemical mechanisms that contribute to alcohol-induced hypogonadism in the male. Alcohol. Clin. Exp. Res. **7:** 131-134.
26. HUGUES, J. N., T. COSTE, G. PERRET, M. S. JAYLE, J. SEBAOUN & E. MODIGLIANI. 1980. Hypothalamo-pituitary ovarian function in 31 women with chronic alcoholism. Clin. Endocrinol. **12:** 543-551.
27. MOSKOVIC, S. 1975. Effect of chronic alcohol intoxication on ovarian dysfunction. Srp. Arh. Celok. Lek. **103:** 751-758.
28. RYBACK, R. S. 1977. Chronic alcohol consumption and menstruation. J. Am. Med. Assoc. **238:** 2143.
29. VALIMAKI, M., R. PELKONEN, M. SALASPORO, M. HARKONEN, E. HIRVONEN & R. YLIKAHRI. 1984. Sex hormones in amenorrheic women with alcoholic liver disease. J. Clin. Endocrinol. Metab. **59:** 133-138.
30. GAVALER, J. S. 1985 A review of alcohol effects on endocrine function in postmenopausal women: What we know, what we need to know, and what we do not yet know. J. Stud. Alcohol. **46:** 495-516.
31. GAVALER, J. S. 1988. Effects of moderate consumption of alcoholic beverages on endocrine function in post-menopausal women: Bases for hypotheses. *In* Recent Developments in Alcoholism. M. Galanter, Ed. Vol. 6: 229-251. Plenum Press. New York, NY.
32. MELLO, N. K., M. P. BREE, J. H. MENDELSON & J. ELLINGBOE. 1983. Alcohol self-

administration disrupts reproductive function in female Macaque monkeys. Science **221**: 677-679.

33. MELLO, N. K., J. H. MENDELSON, N. W. KING, M. P. BREE, A. SKUPNY & J. ELLINGBOE. 1988. Alcohol self-administration by female macaque monkey: A model for study of alcohol dependence, hyperprolactinemia and amenorrhea. J. Stud. Alcohol. **49**: 551-560.
34. SANCHIS, R., A. ESQUIFINO & C. GUERRI. 1985. Chronic ethanol intake modifies estrous cyclicity and alters prolactin and LH levels. Pharmacol. Biochem. Behav. **23**: 221-224.
35. ESKAY, R. L., R. S. RYBACK, M. GOLDMAN & E. MAJCHROWICZ. 1981. Effect of chronic ethanol administration on plasma levels of LH and the estrous cycle in the female rat. Alcohol. Clin. Exp. Res. **5**: 204-206.
36. KRUEGER, W. A., J. B. WALTER & P. K. RUDEEN. 1983. Estrous cyclicity in rats fed an ethanol diet for 4 months. Pharmacol. Biochem. Behav. **19**: 583-585.
37. VAN THIEL, D. H., J. S. GAVALER & R. LESTER. 1978. Alcohol-induced ovarian failure in the rat. J. Clin. Invest. **61**: 624-632.
38. GAVALER, J. S., D. H. VAN THIEL & R. LESTER. 1980. Ethanol: A gonadal toxin in the mature rat of both sexes. Alcohol. Clin. Exp. Res. **4**: 271-276.
39. MENDELSON, J. H. & N. K. MELLO. 1988. Chronic alcohol effects on anterior pituitary and ovarian hormones in healthy women. J. Pharmacol. Exp. Ther. **245**: 407-412.
40. JUNG, Y. & A. B. RUSSFIELD. 1972. Prolactin cells in the hypophysis of cirrhotic patients. Arch. Pathol. **94**: 265-269.
41. CROWLEY, W. F., JR., M. FILICORI, D. I. SPRATT & N. F. SANTORO. 1985. The physiology of gonadotropin-releasing hormone (GnRH) secretion in men and women. Recent Prog. Horm. Res. **41**: 473-526.
42. SANTORO, N., M. FILICORI & W. F. CROWLEY, JR. 1986. Hypogonadotropic disorders in men and women: Diagnosis and therapy with pulsatile low-dose gonadotropin-releasing hormone. Endocr. Rev **7**: 11-23.
43. HURLEY, D. M., R. BRIAN, K. OUTCH, J. STOCKDALE, A. FRY, C. HACKMAN, I. CLARKE & H. G. BURGER. 1984. Induction of ovulation and fertility in amenorrheic women by pulsatile low-dose gonadotropin-releasing hormone. N. Engl. J. Med. **310**: 1069-1074.
44. HAMMOND, C., R. H. WIEBE, A. F. HANEY & S. G. YANCY. 1979. Ovulation induction with luteinizing hormone-releasing hormone in amenorrheic infertile women. Am. J. Obstet. Gynecol. **135**: 924.
45. LEYENDECKER, G. & L. WILDT. 1984. Pulsatile administration of GnRH in hypothalamic amenorrhea. Upsala J. Med. Sci. **89**: 19.
46. DIZEREGA, G. S. & G. D. HODGEN. 1981. Luteal phase dysfunction infertility: A sequel to aberrant folliculogenesis. Fertil. Steril. **35**: 489-499.
47. GOODMAN, A. L. & G. D. HODGEN. 1983. The ovarian triad of the primate menstrual cycle. Recent Prog. Horm. Res. **39**: 1-67.
48. SHERMAN, B. M. & S. G. KORENMAN. 1974. Measurement of plasma LH, FSH, estradiol and progesterone in disorders of the human menstrual cycle: The short luteal phase. J. Clin. Endocrinol. Metab. **38**: 89-93.
49. HALMESMAKI, E., I. AUTTI, M.-L. GRANSTROM, U.-H. STENMAN & O. YLIKORKALA. 1987. Estradiol, estriol, progesterone, prolactin, and human chorionic gonadotropin in pregnant women with alcohol abuse. J. Clin. Endocrinol. Metab. **64**: 153-156.
50. WILSNACK, S. C., A. D. KLASSEN & R. W. WILSNACK. 1984. Drinking and reproductive dysfunction among women in a 1981 national survey. Alcohol. Clin. Exp. Res. **8**: 451-458.
51. MELLO, N. K. & J. H. MENDELSON. 1972. Drinking patterns during work-contingent and non-contingent alcohol acquisition. Psychosom. Med. **34**: 139-164.
52. YEN, S. S. C. 1983. Clinical applications of gonadotropin-releasing hormone and gonadotropin-releasing hormone analogs. Fertil. Steril. **39**: 257-266.
53. YEN, S. S. C., M. E. QUIGLEY, R. L. REID, J. F. ROPERT & N. S. CETEL. 1985. Neuroendocrinology of opioid peptides and their role in the control of gonadotropin and prolactin secretion. Am. J. Obstet. Gynecol. **4**: 485-493.
54. REBAR, R. W. 1986. Practical evaluation of hormonal status. *In* Reproductive Endocrinology: Physiology, Pathophysiology and Clinical Management. 2nd edit. S. S. C. Yen & R. B. Jaffe, Eds.: 683-733. W. B. Saunders. Philadelphia, PA.

55. MARTIN, J. B. & S. REICHLIN, Eds. 1987. Clinical Neuroendocrinology. 2nd edit. F. A. Davis. Philadelphia, PA.

56. MURAD, F. & R. C. HAYNES. 1985. Adenohypophyseal hormones and related substances. In The Pharmacological Basis of Therapeutics. 7th edit. A. G. Gilman. L. S. Goodman, T. W. Rall & F. Murad, Eds.: 1362-1368. Macmillan. New York, NY.

57. MURAD, F. & R. C. HAYNES. 1985. Estrogens and progestins. In The Pharmacological Basis of Therapeutics. 7th edit. A. G. Gilman, L. S. Goodman, A. Gilman, T. W. Rall & F. Murad, Eds.: 1412-1439. Macmillan. New York, NY.

58. FILICORI, M., N. SANTORO, G. R. MERRIAM & W. F. CROWLEY, JR. 1986. Characterization of the physiological pattern of episodic gonadotropin secretion throughout the human menstrual cycle. J. Clin. Endocrinol. Metab. 62: 1136-1144.

59. MELLO, N. K., J. H. MENDELSON, M. P. BREE & A. S. T. SKUPNY. 1986. Alcohol effects on LHRH stimulated LH and FSH in female rhesus monkeys. J. Pharmacol. Exp. Ther. 236: 590-595.

60. MELLO, N. K., J. H. MENDELSON, M. P. BREE & A. SKUPNY. 1986. Alcohol effects on LHRH-stimulated LH and FSH in ovariectomized female rhesus monkeys. J. Pharmacol. Exp. Ther. 239: 693-700.

61. PHIPPS, W. R., S. E. LUKAS, J. H. MENDELSON, J. ELLINGBOE, S. L. PALMIERI & I. SCHIFF. 1987. Acute ethanol administration enhances plasma testosterone levels following gonadotropin stimulation in men. Psychoneuroendocrinology 12: 459-465.

62. MENDELSON, J. H., J. ELLINGBOE, J. C. KUEHNLE & N. K. MELLO. 1979. Effects of naltrexone on mood and neuroendocrine function in normal adult males. Psychoneuroendocrinology 3: 231-236.

63. MIRIN, S. M., J. H. MENDELSON, J. ELLINGBOE & R. E. MEYER. 1976. Acute effects of heroin and naltrexone on testosterone and gonadotropin secretion: A pilot study. Psychoneuroendocrinology 1: 359-369.

64. MORLEY, J. E., N. G. BARANETSKY, T. D. WINGERT, H. E. CARLSON, J. M. HERSHMAN, S. MELMED, S. R. LEVIN, K. R. JAMISON, R. WEITZMAN, R. J. CHANG & A. A. VARNER. 1980. Endocrine effects of naloxone-induced opiate receptor blockade. J. Clin. Endocrinol. Metab. 50: 252-257.

65. MENDELSON, J. H., N. K. MELLO, P. CRISTOFARO, A. SKUPNY & J. ELLINGBOE. 1986. Use of naltrexone as a provocative test for hypothalamic-pituitary hormone function. Pharmacol. Biochem. Behav. 24: 309-313.

66. SHERMAN, B. M. 1984. Hypothalamic control of the menstrual cycle: Implications for the study of anorexia nervosa. In Neuroendocrinology and Psychiatric Disorders. G. M. Brown, S. H. Koslow & S. Reichlin, Eds: 315-323. Raven Press. New York, NY.

67. FRISCH, R. E. 1982. Fatness, puberty, menstrual periodicity and fertility. In Clinical Reproductive Neuroendocrinology. J. L. Vaitukaitis, Ed.: 105-135. Elsevier. New York, NY.

68. FRISCH, R. E. & J. W. MCARTHUR. 1974. Menstrual cycles: Fatness as a determinant of minimum weight for height necessary for their maintenance or onset. Science 185: 949-951.

69. MCARTHUR, J. W., B. A. BULLEN, I. Z. BEITINS, M. PAGANO, T. M. BADGER & A. KLIBANSKI. 1980. Hypothalamic amenorrhea in runners of normal body composition. Endocrinol. Res. Commun. 7: 13.

70. KNOBIL, E. 1974. On the control of gonadotropin secretion in the rhesus monkey. Recent Prog. Horm. Res. 30: 1-46.

71. KNOBIL, E. 1980. The neuroendocrine control of the menstrual cycle. Recent Prog. Horm. Res. 36: 53-88.

72. KNOBIL, E. & J. HOTCHKISS. 1988. The menstrual cycle and its neuroendocrine control. In The Physiology of Reproduction. E. Knobil, J. N. Neill, L. L. Ewing, G. S. Greenwald, C. L. Makert & D. W. Pfaff, Eds. Vol. 2: 1971-1994. Raven Press. New York, NY.

73. REAME, N. E., S. E. SAUDER, G. D. CASE, R. P. KELCH & J. C. MARSHALL. 1985. Pulsatile gonadotropin secretion in women with hypothalamic amenorrhea: Evidence that reduced frequency of gonadotropin-releasing hormone secretion is the mechanism of persistent anovulation. J. Clin. Endocrinol. Metab. 61: 851-852.

74. SANTORO, M., M. E. WIESMAN, M. FILICORI, J. WALDSTREICKER & W. F. CROWLEY, JR. 1986. Intravenous administration of pulsatile gonadotropin-releasing hormone in hypothalamic amenorrhea: Effects of dosage. J. Clin. Endocrinol. Metab. **61:** 109-116.

75. BUCHANAN, G. C. & D. R. TREDWAY. 1979. Hyperprolactinemia and ovulatory dysfunction. *In* Human Ovulation. E. S. E. Hafez, Ed.: 255-277. Elsevier/North Holland. New York, NY.

76. SAUDER, S. E., M. FRAGER, G. D. CASE, R. P. KELCH & J. C. MARSHALL. 1984. Abnormal patterns of pulsatile luteinizing hormone secretion in women with hyperprolactinemia and amenorrhea: Responses to bromocriptine. J. Clin. Endocrinol. Metab. **59:** 941-948.

77. TOLIS, G. 1980. Prolactin: Physiology and pathology. *In* Neuroendocrinology. D. T. Krieger & J. C. Hughes, Ed.: 321-328. Sinauer Associates. Sunderland, MA.

78. DHONT, M. & D. VANDEKERCKHOVE. 1984. Prolactin secretion in normoprolactinaemic amenorrhea. *In* First Symposium of the European Neuroendocrine Association. E. delPozo & E. Fluckiger, Eds. Abstract 163. Basle.

79. JAFFE, R. B. & W. R. KEYE. 1974. Estradiol augmentation of pituitary responsiveness to gonadotropoin-releasing hormone in women. J. Clin. Endocrinol. Metab. **39:** 850-855.

80. EDWARDS, C. R. W. & C. M. FEEK. 1981. Prolactinemia: A question of rational treatment. Br. Med. J. **283:** 1561-1562.

81. TOLIS, G., M. SOMMA, J. VAN CAMPENHOUT & H. FRIESEN. 1974. Prolactin secretion in sixty-five patients with galactorrhea. Am. J. Obstet. Gynecol. **118:** 91-101.

82. VALIMAKI, M., M. HARKONEN & R. YLIKAHRI. 1983. Acute effects of alcohol on female sex hormones. Alcohol. Clin. Exp. Res. **7:** 289-293.

83. MENDELSON, J. H., N. K. MELLO & J. ELLINGBOE. 1981. Acute alcohol intake and pituitary gonadal hormones in normal human females. J. Pharmacol. Exp. Ther. **218:** 23-26.

84. ELLINGBOE, J., J. H. MENDELSON, J. C. KUEHNLE, A. S. T. SKUPNY & K. D. MILLER. 1980. Effect of acute ethanol ingestion on integrated plasma prolactin levels in normal men. Pharmacol. Biochem. Behav. **12:** 297-301.

85. VALIMAKI, M. J., M. HARKONEN, C. J. P. ERIKSSON & R. H. YLIKAHRI. 1984. Sex hormones and adrenocortical steroids in men acutely intoxicated with alcohol. Alcohol **1:** 89-93.

86. REDEI, E., B. J. BRANCH & A. N. TAYLOR. 1986. Direct effect of ethanol on adrenocorticotropic (ACTH) release *in vitro*. J. Pharmacol. Exp. Ther. **237:** 59-64.

87. RIVIER, C., T. BRUHN & W. VALE. 1984. Effect of ethanol on the hypothalamic-pituitary-adrenal axis in the rat: Role of corticotropin-releasing factor (CRF). J. Pharmacol. Exp. Ther. **229:** 127-131.

88. RIVIER, C., J. RIVIER & W. VALE. 1986. Stress-induced inhibition of reproductive functions: Role of endogenous corticotropin-releasing factor. Science **31:** 607-609.

89. OLSTER, D. H. & M. FERIN. 1987. Corticotropin-releasing hormone inhibits gonadotropin secretion in the ovariectomized rhesus monkey. J. Clin. Endocrinol. Metab. **65(2):** 262-267.

90. XIAO, E. & M. FERIN. 1988. The inhibitory action of corticotropin-releasing hormone on gonadotropin secretion in the ovariectomized rhesus monkey is not mediated by adrenocorticotropic hormone. Biol. Reprod. **38:** 763-767.

91. PETRAGLIA, F., S. SUTTON, W. VALE & P. PLOTSKY. 1987. Corticotropin-releasing factor decreases plasma luteinizing hormone levels in female rats by inhibiting gonadotropin-releasing hormone release into hypophysial-portal circulation. Endocrinology **120:** 1083-1088.

92. ROSS, G. T. 1985. Disorders of the ovary and female reproductive tract. *In* Williams Textbook of Endocrinology. 7th edit. J. D. Wilson & D. W. Foster, Eds.: 106-258. W. B. Saunders. Philadelphia, PA.

93. DiZEREGA, G. S. & J. W. WILKS. 1984. Inhibition of the primate ovarian cycle by a porcine follicular fluid protein (s). Fertil. Steril. **41:** 635-638.

94. WILKS, J. W., G. D. HODGEN & G. T. ROSS. 1977. Anovulatory menstrual cycles in the rhesus monkeys, the significance of serum, follicle stimulating hormone/luteinizing hormone ratios. Fertil. Steril. **28:** 1094-1100.

95. HODGEN, G. D. 1982. The dominant ovarian follicle. Fertil. Steril. **38**: ;281-300.
96. CHANNING, C. P., W. L. GORDON, W.-K. LIU & D. N. WARD. 1985. Physiology and biochemistry of ovarian inhibin. Proc. Soc. Exp. Biol. Med. **178**: 339-361.
97. MCLACHLAN, R. I., D. M. ROBERTSON, D. L. HEALY, H. G. BURGER & D. M. DE KRETSER. 1987. Circulating immunoreactive inhibin levels during the normal human menstrual cycle. J. Clin. Endocrinol. Metab. **65**: 954-961.
98. DIERSCHKE, D. J., R. J. HUTZ & R. C. WOLF. 1985. Induced follicular atresia in rhesus monkeys. Strength-duration relationships of the estrogen stimulus. Endocrinology **117**: 1397-1403.
99. DIERSCHKE, D. J., R. J. HUTZ & R. C. WOLF. 1987. Atretogenic action of estrogen in rhesus monkeys: Effects of repeated treatment. Am. J. Primatology **12**: 251-261.
100. ZELEZNEK, A. J. 1981. Premature elevation of systemic estradiol reduces serum levels of FSH and lengthens the follicular phase of the menstrual cycle in rhesus monkeys. Endocrinology **109**: 352-355.
101. MENDELSON, J. H., N. K. MELLO, P. CRISTOFARO, J. ELLINGBOE, A. SKUPNY, S. L. PALMIERI, R. BENEDIKT & I. SCHIFF. 1987. Alcohol effects on naloxone-stimulated luteinizing hormone, prolactin and estradiol in women. J. Stud. Alcohol. **48**: 287-294.
102. TEOH, S. K., J. H. MENDELSON, N. K. MELLO & A. SKUPNY. 1988. Alcohol effects on naltrexone-induced stimulation of pituitary, adrenal, and gonadal hormones during the early follicular phase of the menstrual cycle. J. Clin. Endocrinol. Metab. **66**: 1181-1186.
103. MARSHALL, J. C., C. D. CASE, T. W. VALK, K. P. CORLEY, S. E. SAUNDER & R. P. KELCH. 1983. Selective inhibition of follicle-stimulating hormone secretion by estradiol. J. Clin. Invest. **71**: 248-257.
104. MENDELSON, J. H., S. E. LUKAS, N. K. MELLO, L. AMASS, J. ELLINGBOE & A. SKUPNY. 1988. Acute alcohol effects on plasma estradiol levels in women. Psychopharmacology **94**: 464-467.
105. MELLO, N. K., J. ELLINGBOE, M. P. BREE, K. L. HARVEY & J. H. MENDELSON. 1983. Alcohol effects on estradiol in female macaque monkeys. *In* Problems of Drug Dependence 1981. L. S. Harris, Ed. NIDA Research Monograph 43: 210-216. U. S. Government Printing Office. Washington, DC.
106. VAN THIEL, D. H. 1983. Ethanol: Its adverse effects upon the hypothalamic-pituitary-gonadal axis. J. Lab. Clin. Med. **101**: 21-23.
107. VAN THIEL, D. 1984. Ethyl alcohol and gonadal function. Physiology in medicine. Hosp. Prac. **19**: 152-158.
108. MELLO, N. K., J. H. MENDELSON, M. P. BREE, J. ELLINGBOE & A. S. T. SKUPNY. 1985. Alcohol effects on LH and testosterone in male macaque monkeys. J. Pharmacol. Exp. Ther. **223**: 588-596.
109. KARSCH, F. H., R. F. WEICK, W. R. BUTLER, D. J. DIERSCHKE, L. C. KREY, G. WEISS, J. HOTCHKISS, T. YAMAJI & E. KNOBIL. 1973. Induced LH surges in the rhesus monkey: Strength-duration characteristics of the estrogen stimulus. Endocrinology **91**: 1740-1747.
110. KREY, L. C., W. R. BUTLER, G. WEISS, R. F. WEICK, D. J. DIERSCHKE & E. KNOBIL. 1973. Influence of endogenous and exogenous gonadal steroids on the action of synthetic RF in the rhesus monkey. Excerpta Med. Int. Congr. Ser. **263**: 39-47.
111. LASLEY, B. L., C. F. WANG & S. S. C. YEN. 1975. The effects of estrogen and progesterone on the functional capacity of the gonadotrophs. J. Clin. Endocrinol. Metab. **1**: 820-831.
112. ARIMURA, A. & A. V. SCHALLY. 1971. Augmentation of pituitary responsiveness to LH-releasing hormone (LHRH) by estrogen. Proc. Soc. Exp. Biol. Med. **136**: 290-298.
113. CRONHOLM, T. & J. SJOVALL. 1968. Effect of ethanol on the concentrations of solvolyzable plasma steroids. Biochim. Biophys. Acta **152**: 233-236.
114. CRONHOLM, T., J. SJOVALL & K. SJOVALL. 1969. Ethanol induced increase of the ratio between hydroxy- and ketosteroids in human pregnancy plasma. Steroids **13**: 671-678.
115. MURONO, E. P. & V. FISCHER-SIMPSON. 1984. Ethanol directly increases dihydrotestosterone conversion to 5α-androstan-3β. 17β-diol and 5α-androstan-3α, 17β-diol in rat Leydig cells. Biochem. Biophys. Res. Commun. **121**: 558-565.
116. MURONO, E. P. & V. FISCHER-SIMPSON. 1985. Ethanol directly stimulates dihydrostestosterone conversion to 5α-androstan-3α, 17β-diol and 5α-androstan-3β, 17β-diol in rat liver. Life Sci. **26**: 1117-1124.

117. MENDELOFF, A. I. 1954. Effects of intravenous infusions of ethanol upon estimated hepatic blood flow in man. J. Clin. Invest. **33:** 1298-1302.
118. CASTENFORS, H., E. HULTMAN & B. JOSEPHSON. 1960. Effect of intravenous infusions of ethyl alcohol on estimated hepatic blood flow in man. J. Clin. Invest. **39:** 776-781.
119. STEIN, S. W., C. S. LIEBER, C. M. LEERY, G. R. CHERRICK & W. H. ABELMANN. 1963. The effect of ethanol upon systemic and hepatic blood flow in man. Am. J. Clin. Nutr. **13:** 68-74.
120. FORSANDER, O., N. RAIHA & H. SUMALAINEN. 1958. Alkoholoxydation and bildung von acetoacetat in normaler und glykogenarmer intaker rattenleber. Hoppe Seyler's Z. Physiol. Chem. **312:** 243-248.
121. SLATER, T. F., B. C. SAWYER & U. D. STRAULI. 1964. Changes in liver nucleotide concentrations in experimental liver injury. Biochem. J. **93:** 267-270.
122. Alcohol and Health. Sixth Special Report to the U.S. Congress on Alcohol and Health from the Secretary of Health and Human Services, 1987. DHHS Publ. No. (ADM) 87-1519. U.S. Government Printing Office. Washington, DC.
123. NORA, J. J., A. H. NORA, A. G. PERINCHIEF, J. W. INGRAM, A. K. FOUNTAIN & M. J. PETERSON. 1976. Congenital abnormalities and first-trimester exposure to progestogen/oestrogen. Lancet **1:** 313-314.
124. SCHARDEIN, J. L. 1980. Congenital abnormalities and hormones during pregnancy: A clinical review. Teratology **22:** 251-270.
125. HEINONEN, O. P., D. SLONE, R. R. MONSON, E. B. HOOK & S. SHAPIRO. 1977. Cardiovascular birth defects and antenatal exposure to female sex hormones. N. Engl. J. Med. **296:** 67-70.
126. SMITH, A. W. 1948. Diethylstilbesterol in prevention and treatment of complications of pregnancy. Am. J. Obstet. Gynecol. **56:** 821-834.
127. KAPLAN, N. M. 1959. Male pseudohermaphrodism: Report of a case, with observations on pathogenesis. N. Engl. J. Med. **261:** 641-644.
128. WEINBERG, J. & S. BEZIO. 1987. Alcohol-induced changes in pituitary-adrenal activity during pregnancy. Alcohol. Clin. Exp. Res. **11**(3): 274-280.
129. TAYLOR, A. N., B. J. BRANCH, S. LIU & N. KOKKA. 1982. Long-term effects of fetal ethanol exposure on pituitary-adrenal responses to stress. Pharmacol. Biochem. Behav. **16:** 585-590.
130. TAYLOR, A. N., B. J. BRANCH, S. LIU, A. F. WEICHMANN, M. A. HILL & N. KOKKA. 1981. Fetal exposure to ethanol enhances pituitary-adrenal and temperature responses to ethanol in adult rats. Alcohol. Clin. Exp. Res. **5:** 237-246.
131. TAYLOR, A. N., L. R. NELSON, B. J. BRANCH, N. KOKKA & R. E. POLAND. 1984. Altered stress responsiveness in adult rats exposed to ethanol *in utero:* Neuroendocrine mechanisms. *In* Mechanisms of Alcohol Damage *In Utero*. M. O'Connor, Ed.: 47-65. Ciba Found. Symp. 1095. Pitman. London.
132. CUMMING, D. C., M. E. QUIGLEY & S. S. C. YEN. 1983. Acute suppression of circulating testosterone levels by cortisol in men. J. Clin. Endocrinol. Metab. **57:** 671-673.
133. HARLAP, S. & P. H. SHIONO. 1980. Alcohol, smoking, and incidence of spontaneous abortions in the first and second trimester. Lancet **2:** 173-176.
134. KLINE, J., Z. STEIN, P. SHROUT, M. SUSSER & D. WARBURTON. 1980. Drinking during pregnancy and spontaneous abortion. Lancet **2:** 176-180.
135. WARNER, R. H. & H. L. ROSETT. 1975. Effects of drinking on offspring: An historical survey of the American and British literature. J. Stud. Alcohol. **36:** 1395-1420.
136. JONES, K. L., D. W. SMITH, C. N. ULLELAND & A. P. STREISSGUTH. 1973. Pattern of malformation in offspring of chronic alcoholic mothers. Lancet **1:** 1267-1271.
137. SOKOL, R. J., S. I. MILLER & G. REED. 1980. Alcohol abuse during pregnancy: An epidemiologic study. Alcohol. Clin. Exp. Res. **4:** 135-145.
138. MENDELSON, J. H. 1987. Marijuana. *In* Psychopharmacology: The Third Generation of Progess. H. Y. Meltzer, Ed.: 1565-1571. Raven Press. New York, NY.
139. BRAUDE, M. C. & J. P. LUDFORD, Eds. 1984. Marijuana Effects on the Endocrine and Reproductive Systems. RAUS Review Report. NIDA Research Monograph 44, DHEW Publ. No. (ADM) 84-1278. U.S. Government Printing Office. Washington, DC.
140. STOFFER, S. S. 1968. A gynecologic study of drug addicts. Am. J. Obstet. Gynecol. **101**(6): 779-783.

141. COCORES, J. A., C. A. DACKIS & M. S. GOLD. 1986. Sexual dysfunction secondary to cocaine abuse in two patients. J. Clin. Psychiatry **47:** 384-385.
142. COCORES, J. A., N. S. MILLER, A. C. POTTASH & M. S. GOLD. 1988. Sexual dysfunction in abusers of cocaine and alcohol. Am. J. Drug Alcohol Abuse **14:** 169-173.
143. DACKIS, C. A. & M. S. GOLD. 1985. Pharmacological approaches to cocaine addiction. J. Subst. Abuse Treat. **2:** 139-145.
144. VAN DYKE, C. & R. BYCK. 1983. Cocaine use in man. *In* Advances in Substance Abuse, Behavioral and Biological Research. N. K. Mello, Ed. Vol. 3: 1-24. JAI Press. Greenwich, CT.
145. KREEK, M. J. 1987. Multiple drug abuse patterns and medical consequences. *In* Psychopharmacology: The Third Generation of Progress. H. Y. Meltzer, Ed.: 1597-1604. Raven Press. New York, NY.
146. KREEK, M. J. 1989. Multiple drug abuse patterns: Recent trends and associated medical consequences. *In* Advances in Substance Abuse, Behavioral and Biological Research. N. K. Mello, Ed. Vol. 4. JAI Press. Greenwich, CT. In press.
147. KING, J. C. & S. FABRO. 1983. Alcohol consumption and cigarette smoking: Effect on pregnancy. Clin. Obstet. Gynecol. **26:** 437-448.
148. WRIGHT, J. T., K. D. MACRAE, I. G. BARRISON & E. J. WATERSON. 1984. Effects of moderate alcohol consumption and smoking on fetal outcome. Ciba Found. Symp. **105:** 240-253.
149. FRIED, P. A., B. WATKINSON & A. WILLAN. 1984. Marijuana use during pregnancy and decreased length of gestation. Am. J. Obstet. Gynecol. **150:** 23.
150. ASCH, R. H. & C. G. SMITH. 1987. Effects of delta-9-tetrahydrocannabinol, the principal psychoactive component of marijuana, during pregnancy in the rhesus monkey. J. Reprod. Med. **31:** 1071-1081.

Maternal AIDS: Effects on Mother and Infant

KENNETH C. RICH

Department of Pediatrics (M/C 856)
University of Illinois at Chicago College of Medicine
840 South Wood Street
Chicago, Illinois 60212

HIV infection is a serious and increasingly frequent consequence of maternal substance abuse. Nearly one infant in fifty born in inner-city New York is HIV-infected and a majority of the infected women are either intravenous (iv) substance abusers or have sexual partners who are iv substance abusers.[1] Although the rate of infection is much lower in many parts of the country, the high risk of transmission of the infection to an infant, the high mortality and the close association with substance abuse makes this disease an important topic in discussion of the effects of maternal substance abuse on infants.

Epidemiology

Description of the magnitude of the problem of HIV infection in pregnant women has been hampered by a lack of objective data gathered without selection bias. Recently, an anonymous seroprevalence study of newborn sera in the Commonwealth of Massachusetts showed that 1 of every 476 women (2.1 per 1000) was positive for HIV antibody. The seroprevalence varied according to the type and location of the hospitals were the samples were obtained, ranging from 8.0 per 1000 in inner-city hospitals to 0.9 per 1000 in suburban and rural hospitals.[2] The proportion of these who are iv substance abusers is unknown although among women who are reported to the Center for Disease Control (CDC) with fully developed AIDS. 52% are substance abusers and an additional 26% have sexual contact with an iv drug user.[3]

In addition to being spread through iv substance abuse, HIV infection is a sexually transmitted disease and affects some segments of the population more heavily than others. In the population of young adult men and women entering the armed forces from a high endemic area, the rate of infection is similar between the sexes (male to female, 10.6 to 8.3 per 1000, respectively).[4] It affects minority populations more than the white majority. When adjusted for population size, the rates of AIDS are much higher in black and Hispanic women than in whites (13 and 11 times, respectively),[5] undoubtedly reflecting societal ills such as poverty and impediments to medical care.

Over one thousand infants and children have been reported to the CDC as patients with AIDS. The prevalence of asymptomatic HIV infection excluding AIDS is surely far greater but no reliable estimates are available. Estimates of the rates of transmission from mother to infant have ranged from a low of 20% of all infants being infected to a high of 65% of infants infected if the mother has had one or more infected infants previously.[6,7] The applicability of data from these studies to the general population, however, is suspect because most of the studies suffer from the lack of sufficient numbers of patients and from a selection bias that emphasizes symptomatic patients. Some idea of the rate of transmission, however, can be gleaned from a preliminary European study showing that up to 75% of infants born to HIV-infected women lose their HIV antibodies by one year of age, implying an infection rate of 25% or greater.[6]

HIV Infection in Women

Factors Affecting Infection and Outcome

The most common risk factors in women for the acquisition of HIV infection are iv substance abuse and having a sexual partner who is HIV infected and/or an iv substance abuser. From epidemiological studies, it has been found that survival in AIDS patients is determined by a number of factors including substance abuse history, race, age and AIDS-related illness history. Survival of substance abusers is reduced in both men and women but there is a complex interplay of the other factors that help determine outcome. From these studies, a profile of patients with particularly short survival can be obtained. For example, mean conditional survival duration in black substance abusing women with a history of pneumocystis pneumonia is roughly 1/4 that of a white gay male with Kaposi's sarcoma (206 and 810 days, respectively).[8] Undoubtedly social and other factors are important in determining the shorter survival, but they remain to be defined in future studies.

We can speculate on the explanations for the adverse effect of substance abuse on survival. Some of the drugs of abuse themselves reduce immune function. For example, natural killer activity, phagocyte function and T-cells are reduced in human experimental opiate use,[9-11] while alcohol abuse causes a myriad of adverse effects, particularly on phagocyte function.[12] In addition, drug use and its surrounding behaviors and stresses indirectly affect immune function through the neuroendocrine connection with the immune system. Finally, substance abuse is also associated with an increased exposure to toxic or infectious agents and with reduced use and access to medical care. These factors all may influence HIV infection and its outcome in women.

Pregnancy and HIV Infection

Early studies suggested that pregnancy was associated with progression of HIV infection and shortened survival.[13] In contrast, a series of patients in which drug use histories were matched between asymptomatic HIV-infected and noninfected women, found similar outcomes.[14] The study did not address the outcome in symptomatic patients and, indeed, it might be expected that pregnancy would have an adverse effect on HIV infection because of the modest reduction of immune function during pregnancy[15] and the observation that other infectious illnesses progress during pregnancy. Further, environmental stresses similar to those found during pregnancy may be associated with reduced immune function, although whether the magnitude of the changes is sufficient to be clinically important is unclear. Whether adverse consequences of pregnancy in the face of HIV infection can be altered by first or second trimester pregnancy termination remains to be determined.

Clinical Care of Women with HIV Infection

Clinical care of HIV-infected pregnant women is complicated by the complex psychosocial issues surrounding HIV infection, the major illnesses that can develop with the necessity of using drugs that can have an adverse effect on the fetus and the risk of nosocomial infection.

The psychosocial problems associated with HIV infection inevitably color the management of the women. Many women are first diagnosed as having HIV infection during pregnancy through prenatal voluntary screening programs. Notification of patients of their diagnosis is often associated with an initial increase in substance abuse behavior, with denial of the diagnosis and with thoughts of suicide. HIV-infected persons also encounter discrimination in the community over the perceived risk of transmission of the virus despite reports of the extremely low risk of casual transmission.[16]

Medical management of HIV-infected pregnant patients may be complex. Symptoms of progressive weight loss, anorexia and fatigue are commonly seen in early pregnancy.[17] These symptoms must be distinguished from signs of progression of HIV infection to prevent a delay in optimal management. Major infections such as Pneumocystis carinii pneumonia and toxoplasmosis can complicate the pregnancy. Unfortunately, little formal information is available on the safe use during pregnancy of drugs such as zidovudine for HIV infection or sulfamethoxazole and trimethoprim for Pneumocystis. Additionally, some infections in the mother such as cytomegalovirus and toxoplasmosis may have devastating consequences in the fetus.[18]

The risk of nosocomial infection during delivery has received considerable attention and is a source of concern for health care workers despite objective data documenting the low risk.[16] It has brought about recommendations for universal precautions in all patients in order to reduce the risk of spread from the patient who has not been HIV tested or the patient who is infected but has not yet made detectable antibodies.

Infants and HIV Infection

Factors Affecting Transmission and Progression

A number of factors may influence the development and progression of HIV infection in infants. The presence of symptoms in the mother during pregnancy carries an increased risk of infection in the infant.[6] The reason has not yet been elucidated. It is known that HIV antigen becomes detectable in advancing HIV infection,[19] and it can be speculated that free antigen in the mother's circulation may increase the risk of infection in the fetus.

It is likely that the fetus usually becomes infected during intrauterine life. This is based on finding infected fetuses in early or midtrimester abortions,[20] demonstration of HIV in cord blood[21] and infected infants from Caesarean section deliveries[22] as well as on the description of a fetopathy thought to be characteristic of infants exposed to HIV infection in utero (see below). Whether infection can occur in addition by exposure to HIV known to be present in blood and secretions in the birth canal[23] in a vaginal delivery is a matter for speculation until more definitive data are available. At present the data do not warrant routine Caesarean deliveries.[24]

HIV infection has also been reported to have been passed to an infant by breast feeding.[25] Breast milk can carry the virus in the cell free fraction.[26] It is also of interest that a monozygotic twin pair was born to an infected mother in which only one was infected.[27]

It is not known whether maternal drug use will reduce the fetal immune response, thereby possibly affecting the HIV infection and progression. In our preliminary studies, we found that infants exposed to iv administered drugs in utero which were primarily opiates, had an increased incidence of infections during the first year of life compared to those exposed to orally administered drugs or nondrug exposed.[28]

Diagnosis of HIV Infection in Infants

The diagnosis of HIV infection in infants is complicated by the presence of transplacentally acquired IgG anti-HIV antibodies. Since IgG has a half-life of roughly 21 days, the maternal antibody can remain detectable for considerable periods of time, particularly if a sensitive assay system is used. After infection, the production of antibody may also be delayed for weeks to months. Thus, an infant during the first year of life may initially have antibodies, lose them and later develop them again. It has also been found that some infants may have no antibody detectable by ELISA techniques but have detectable antibodies by Western blot and/or have antigen detectable.[29] Therefore, the CDC has recommended that, in the absence of a positive HIV culture or antigen assay or clinical evidence of fully developed AIDS, a diagnosis of HIV infection not be made until 15 months of age.

Other techniques are being evaluated to assist in the early diagnosis of HIV infection in the newborn. Some that may prove useful are IgM-Western blot assays[30] and assay of lymphocyte culture supernatants for secreted HIV antibodies.[31] Another promising technique is examination of lymphocytes for HIV genome by the very sensitive polymerase chain reaction.[32]

Clinical Manifestations of HIV Infection in Infants

The pattern of infections in infants varies from those observed in adults. Although the pattern of opportunistic infections and the nonspecific findings of fever and weight loss are similar between infants and adults, infants differ in an increased incidence of bacterial sepsis, the presence of lymphoid interstitial pneumonitis and the low risk of Kaposi's sarcoma.[33] An early immunologic manifestation of HIV infection is loss of ability to respond to neoantigens such as the standard bacterial toxoids[34] or unique antigens such as bacteriophage 0X174.[35] Therefore, infants are at risk for the development of recurrent bacterial sepsis due to defective ability to make a primary antibody response. In contrast, adults who have preexisting antibodies to the common antigens are often protected. Lymphoid interstitial pneumonitis is another manifestation seen rarely if ever in adult patients. Interstitial collections of lymphoid and plasmacytoid cells are seen as well as nodular aggregates of lymphoid cells with germinal centers.[36] Most malignancies that develop in HIV-infected children are lymphoreticular in origin such as non-Hodgkins lymphoma. The neurologic findings in children can include static or progressive encephalopathy with loss of developmental milestones or intellectual ability, progressive weakness with pyramidal tract signs and impaired brain growth. HIV antigen is frequently observed in the CSF as well as local production of antibodies to HIV.[37] An AIDS fetopathy has also been described with characteristic dysmorphic features.[38] However, further studies will need to be performed to ensure that the features are not those of an associated condition such as intrauterine drug exposure.

Treatment of HIV Infection in Infants and Children

The battery of treatment modalities available for the treatment of infants is limited. AZT is in the early stages of testing for children. Preliminary studies suggest improvement in clinical, immunologic and neuropsychologic status with acceptable toxicity.[39] Other supportive modalities may be indicated. Administration of immune serum globulin may help protect infants from infection with major bacterial and viral illnesses.

Prognosis of HIV Infection in Infants and Children

Little data is available on the prognosis. A rough indication of the prognosis can be gleaned by New York City data on the age of death of patients diagnosed as having pediatric AIDS.[40] It was found that 50% died by the age of 15 months while 15% were still alive at 5 years of age. The factors that influence prognosis have also been poorly described. It has been shown that those who develop lymphoid interstitial pneumonitis have a better overall prognosis than those who develop Pneumocystis carinii pneumonia. Similarly, a better prognosis is seen in patients who have specific antigen reactivity in *in vitro* blastogenic assays compared to those who do not.[41]

CONCLUSIONS

It has been only a few years that HIV infection has been present in the general community. It is now spreading more into the heterosexual community using the vehicle of iv drug use. A special segment of the newly affected population are women and their infants who present major medical and psychosocial challenges. There are wide gaps in our knowledge of the risks and factors affecting vertical transmission of HIV infection and optimal medical management of the mother and infant dyad. It is the challenge of this era to provide quality, compassionate care for the ever increasing number of these patients.

REFERENCES

1. LANDSMAN, S., H. MINKOFF, S. HOLMAN, S. MCCALLA, & O. SIJIN. 1987. Serosurvey of human immunodeficiency virus in parturients. J. Am. Med. Assoc. **258:** 2701-2703.
2. HOFF, R., V. P. BERARDI, B. J. WEIBLEN, L. MAHONEY-TROUT, M. L. MITCHESS & G. F. GRADY. 1988. Seroprevalence of human immunodeficiency virus among childbearing women: Estimation by testing samples of blood from newborns. N. Engl. J. Med. **318:** 525-530.
3. GUINAN, M. E. & A. HARDY. 1987. Epidemiology of AIDS in women in the United States: 1981 through 1986. J. Am. Med. Assoc. **257:** 2039-2042.
4. BURKE, D. S., J. F. BRUNDAGE, W. BERNIER et al. 1987. Demography of HIV infections among civilian applicants for military service in four counties in New York City. N. Y. State J. Med. **87:** 262-264.
5. Center for Disease Control. 1986. Acquired immunodeficiency syndrome (AIDS) among black and Hispanics—United States. Morbidity and Mortality Weekly Report **35:** 655-666.
6. MOK, J. Q., C. GIAQUINTO, A. DEROSSI, I. GROSCH-WORNER, A. E. ADES & C. S. PECKHAM. 1987. Infants born to mothers seropositive for human immunodeficiency virus: Preliminary findings from a multicentre European study. Lancet **1:** 1164-1168.
7. WILLOUGHBY, A., H. MENDEZ, H. MINKOFF et al. 1987. Human immune deficiency virus in pregnant women and their offspring. Presented at the Third International Conference on AIDS, Washington, DC. June 1-5.
8. ROTHENBERG, R., M. WOELFEL, R. STONEBURNER, J. MILBERG, R. PARKER & B. TRUMAN. 1987. Survival with the acquired immunodeficiency syndrome: Experience with 5833 cases in New York City. N. Engl. J. Med. **317:** 1297-1302.
9. MCDONOUGH, R. J., J. J. MADDEN, A. FALEK, D. A. SHAFER, M. PLINE, D. GORDON, P. BOKOS, J. O. KUEHNLE & J. MENDELSON. 1980. Alteration of T and null lymphocyte frequencies in the peripheral blood of human opiate addicts: in vivo evidence for opiate receptor sites on T lymphocytes. J. Immunol. **125:** 2539-2543.
10. POLI, G., M. INTRONA, F. ZANABONI, G. PERI, M. CARBONARI, F. AUTI, A. LAZZARIN, M. MORONI & A. MANTOVANI. 1985. Natural killer cells in intravenous drug abuse with lymphadenopathy syndrome. Clin. Exp. Immunol. **62:** 128-135.
11. TUBARO, E., U. AVICO, C. SANTIANGELI, P. ZUCCARO, G. CAVALLO, R. PACIFICI, C. CROCE & G. BORELLI. 1985. Morphine and methadone impact on human phagocytic physiology. Int. J. Immunopharmacol. **7:** 865-874.
12. MACGREGOR, R. R., M. SAFFORD & M. SHALIT. 1988. Effect of ethanol on functions required for the delivery of neutrophils to sites of inflammation. J. Infect. Dis. **157:** 682-689.
13. SCOTT, G. B., M. A. FISCHL, N. KLIMAS, M. A. FLETCHER, G. M. DICKINSON, R. S. LEVINE & W. P. PARKS. 1985. Mothers of infants with the acquired immunodeficiency syndrome: Evidence for both symptomatic and asymptomatic carriers. J. Am. Med. Assoc. **253:** 363-366.
14. JOHNSTONE, F. D., L. MACCALLUM, R. BRETTLE, J. M. INGLIS & J. F. PEUTHERER. 1988. Does infection with HIV affect the outcome of pregnancy? Br. Med. J. **296:** 467.
15. TALLON, D. F., D. CORCORAN, D. J. O'DWYER & J. F. GREALLY. 1984. Circulating lymphocyte subpopulations in pregnancy: A longitudinal study. J. Immunol. **132:** 1784-1787.
16. FRIEDLAND, G. H. & R. S. KLEIN. 1988. Transmission of the human immunodeficiency virus. N. Engl. J. Med. **317:** 1125-1135.
17. MINKOFF, H. L. 1987. Care of pregnant women infected with human immunodeficiency virus. J. Am. Med. Assoc. **258:** 2714-2717.
18. REMINGTON, J. S. & G. DESMONTS. 1983. Toxoplasmosis. In Infectious Diseases of the Fetus and Newborn Infant. J. S. Remington & J. O. Klein, Eds.: 143-263. W. B. Saunders. Philadelphia, PA.
19. ALLAIN, J. P., Y. LAURIAN, D. A. PAUL, F. VERROUST, M. LEUTHER, C. GAZENGEL, D. SENN, M. J. LARRIEU & C. BOSSER. 1987. Long-term evaluation of HIV antigen and antibodies to p24 and gp41 in patients with hemophilia: Potential clinical importance. N. Engl. J. Med. **317:** 1114-1121.

20. JOVAISAS, E., M. A. KOCH, A. SCHAFER, M. STAUBER & D. LOWENTHAL. 1985. LAV/ HTLV-III in 20-week fetus. Lancet 2: 1129.
21. MACCHI, B., P. VERANI, A. LAZAARIN et al. 1986. Evidence of HTLV-III/LAV intrauterine infection. Presented at the Second International Conference on AIDS, Paris, June 1986.
22. LAPOINTE, N., J. MICHAND, D. PEKOVIC, J. P. CHAUSSEAU & J. M. DUPUY. 1985. Transplacental transmission of HTLV-III virus. N. Engl. J. Med. 312: 1325-1326.
23. WOFSY, C. B., J. B. COHEN, L. B. HAUER, N. S. PADIAN, L. B. MICHAELIS, L. A. EVANS & J. A. LEVY. 1986. Isolation of AIDS-associated retrovirus from genital secretions of women with antibodies to the virus. Lancet 1: 527-529.
24. PECKHAM, C. S., Y. D. SENTURIA & A. E. ADES. 1987. Obstetric and perinatal consequences of human immunodeficiency virus (HIV) infection: A review. Br. J. Obstet. Gynecol. 94: 403-407.
25. ZIEGLER, J. B., D. A. COOPER, R. O. JOHNSON & J. GOLD. 1985. Postnatal transmission of AIDS-associated retrovirus from mother to infant. Lancet 1: 896-899.
26. THIRY, L., S. SPRECHER-GOLDBERGER, T. JONCKHEER et al. 1985. Isolation of AIDS virus from cell free breast milk of three healthy virus carriers. Lancet 2: 891-892.
27. MENEZ-BAUTISTA, R., S. M. FIKRIG, S. PAHWA, M. G. SARANGADHARAN & R. L. STONEBURNER. 1986. Monozygotic twins discordant for the acquired immunodeficiency syndrome. Am. J. Dis. Child. 140: 678-679.
28. RICH, K. C. 1986. Immunologic function and AIDS in drug-exposed infants. In Drug use in pregnancy: Mother and child. I. J. Chasnoff, Ed. MTP Press Ltd. Lancaster, England.
29. BORKOWSKY, W., K. KRASINSKI, D. PAUL, T. MOORE, D. BEHENROTH & S. CHANDWANI. 1987. Human immunodeficiency virus infections in infants negative for anti-HIV by enzyme-linked immunoassay. Lancet 1: 1168-1171.
30. MULLER, F. & K. H. MULLER. 1988. Detection of anti-HIV-1 immunoglobulin M antibodies in patients with serologically proved HIV-1 infection. Infection 16: 115-118.
31. JOHNSON, J. P. & P. NAIR. 1987. Early diagnosis of HIV infection in the neonate. N. Engl. J. Med. 316: 273-274.
32. OU, C. Y., S. KWOK, S. W. MITCHELL, D. H. MACK, J. J. SNINSKY, J. W. KREBS, P. FEORINO, D. WARFIELD & G. SCHOCHETMAN. 1988. DNA amplification for direct detection of HIV-1 in DNA of peripheral blood mononuclear cells. Science 239: 295-297.
33. PAHWA, S., M. KAPLAN, S. FIKRIG, R. PAHWA, M. G. SARNGADHARAN, M. POPOVIC & R. C. GALLO. 1986. Spectrum of human T-cell lymphotropic virus type III infection in children: Recognition of symptomatic, asymptomatic, and seronegative patients. J. Am. Med. Assoc. 255: 2299-2305.
34. BORKOWSKY, W., C. J. STEELE, S. GRUBMAN, T. MOORE, P. LaRUSSA & K. KRASINSKI. 1987. Antibody responses to bacterial toxoids in children infected with human immunodeficiency virus. J. Pediatr. 110: 563-566.
35. BERNSTEIN, L. J., H. D. OCHS, R. J. WEDGWOOD & A. RUBINSTEIN. 1985. Defective humoral immunity in pediatric acquired immune deficiency syndrome. J. Pediatr. 107: 352-357.
36. JOSHI, V. V., J. M. OLESKE, A. B. MINNEFOR, K. M. KLEIN, R. SINGH, M. ZABALA, C. DADZIE, M. SIMPSER & R. H. RAPKIN. 1985. Pathologic pulmonary findings in children with the acquired immunodeficiency syndrome: A study of ten cases. Hum. Pathol. 16: 241-246.
37. EPSTEIN, L. G., J. GOUDSMIT, D. A. PAUL, S. H. MORRISON, E. M. CONNOR, J. M. OLESKE & B. HOLLAND. 1987. Expression of human immunodeficiency virus in cerebrospinal fluid of children with progressive encephalopathy. Ann. Neurol. 21: 397-401.
38. MARION, R. W., A. A. WIZNIA, R. G. HUTCHEON et al. 1986. Human T-cell lymphotropic virus type III (HTLV-III) embryopathy. Am. J. Dis. Child. 140: 638-640.
39. PIZZO, P. A., J. EDDY, J. FALLOON, F. BALIS, M. MAHA, S. LEHRMAN, R. YARCHOAN, S. BRODER & D. G. POPLAK. 1988. Continuous intravenous administration of AZT to children with symptomatic HIV infection. Presented at the Fourth International Conference on AIDS, Oslo.
40. BLANCHE, S., F. LeDEIST, A. FISCHER, F. VEBER, M. DEBRE, S. CHAMARET, L. MONTAGNIER & C. GRISCELLI. 1986. Longitudinal study of 18 children with perinatal LAV/ HTLV III infection: Attempt at prognostic evaluation. J. Pediatr. 109: 965-970.

Maternal-Fetal Conflicts: Ethical and Legal Considerations

Department of Pediatrics
Program in Medical Ethics
University of Wisconsin-Madison Medical School
H4/442 Clinical Science Center
600 Highland Avenue
Madison, Wisconsin 53792

INTRODUCTION

I would like to address three ethical questions involved in maternal use of drugs which may be harmful to the fetus:

1. Does a woman have a duty to abstain from using drugs which are likely to harm the fetus?
2. Does the state have an obligation to protect the fetus/newborn from harm?
3. Should there be legal measures to reduce the incidence of or to prevent such harm from occurring?

For the purpose of this discussion I will not address the difficult balancing judgments that must be made when a woman considers using a drug which is intended to have some medical therapeutic benefit for herself and/or the fetus, with an associated risk for her or the fetus. I will be concerned primarily with illicit drug use, intended primarily for so-called "recreational" use, such as cocaine and heroin. I will make a few comments at the end regarding legal hazardous drugs such as tobacco, alcohol and the related issue of phenylalanine intake in pregnant women who themselves have phenylketonuria (PKU).

I will also not address the difficult and important question of whether the *fetus* is entitled to protection, but rather, will focus on pregnancies in which there is a high likelihood of a live birth, with a risk of injury, suffering or death to an infant, who may also live a long life of disability due to prenatal events.

One final preliminary comment: as a physician and human being I feel great empathy for women who find themselves taking illicit drugs. The social antecedents of drug abuse are not generally chosen by the people involved, and the continued use of such drugs, once begun, is a complex mixture of voluntary behavior, psychological and physical addiction, and varying opportunities for treatment programs that help women abstain from harmful drugs. As a pediatrician, I also regret the children born dying or damaged as a result of maternal addiction. My analysis of the issues implies no pejorative judgments about the character of the women involved. It is an attempt to analyze the difficult balancing that must be done, and to suggest policies that seem to follow from that analysis.

Historical Trends

The past 15 years have seen a strong trend in American attitudes, practice and law towards fetal protection, particularly when a live birth results.[1] In 1973, the same year in which the U.S. Supreme Court gave women nearly total discretion to end the life of the fetus prior to viability, another federal agency—the National Commission for the Protection of Human Subjects—was beginning deliberations which would result in extremely strict prohibitions against research which could harm pre-viable fetuses. These proposals eventually became part of federal law when they were incorporated into the still extant research regulations of the U.S. Department of Health and Human Services.[2] By 1975, therefore, the federal government was taking the apparently paradoxical position of allowing a woman to kill a fetus for any or no reason, but prohibiting her from exposing it to almost any risk at all in the course of nontherapeutic research.[3] It is noteworthy that the Commission was persuaded to support the principle that the moral status of the fetus should not be affected by its destiny: fetuses about to be aborted were entitled to the same protection as fetuses going to term. It should also be noted that the Commission was not dominated by "pro-life" views. Its members included many who were outspoken advocates of abortion-on-demand.

The ensuing decade saw an increase in the number and extent of "wrongful birth" suits, tort actions against physicians and others whose negligent conduct resulted in harm incurred *in utero* but which resulted in injury to a live-born infant. The purpose of these suits was primarily to obtain monetary damages to provide for the necessary care and treatment of the affected children. The moral basis of such tort actions is the principle of reparations, the notion that a person has a duty to help repair injuries caused by his own negligent action. Such lawsuits also have the effect of deterring others from behaving in ways which jeopardize fetal, and particularly neonatal well-being.

The decade also saw erosion in the long-established doctrine of intrafamilial tort immunity, the notion that a child could not sue his own mother. The celebrated case of *Grodin v Grodin* involved a woman who took tetracycline during pregnancy, despite being informed that it could stain her baby's teeth. The baby was in fact born with stained teeth; as the judge put it—the mother had taken the baby's smile away. An action for damages was brought against the mother on behalf of the baby and the appellate court ruled that the suit was proper. The case achieved particular notoriety when it was revealed that the mother was a willing participant in the lawsuit, having been advised that a judgment for damages could result in shifting a substantial part of her estate to the infant, with favorable tax consequences that could not be achieved otherwise.

In some jurisdictions, there was criminal as well as civil liability for prenatal injuries causing harm or death to live-born children. There were even jurisdictions in which deaths *in utero,* after viability, could result in homocide actions against the offending person.

Finally, in the 1980s there have been reports of increasing use of the courts to order women to undergo cesarean section for the benefit of the newborn. The most common scenario is a woman near term, with a presumably normal fetus, who refuses C-section for placenta previa, a condition with nearly universal catastrophic consequences for the infant, harms which can be prevented in nearly all cases with C-section. Vaginal delivery also entails a very high risk of serious harm to the mother, but it is clear that the courts were intervening primarily on behalf of the expected infant. There is a longstanding and growing consensus that competent adults should have very broad freedom to refuse lifesaving medical treatment for themselves. At least two state supreme courts have upheld such orders.[4] These decisions have been criticized for several reasons, including questionable medical facts in some of the more publicized cases,[5] but the point is that the law has increasingly accepted the principle that women have less than total discretion to make judgments in the third trimester when there are serious health implications for an expected infant.

In summary, *Roe v Wade* and the related cases stand almost alone in the law's approach to maternal-fetal conflict. The general trend has been to protect fetal interest, particularly when a live-birth results or is expected.

Do the Fetal Protection Cases Conflict with Roe v Wade ?

Roe v Wade seemed to provide women with nearly absolute immunity from state action for decisions regarding pre-viable fetuses. The federal research regulations appeared to conflict with *Roe,* but have not been tested in the courts. Whether or not the U.S. Supreme Court will find the fetal protection cases to be consistent with *Roe* is conjectural and dependent on many variables, including the composition of the Court itself. I would only suggest that the Court could defend these cases without necessarily violating the principles established in *Roe.*

I will consider the most controversial cases, those involving forced fetal treatment. The paradigm case, as mentioned, involves a woman with a presumably healthy fetus, near term, refusing a C-section for placenta previa. A court finding that a woman may be compelled to undergo such a procedure is not necessarily violating the moral principles underlying *Roe v Wade* for three reasons.

First, the fight for freedom of choice in decisions regarding abortion was primarily on behalf of women who do not want to be pregnant, to have children, to be mothers, or to have their offspring raised by others. None of these issues is present in the C-section cases. The women involved have generally chosen to be pregnant or to continue a pregnancy. They typically want to have a baby, and to be mothers.

Second, the state's interest in the C-section cases is primarily that of protecting newborns, not fetuses. Whether or not fetuses are deserving of the full protection of society is controversial and unlikely to attract consensus. But there is a strong consensus that infants, born alive, are entitled to the protection of the state against abuse or neglect by their parents. It is this consensus that underlies that the wrongful birth suits mentioned earlier. Whether or not this interest is strong enough to justify an unconsented surgical intrusion on the mother is a separate matter, to be discussed later. The point here is that the state could consistently seek to protect the interests of an imminent newborn while conceding the autonomy of the woman earlier in pregnancy. Few if any requests for abortion would be jeopardized by laws which limited discretion in the last few weeks of pregnancy.

Third, the immunity to state action established in *Roe v Wade* was limited to pre-viable fetuses. The court acknowledged that in the third trimester the state had sufficient interests in the well-being of the fetus that it could even prohibit abortions, unless necessary for the woman's health. That is, regardless of whether birth is imminent or the woman intends to go to term, the legal limits of *Roe* are compatible with state involvement in protecting fetal life in the third trimester.

Is There a Moral Basis for Maternal Duty Towards a Third-Trimester Fetus?

In her classic "A Defense of Abortion" the philosopher Judith Thomson argued that even if her opponents' strongest claim were true—that the fetus is a person—a woman had no duty to carry a pregnancy to term.[6] She used the analogy of someone finding himself connected by a lifeline—an umbilical cord—to a famous violinist whose life was absolutely dependent on the willingness of the other to maintain the connection. While conceding it would be morally desirable and praiseworthy to do so, she argued that there would be no duty to support the life of another. Her argument depended, however, on the connection being involuntary. She conceded that a person who invited the violinist into the arrangement would have a duty to support him.

The implication of Thomson's analysis is that a woman who chooses to create a life is in a morally different position than one who finds herself connected with such a life involuntarily. Most abortions are chosen by women in the latter category. In contrast, a woman who voluntarily creates a life, rejects opportunities to terminate a pregnancy, and declares her interest in giving birth to and rearing a child incurs some obligation to the person so created. From the perspective of the child or adult who finds himself suffering or disabled due to the conduct of his mother, when such injury was avoidable without substantial risk to the mother, he has a morally legitimate claim that he was wronged. The usual remedy for injuries caused by the negligence of another is reparations—monetary damages. This is of little help in such cases since the mother would be financially obligated to provide for the child's needs in any case. More important, it is of little consolation to the person whose life is cut short or filled with disability or suffering which could have been prevented.

Is a Woman Required to be a "Procreative Saint?"

The claim that a woman has *some* responsibility to avoid damaging an infant brought into the world voluntarily has led some to the *reductio ad absurdum* of a slippery slope which would hold women liable for any and all prenatal behaviors associated with fetal harm. According to this view, forcing C-sections will inevitably lead to incarceration to prevent smoking, drinking or failing to keep prenatal appointments.[5] These conclusions are not implicit in the argument.

The C-section cases differ from many other maternal choices in four important ways. First, they typically arise late in the third trimester when there is a high probability of a live birth of an infant who is otherwise expected to be normal. Second, there is an extremely high probability of death or serious harm to the infant. Third, there is a high probability that standard treatment will prevent the harm from occurring. And fourth, the risk of serious harm to the mother is low.

In contrast, consider the woman who is found to be consuming large amounts of alcohol in the first trimester, refusing to comply with advice to stop drinking. The probability of a live birth is uncertain. The benefits of forced cessation are unclear, in that the risk of permanent fetal damage is already past and cannot be reduced by abstinence from that point on. And forced abstinence would require incarceration, possibly for months.

A similar analysis would apply to the less common but more dramatic problem involving women with phenylketonuria who choose to become pregnant but adamantly refuse to comply with the special diet that is necessary to prevent fetal damage. The risk of serious malformation in such cases is very high. The benefits of strict dietary control are reasonably clear, though not absolute, but apparently require maintenance of normal blood phenylalanine levels at the time of conception, if not before. As with the case of alcohol, enforcement of dietary control might require incarceration and forced feeding throughout pregnancy. If dietary control is indeed required before conception it is difficult to imagine how conception could even occur under such circumstances.

In summary, if there is ever a justification for compelling a woman to behave in a way that avoids fetal risk, this analysis suggests that it would be confined to circumstances in which all of the following conditions were met:

1. There is a high probability of a live birth.
2. There is a high probability of serious physical harm occurring to the infant-to-be.
3. There is a high probability that the harm can be prevented using standard, established treatment.
4. There is a low probability of serious harm to the mother.

These criteria would not support forced intervention on women who abused drugs of the kind discussed in this volume, nor would they support intervention for most maternal behaviors which expose the fetus or newborn to risk. The discussion does support the view that it is morally irresponsible to voluntarily bring an infant into the world but refuse to make reasonable efforts to allow that child to be born healthy.

What Kind of "Force" is Justified?

While court-ordered treatment may only be justifiable in a limited number of cases, questions remain about the sanctions that could be imposed to modify maternal behavior. Discussions of this problem commonly refer to "forced" treatment, suggesting physical force, but there are other methods of modifying behavior that are less draconian.

First, there is persuasion and moral pressure. The preeminence of the principle of autonomy in contemporary medical ethics sometimes leads physicians to think it is always improper to give directive counseling. This tolerance may allow some patients to believe falsely that they are being supported in a decision which many, including the physician, consider outrageous. In that sense, an appearance of value-neutrality is deceptive and dishonest. Many patients look to their physicians for moral guidance, and many others are heavily influenced by even subtle pressures. The author was involved in a lawsuit in which a woman successfully sued her obstetrician for failing to be more persuasive in his efforts to get her consent to a C-section for fetal distress.

Second, court orders are a powerful way of sending messages to patients about their responsibilities. Laws reflect prevailing moral consensus, however imperfectly, and most of us are predisposed to obeying the law. I am aware of no cases in which physical force was used to achieve a court-ordered C-section, but most women confronted with such orders have acquiesced. Physical force is only rarely required to promote compliance with the law. It may be that the threat of force lies behind such compliance, but whether or how often such threats must be carried out will depend on many complex variables.

Finally, there are post-hoc sanctions which the law could impose that would affect maternal decisions. These would include various interventions under child abuse and neglect statutes, as well as possible criminal prosecutions for homicide or lesser offenses.

Many who would support moral and legal pressures to discourage pregnant women from abusing drugs or jeopardizing neonatal well-being in other ways would oppose physical force. No sanction will be completely effective in achieving the desired end.

What are the Likely Costs of Requiring Women to Protect the Interests of Their Expected Infants?

It should go without saying that the overwhelming majority of women want healthy babies, and many will undergo considerable deprivation and even risk to achieve that end. Others are similarly motivated but unable or unwilling to abstain from behaviors which they know will be harmful. Willful disregard of neonatal well-being, whatever the reasons, is likely to constitute a small percentage of cases, but obviously evokes the greatest outrage. It is more difficult to raise concern for the far larger number of women who desire healthy babies but are unable to find the support and care which would help them achieve that goal. One of the strongest objections to pressure or coercion is the risk of driving women out of the health care system, particularly women who may have the greatest need for medical attention because of drug abuse or other risk factors. Whether or not policies of forced treatment would result in an increase or decrease of healthy babies is an empirical question of considerable importance, but how large a role such calculations should play is complex. Traditional child abuse laws, for example, surely deter some parents from seeking medical care for their injured children, with adverse consequences for the child, but that alone would not argue for abolition of child abuse laws or prosecution of some parents who inflict injury on their children.

Even if policies to compel healthy prenatal behavior were effective, there would be concerns about equity, since the women subject to such pressures would be predominantly indigent, with a high proportion of racial minorities. Educated women are less likely to be subject to such pressures, and are more likely to have access to legal counsel and the financial means to resist such pressures.

Inequity alone would not be a sufficient argument for resisting policies which protected newborns from harm. Few benefits or burdens are distributed fairly in a society. Such inequities call for corrective and compensatory measures, but not for the elimination of efforts to prevent harmful behavior which is considered morally indefensible on other grounds.

CONCLUSION

Moral and legal questions about maternal drug abuse involve conflicts between the interests of mothers and the interests of newborns, not just fetuses. There is a trend in the law towards protecting fetuses from injury, particularly when a live birth results or is likely to result. Holding a woman responsible for the health of such infants when the pregnancy is voluntary is not inconsistent with moral and legal support for abortion. Whether or not moral responsibility should lead to legal responsibility would depend on many variables. A proposal has been offered for state involvement limited to such cases in which there is a high probability of serious preventable harm to a newborn. According to this analysis, drug abuse during pregnancy could be considered morally irresponsible in some circumstances without necessarily leading to a conclusion that forced prenatal treatment would be justified. Such behavior might, however, justify postnatal sanctions.

REFERENCES

1. CALLAHAN, D. 1986. How technology is reframing the abortion debate. Hastings Center Report **16**(#1): 33-42.
2. U.S. Department of Health and Human Services. 45 CFR 46. Protection of human subjects. Subpart B—Additional protections pertaining to research development, and related activities involving fetuses, pregnant women, and human *in vitro* fertilization.
3. FOST, N. 1974. Our curious attitude toward the fetus. Hastings Center Report **4**(#1): 4-5.
4. BOWES, W. A. & B. SELGESTAD. 1981. Fetal vs maternal rights: medical and legal perspectives. Obst. Gyn. **58**(2): 209-214.
5. ANNAS, G. J. 1982. Forced cesareans: the most unkindest cut of all. Hastings Center Report **12**(3): 45.
6. THOMSON, J. J. 1971. A defense of abortion. Philosophy and Public Affairs **1**: 47-66.

Public Health Policy: Maternal Substance Use and Child Health[a]

ERNESTINE VANDERVEEN

National Institute on Drug Abuse
Division of Clinical Research
5600 Fishers Lane
Room 10A-38
Rockville, Maryland 20857

Research in the field of maternal substance abuse has become a respected scientific endeavor in a few short years. As our knowledge accrues so must our involvement in public health issues where such knowledge is relevant to the recognition and ultimate resolution of society's problems. No one denies that drug abuse is an enormous problem with widespread implications and dimensions, including health and social consequences. In the case of maternal drug use and fetal outcome, what has been learned must become integrated with child care and child health concerns as these issues are publicly debated and ultimately evolve as policies at the community, state and federal levels. As scientists most of us are not politicians and we have little inclination to become active in political arenas. We can, however, and we should, help decision makers in public life to recognize that the determinants of health problems include social, economic, and psychological as well as biological phenomena. Substance abuse and its array of associated detrimental effects on human life make it a public health issue that needs to be addressed using science, political action, diplomacy, ethics and common sense.[1]

In the public arena scientists and those who pursue knowledge through research walk a thin line. We face on the one hand the ever-present temptation to overinterpret our data and thus risk negative impacts on the credibility of our work. In the world of science, no judge is more harsh than one's own peers. The other risk is the overly cautious interpretation of limited or incomplete findings. Here, when we are totally honest with the limitations of early or new knowledge we are not infrequently accused of the "we don't know everything yet" approach, translated into a justification for more research. Faced with this dilemma it is of course much safer for scientists not to get involved, choosing instead, the "safe position." This course however, serves to limit or curtail the opportunity to influence decisions in policy and matters of public health importance.

This discussion will cite only a few examples of drug-abuse-related concerns and issues and try to provide some rationale for their inclusion in the formulation of health policies.

---

[a] The opinions expressed herein are the views of the author and do not necessarily reflect the official position of the National Institute on Drug Abuse or any other part of the U.S. Department of Health and Human Services.

Maternal drug use effects are incremental and cumulative in the child's life; prenatally through risk of in utero drug exposure, postnatally through inadequate care or neglect imposed by maternal functioning decriments associated with drug use, and in developmental stages through the detrimental environment that is frequently part of the drug abusing woman's chaotic life. An important factor here is the impact of poor parenting skills on the child who may be in need of enhanced care and nurture to compensate for possible in utero exposure effects. Widespread use and acceptance of licit and illicit drugs has intensified concerns about maternal drug use during pregnancy. Women who are of childbearing age are also in the age group most likely to be drug users and abusers, a phenomenon that cuts across traditionally defined sectors of society. Cocaine users, for example, now include members from all socioeconomic groups.

Society perceives illicit drug use as a criminal behavior problem. Inappropriate alcohol use is also viewed as criminal activity when associated with a consequence involving the law such as alcoholic beverage consumption by underage persons, driving while intoxicated and other potentially harmful behaviors. This not only makes research more complicated and much more subject to public scrutiny but also challenges our ability to convince people that drug abuse is a health issue. Far too many people still think of cocaine as a "harmless" and "acceptable" drug.[2] Thus far the harmful consequence message has not been sufficiently convincing to effect a downward trend in cocaine use, while, on the other hand, the leveling off observed in gross per capita alcohol consumption is reason for optimism. However, the groups most at risk for heavy or abusive drinking, including women of child bearing age, may not be decreasing their alcohol use.

The legal status of some drugs as opposed to illegal status of other drugs often hinders the credibility and acceptability of health-related messages. Since the very attraction of drugs may be imbedded in their addictive properties, drug seeking behavior, whether the user is drug dependent or merely using an illicit substance, and acquisition of the drug constitutes criminal behavior as does the act of consuming it. Some would argue that the inconsistent legal sanctions surrounding psychoactive substance use serve to weaken the case for credibility regarding the health injurious aspects of sustained or sporadic use of various drugs. Relaxation of certain penalties for certain drugs is believed by some to promise indirect and ultimately beneficial effects in terms of reducing law enforcement efforts and the associated costs to society.[3,4]

Existence of drug cultures and subcultures together with emergence of new drug-using patterns generate additional cause for concern about maternal substance use. Persons whose lives are destabilized, runaway adolescents and youth, homeless persons of all ages as well as intact families, present an entire spectrum of health problems including substance abuse. Survival among the teenage homeless is intricately entwined with a life characterized by fear, loneliness, violence, sex, drugs, and constant escape from authority. While the actual size of the runaway population is unknown, every city of any size has a runaway youth population as evidenced by news media listings of agencies that provide services and solace to homeless young people.

Societal costs directly and indirectly associated with maternal drug abuse cannot be calculated. If such computations were to be made, since we have the technology even if we do not have the data on affected persons, the calculations would at a minimum have to include intensive neonatal care for addicted and high-risk, drug-exposed infants, custodial care for infants and children of dysfunctional mothers, treatment and rehabilitation for addicted mothers, long-term specialized services for impaired children who survive precarious neonatal beginnings, and possibly a range of specialized services for the more subtley affected child who becomes an adult.

Abel and Sokol have estimated the economic cost of providing treatment for some of the disorders related to Fetal Alcohol Syndrome (FAS) at approximately $321 million annually. They estimate that FAS alone accounts for about 11% of the $11.7 billion per year cost for residential and support services for mentally retarded persons in the U.S.[5] Costs in human suffering and anguish, lost human potential, lost productivity and a weakened society with large numbers of unproductive citizens cannot be calculated. In the worst case scenario there may be a point in time where more persons will be recipients of care, because they cannot function and contribute, than persons who are sufficiently productive to provide the resources needed to sustain the impaired.

Individual freedom along with the right to choose what is in one's own best self-interest is a valued concept in our society. With increased awareness of maternal substance abuse effects on the fetus, the issue of fetal rights looms in our land and in our courts. A literature is emerging on this issue and has the potential to bring the whole relationship between mother and child in utero out of the health care arena, i.e., the clinician's domain, into the courtroom. Arguments are in progress that purport to examine the need to "readjust the balance between the rights of women and the evolving rights of the fetus as their rights become diametrically opposed when a woman willfully abuses substances during pregnancy."[6] What is interesting is the legal interpretation that there is a conflict between the right of a fetus to be born free of substance-abuse-inflicted damage and the mother's right to pursue use of alcohol, tobacco and narcotics. In the interpretation cited, the use of substances is not a fundamental right, alcohol and tobacco use are merely a privilege, and narcotic use is a crime.[6]

The appropriate role of health care professionals when medical matters become arguments in legal arenas raises more issues than can be addressed in this discussion. The question or assertion of legal obligation to the fetus has many implications for health professionals and health care systems. Some involve truthfulness in reporting drug use, by both physician and patient. Confidentiality, right to privacy, as well as criminal child neglect and endangerment charges are related issues of grave concern.

Product liability activity in the public health area indicates that regulatory action has not been totally successful in the prevention of injury and disease. Public health advocates have turned to the courtroom for progress in protection of the public from unsafe products, one of which is tobacco.[7] Can other injurious drugs be far behind? And are we moving from a health issue to a legal issue in maternal substance abuse? A new dyad, the drug-using mother and the affected infant is challenging the medical profession in many ways.

If a new role is emerging for the health care professional in the care and management of the drug-using pregnant woman it needs to be taken seriously in the context of reality. Injury from in utero drug exposure is preventable. Will physicians who are healers by tradition and training become educators in a role that seeks to prevent rather than to cure? This assumes, of course, that physicians are the primary source of health information and that patients are compliant in adhering to advice prescribed in the medical setting. How to get information from the researcher to the advising clinician and ultimately to the patient in a way that will result in positive behaviors would seem to be among the more significant challenges of our time.

This brings us to intervention and a brief look at a narrow range of options. Advances in the technical aspects of sustaining human life have posed challenges and dilemmas in almost every facet of medicine. The question of society's commitment to a "rescue mentality" in the management of high-risk infants as opposed to a "strategy of prevention" has been raised. Technology-based intervention in early life is possible through modern neonatal medicine and may indeed be achievable but brings new ethical dilemmas to those responsible for the care of pregnant women and infants.[8]

Prevention as a basis for national public health policy formulation is logical to those who recognize that children born to substance-abusing mothers are likely to place growing demands on the nation's capacity to provide health and social services.

The questions surrounding prevention are numerous: 1) What kind of preventive treatment intervention, 2) when and at what stage of drug use or drug dependence should it be effected, 3) by whom shall the intervention be delivered, and 4) by what kind or mix of messages and message givers? Should prevention efforts be in the domain of health professionals or should we aim for a communitywide or nationwide approach? Should it be a holistic approach that attempts to promote a life style that lifts poor women from fragmented, socially and economically deprived circumstances to an environment that minimizes drug using behavior, reduces fetal and neonatal risk, and supports growth of self-esteem along with coping and maternal functioning skills? These are truly complex issues that reach beyond traditional health care but serve to remind us that the likelihood of effective intervention when only health professionals and the health community are involved may be minimal.

Education as a cornerstone of prevention and a positive health intervention deserves special mention. In the past we have probably failed to clarify misperceptions about health-related harmful effects of drug use. Moral issues and health issues may need to become separated agenda items. In our efforts to educate about drug use it would seem we need to enable people to make informed decisions as opposed to rules and slogans that are interpreted as paternalistic and without sufficient grounding in reality. In education for the health professions, integration of current scientific knowledge into academic preparation curricula is exceedingly urgent.

SUMMARY

Maternal substance use and abuse is a public health issue. Much of what researchers have discovered in this field has been achieved through support of funds appropriated by Congress to the Public Health Service agencies and institutes whose mandates include stimulating and supporting this research in the scientific community. In this same vein the research institutes have a responsibility for disseminating new knowledge and encouraging its application in real-life settings.

Individual freedom, social justice and public health relationships need to be carefully weighed by the architects of public policy. We elect those architects through our system of citizen participation in government. However, how to effectively incorporate the relevance of what has been learned about harmful effects of substance abuse into policy that will enable society to deal with emerging maternal and child health issues remains unresolved.

Health-policy-relevant issues, as they impact the lives and well-being of our children, including the increasing number who are children of drug-abusing parents, are too important for politicians to ignore and too complex for health professionals to resolve alone. Participation by the research community in policy development is critical.

It is clear that a policy of preventive intervention will need widespread public support. It will need to be feasible, effective and affordable in relation to other public demands. Society will ultimately need to make choices among those options that can be implemented and sustained in a political climate characterized by conflicting values.

REFERENCES

1. WALKER, B. 1986. Public health responsibilities, roles and realities. Am. J. Public Health 76(5): 555.
2. RYAN, L., S. EHRLICH & L. FINNEGAN. 1987. Cocaine abuse in pregnancy: Effects on the fetus and newborn. Neurotoxicol. Teratol. 9(4): 295-299.
3. BAKALOR, J. B. & L. GRINSPOON. 1984. Drug control: Three analogies. J. Psychoactive Drugs 16(2): 107-118.
4. Drug wars: Legalization gets a hearing. 1988. Science 241(4870): 1157-1159.
5. ABEL, E. L. & R. J. SOKOL. 1987. Incidence of fetal alcohol syndrome and economic impact of FAS-related anomalies. Drug and Alcohol Depend. 19: 51-70.
6. SHELLEY, B. 1988. Maternal substance abuse: The next step in the protection of fetal rights? Dickinson Law Review 92(N3): 691-715.
7. TERET, S. P. 1986. Litigating for the public's health. Am. J. Public Health 76(8): 1027-1029.
8. FLEISCHMAN, A. R. 1988. Ethical issues in neonatology: A U.S. perspective. In Biomedical Ethics: An Anglo-American Dialogue. D. Callahan & G. Dunstan, Eds. Vol. 530: 83-91. Ann. N. Y. Acad. Sci. New York, NY.

Cocaine: Clinical Studies of Pregnancy and the Newborn

IRA J. CHASNOFF

AND DAN R. GRIFFITH

*Perinatal Center for Chemical Dependence
and
Departments of Pediatrics and Psychiatry
Northwestern University Medical School
215 East Chicago Avenue, Suite 501
Chicago, Illinois 60611*

The impact of cocaine on the health of adult users and on American society in general has been documented repeatedly in the past 5 years,[1-3] but its effect on human reproduction has only relatively recently been appreciated. The first published report on the effects of cocaine on pregnancy and neonatal outcome documented the high rate of spontaneous abortions, abruptio placentae, and neonatal neurobehavioral deficiencies.[4] Subsequent studies by our group confirmed these preliminary findings and in addition documented a high rate of premature labor and delivery,[5,6] intrauterine growth retardation,[5] sudden infant death syndrome (SIDS),[6] and malformations of the genitourinary tract[7] in cocaine-exposed infants, as well as a possible risk for intrauterine cerebrovascular accidents associated with maternal cocaine use.[8] Bingol *et al.*[9] found an increased rate of malformations and intrauterine growth retardation in a population of cocaine-exposed infants. Oro and Dixon[10] found a high rate of prematurity, intrauterine growth retardation, altered neonatal behavior patterns and a small head circumference in neonates exposed perinatally to cocaine or methamphetamines. At the recent meetings of the Society for Pediatric Research, Shih *et al.*[11] reported harmful effects of maternal cocaine use on neonatal brainstem auditory system development, Dixon and Bejar[12] reported that 39% of 28 cocaine-exposed neonates exhibited hemorrhagic cerebral infarctions documented on cranial ultrasound at birth, and Riley *et al.*[13] reported a rate of SIDS in cocaine-exposed neonates at 10 to 20 times the average national incidence. Thus, it is becoming clear that cocaine use in pregnancy places the pregnancy and the neonate at high medical and neurobehavioral risk.

Information thus far has viewed cocaine users as a group. Preliminary information from our program specifically analyzes the differing effect of patterns of cocaine use on pregnancy and the neonate.

METHODS

The Perinatal Center for Chemical Dependence at Northwestern University Medical School was established in 1976 to provide a comprehensive program of psychiatric, obstetric and follow-up pediatric care to substance-abusing pregnant women and their infants. All women receive intensive obstetric care during their pregnancies and participate in individual and group therapy sessions as well as education classes. The goal of psychotherapeutic intervention is to achieve abstinence. Urine toxicology through EMIT screening is performed at admission with positive results confirmed by gas chromatography/mass spectrometry. At each prenatal obstetric visit, current substance-abuse history is reviewed and urines for toxicology are regularly obtained. History and toxicology studies covered the following substances: caffeine, nicotine, barbiturates, cocaine and its metabolites, opiates, benzodiazepenes, propoxyphene, phencyclidine, amphetamines, alcohol, and marijuana.

Two groups of cocaine-using women were studied. The first group consisted of 23 women who conceived during a period when cocaine was used, but reached abstinence by the end of the first trimester and had no further cocaine use during their pregnancy (Group I), as documented by ongoing chemical dependence evaluation and urine toxicologies. The second group (Group II) consisted of 52 women who used cocaine during the period of conception and, despite being enrolled in the comprehensive program, continued to use cocaine throughout their pregnancy.

All neonates were examined at birth by a physician blinded to the infants' prenatal history. Weight, crown to heel length, and fronto-occipital head circumference were recorded. Gestational age assessment was performed using the Ballard evaluation,[14] and each infant birth weight was plotted against gestational age on neonatal birth weight curves developed by Brenner et al.[15] When the infants were 12 to 72 hours old the Neonatal Behavioral Assessment Scale (NBAS)[16] was administered by trained examiners who were blinded to the infants' prenatal history. Infants delivered prior to 38 weeks gestation were not included in NBAS data analysis.

Pregnancy and neonatal data were analyzed by the use of Chi square analysis for nonparametric data or by Student t test or by a 2 way analysis of variance (ANOVA) for parametric data.

RESULTS

Maternal demographic data for the two groups of patients are summarized in TABLE 1. The two groups were similar for maternal age, gravidity, parity, and prenatal weight gain. Racial distribution (Group I: 6 white, 11 black, 6 Hispanic; Group II: 18 white, 28 black, 6 Hispanic) was similar.

Quantitative drug use patterns for the two cocaine groups were also similar (TABLE 1). Women in each group used approximately ½ gram of cocaine (range ¼ gram to 5 grams) with each use. The majority of women in each group snorted and/or free-based the cocaine, with similar numbers using cocaine intravenously. Three (13%) women in Group I and six (11%) women in Group II drank more than 60 ml of alcohol per week in the first trimester. Incidence of marijuana use was similar for the two groups with 10 (43%) women in Group I and 20 (38%) in Group II using marijuana in the first trimester. Only one woman in Group I and two women in Group II used marijuana or alcohol beyond the first trimester. Use of tobacco cigarettes throughout the pregnancy was similar for both groups.

There was no difference in sex distribution or in the incidence of low Apgar scores (<7) at one and five minutes between the two groups. Infants born to women who used cocaine throughout pregnancy (Group II) had a lower mean gestational age (38

TABLE 1. Maternal Demographic and Prenatal Data

	I N = 23		II N = 52	
	$\overline{X}$	± SD	$\overline{X}$	± SD
Age	25.4	4.2	27.5	4.4
Gravidity	3.1	1.8	3.9	2.4
Parity	1.1	1.2	1.3	1.1
Weight gain (lb)	27.6	10.0	27.0	12.0
Cigarettes/day	9.8	9.4	10.1	8.1
Alcohol cc/wk (first trimester)	39.9	119.0	19.4	41.0
Marijuana joints/mo (first trimester)	5.0	9.0	6.5	15.7

± 2.8 weeks) than infants in Group I (38.9 ± 1.5 weeks). The incidence of intrauterine growth retardation was increased in the Group II pregnancies (TABLE 2). Use of cocaine in only the first trimester was associated with a rate of abruptio placentae similar to the abruption rate for women who used cocaine throughout pregnancy.

Evaluation of neonatal growth parameters (TABLE 3) for all term (≥ 38 weeks gestation) infants showed that infants born to mothers who used cocaine throughout pregnancy had a lower mean weight, length and head circumference at birth than Group I infants, but this difference was not significant at the 0.05 level (ANOVA).

Neonatal complications were found at a similar rate in the two cocaine-exposed groups. Two infants born to women who used cocaine throughout pregnancy had ileal atresia presenting in the first 24 hours after birth. Six infants born to women who used cocaine throughout pregnancy had seizures during the neonatal period. These six infants were all born with cocaine and active metabolites in the urine at the time of birth. Genitourinary tract abnormalities occurred in three infants born to mothers who used cocaine only in the first trimester of pregnancy and six infants whose mothers used cocaine throughout pregnancy. Two infants whose mothers used cocaine in the 2-3 days prior to delivery suffered perinatal cerebral infarctions.

Infants assessed with the NBAS (TABLE 4) between 12 and 72 hours of age included 16 whose mothers used cocaine during the first trimester of pregnancy only and 36 whose mothers used cocaine throughout pregnancy. These groups were smaller than the groups which were analyzed for the medical variables due to the elimination of

TABLE 2. Perinatal Complications

	I N = 23		II N = 52		
	N	%	N	%	
Preterm delivery[a]	4	17	16	31	N.S.
Low birth weight[c]	0	—	13	25	<0.05
Small for gestational age[d]	0	—	10	19	<0.05
Abruptio placentae	2	9	8	15	N.S.

[a] x^2 analysis.
[b] <38 weeks gestation.
[c] <2500 grams.
[d] <10th percentile by birth weight curve of Brenner et al.

TABLE 3. Neonatal Growth Parameters for Full-Term Infants

	I N = 19		II N = 36	
	$\overline{X}$	SD	$\overline{X}$	SD
Weight (gm)	3160	453	2829	708
Length (cm)	49.3	2.5	48	3.6
Head circumference (cm)	33.4	2.2	32.7	2.3

premature infants (G.A. < 38 weeks) from the sample and the fact that some infants were delivered on the weekend and were released from the hospital before they could be assessed with the NBAS.

Infants' performances on a priori clusters for the NBAS established by Lester *et al.*[17] indicated that both groups exposed to cocaine demonstrated impairment in the areas of orientation, motor ability, state regulation, and number of abnormal reflexes. Group I performance on the motor cluster was significantly below that of Group II.

An examination of the individual orientation cluster scores illustrates the severity of the cocaine-exposed infants' orientation difficulties. Seven of the 16 Group I infants exposed to cocaine during only the first trimester and 8 of the 36 Group II infants exposed to cocaine throughout pregnancy were unable to reach alert states at all during the exam and consequently were unable to engage in any orientation.

Nine supplementary items have been added to the NBAS in an attempt to qualify the responses of the stressed or fragile infant. Significant differences were obtained on three of the nine additional items when the two cocaine groups were compared (TABLE 5). The infants exposed to cocaine for only the first trimester were significantly more fragile and less robust in their ability to complete the exam and displayed greater imbalances in motor tone than the infants exposed to cocaine throughout the pregnancy. In addition, the infants in Group I were rated significantly lower by the examiners in terms of their overall reinforcement value during the course of the exam than were the infants of Group II.

DISCUSSION

In the present study, the data suggest that cessation of cocaine use in the first trimester improved obstetric outcome in that an increased proportion of pregnancies

TABLE 4. NBAS Cluster Score Comparisons for Term Cocaine-Exposed Infants

NBAS Cluster	I N = 16	II N = 36
Habituation	4.5	4.7
Orientation	1.6	2.6
Motor	3.4[a]	4.0
State range	3.5	3.6
State regulation	2.7	3.5
Autonomic regulation	6.1	6.2
Abnormal reflexes	3.6[a]	3.4

[a] Significant difference from Group II (ANOVA, $p \leq 0.05$).

progressed to term. There was also an improvement in intrauterine growth in that fewer infants had growth impairment if the mother stopped using cocaine in early pregnancy. Surprisingly, the rate of abruptio placentae did not decrease despite abstinence from cocaine in the last two trimesters of pregnancy. It has been hypothesized that the high frequency of abruptio placentae in cocaine-exposed pregnancies is related to acute hypertension produced by cocaine use.[4,18] However, the present study suggests that cocaine-induced damage to uteroplacental vascularities may occur in early pregnancy and places these pregnancies at continued risk for abruptio placentae even if cocaine use ceases. Thus, physicians must consider pregnancies to be at increased risk for perinatal morbidity even if cocaine use ceases by the second trimester.

Recent studies have found that maternal cocaine use is associated with intrauterine growth retardation.[5] In the present study, infants exposed to cocaine throughout pregnancy had a clinically apparent decrease in mean birth weight, length and head circumference compared to the control infants. It has been hypothesized[5] that this decrease in intrauterine growth may be related to intermittent diminution of uteroplacental blood flow associated with maternal cocaine use.[19] Infants whose mothers

TABLE 5. Comparison of NBAS Items for the Two Cocaine-Exposed Groups

NBAS Item	I N = 16	II N = 36	Two-Tailed t Values
Alert responsiveness	1.4	2.6	$t_{50} = -1.82$
Cost of attention	2.5	3.6	$t_{50} = -1.76$
Examiner persistence	2.7	3.4	$t_{50} = -1.34$
General irritability	2.9	3.6	$t_{50} = -0.97$
Robustness and endurance	1.2	2.0	$t_{50} = -2.56^a$
Regulatory capacity	2.9	3.5	$t_{50} = -1.50$
State regulation	2.9	4.0	$t_{50} = -1.75$
Balance of motor tone	2.6	3.6	$t_{50} = -2.33^a$
Reinforcement value of infant	2.1	3.3	$t_{50} = -2.70^a$

$^a p \leq 0.05$.

used cocaine only in the first trimester had improved intrauterine growth compared to those whose mothers used cocaine throughout pregnancy. The interactive effect of alcohol, marijuana and tobacco use with cocaine in those pregnancies with significant secondary drug use cannot be completely evaluated in this study.

A recent study completed at the Perinatal Center for Chemical Dependence demonstrated genitourinary tract malformations in infants exposed to cocaine in pregnancy.[7] Among the 50 infants in that study exposed to cocaine in utero, one male infant had prune belly syndrome and one female infant demonstrated female pseudohermaphroditism. In addition, two infants had secondary hypospadius and three infants had hydronephrosis with a normal physical exam. An increased incidence of neural tube defects has been reported by Bingol et al.[9] No infants in either cocaine-exposed group in the present study exhibited neural tube defects, although one infant in our program whose mother used cocaine in the first and third trimesters and thus was not included in the present study, had a myelomeningocoele at birth. Two cases of ileal atresia were documented among the cocaine-exposed infants in the present study. Ileal atresia could be secondary to intrauterine bowel infarction.

The pharmacologic action of cocaine is consistent with the abnormalities found among the cocaine-exposed infants. Cocaine acts at the nerve terminals to prevent dopamine and norepinephrine reuptake producing increased circulating levels of these catecholamines.[20] Subsequent vasoconstriction and tachycardia occur. Placental vasoconstriction is marked,[19] decreasing blood flow to the fetus. Not only could fetal hypoxia and reduced nutrient supply induced by this vasoconstriction explain intrauterine retardation,[19] but also intermittent vascular disruptions could result in an increased rate of malformations.[21,22]

Cocaine use in young adults has been shown to lower the seizure threshold increasing the risk for seizures.[1,3] Six cocaine-exposed infants had seizures in the neonatal period. All six of these infants had cocaine or its metabolites present in their urine at the time of delivery, although the seizures did not necessarily occur when cocaine was present.

Two infants whose mothers used cocaine during the two days prior to delivery suffered cerebral infarctions which were thought to have occurred in the antenatal period.[8] The cardiovascular effects of cocaine have been well documented, and myocardial and cerebral infarctions have occurred in increasing numbers of young adults who use cocaine.[1,2]

Results of the present study confirm earlier findings that exposure to cocaine during the prenatal period leads to significant impairment in neonatal neurobehavioral capabilities.[4,6] The present study further indicates that the neurobehavioral response deficiencies occur in the cocaine-exposed infant whether maternal cocaine use was limited to the first trimester or continued throughout pregnancy.

In normal human fetal development, noradrenaline, serotonin, and dopamine are among the first neurotransmitters present at early stages of brain development, having been shown to be present in the 3-to-4-month fetus.[23] The protective function of the blood-brain barrier is not well developed in the young fetus;[24] thus, cocaine may act on fetal brain neurotransmitters in the first trimester and induce subtle behavioral changes which are evident in the newborn infant. Animal studies using monosodium glutamate (MSG) and diazepam have shown that neonatal rats exposed to MSG early in gestation (day 7 to day 20) demonstrated behavioral deficits in complex discrimination similar to newborn rats exposed to diazepam in late gestation.[24] Cocaine's action in blocking norepinephrine and dopamine reuptake could interfere with some aspects of neuronal development. Grimm[24] has hypothesized that such interference could initiate compensatory neurochemical mechanisms which would partially correct for the abnormalities but still leave the infant impaired in his ability to cope with complex environmental demands later in life. The neurodevelopmental deficiencies exhibited by the infants exposed to cocaine in only the first trimester lend credence to this hypothesis.

The relatively greater impairment found among first trimester-exposed infants as compared to the infants exposed to cocaine throughout pregnancy is difficult to explain. In view of the relatively small size of the groups, the differences may be due, in part, to sampling error. Before drawing firm conclusions from these specific data, it will be necessary to replicate these results with a larger sample and to establish with repeated administrations of the NBAS to each infant whether there are any differences in the neurobehavioral recovery rates of infants exposed to cocaine for varying periods of their prenatal lives.

Current studies have shown that a significant number of women in the prime child-bearing age range of 18-35 years are actively using cocaine.[25] Many of these women conceive and continue to use cocaine without realizing that they are pregnant. Thus, it is important to evaluate the effects of cocaine when use is limited to early pregnancy as well as when it is used throughout pregnancy. In addition, development of intervention programs for cocaine using pregnant women will necessarily rely on information regarding the possibility of improved outcome for pregnancies in which a woman stops using cocaine in the first trimester of pregnancy.

REFERENCES

1. CREGLER, L. & H. MARK. 1986. Medical complications of cocaine abuse. N. Engl. J. Med. **315:** 1495-1500.
2. ISNER, J. M., N. A. M. ESTES III, P. D. THOMPSON, M. A. COSTANZA-NORDIN, R. SUBRAMANIAN, G. MILLER, G. KATSAS, K. SWEENEY & W. Q. STURNER. 1986. Acute cardiac events temporally related to cocaine abuse. N. Engl. J. Med. **315:** 1438-1443.
3. JONSSON, S., M. O'MEARA & J. B. YOUNG. 1983. Acute cocaine poisoning: Importance of treating seizures and acidosis. Am. J. Med. **75:** 1061-1064.
4. CHASNOFF, I. J., W. J. BURNS, S. H. SCHNOLL & K. A. BURNS. Cocaine use in pregnancy. N. Engl. J. Med. **313:** 666-669.
5. MACGREGOR, S. N., L. G. KEITH, I. J. CHASNOFF, M. A. ROSNER, G. M. CHISUM, P. SHAW & J. P. MINOGUE. 1987. Cocaine use during pregnancy: Adverse perinatal outcome. Am. J. Obstet. Gynecol. **157:** 686-690.
6. CHASNOFF, I. J., K. A. BURNS & W. J. BURNS. 1987. Cocaine use in pregnancy: Perinatal morbidity and mortality. Neurobehav. Toxicol. Teratol. **9:** 291-293.
7. CHASNOFF, I. J., G. M. CHISUM & W. E. KAPLAN. 1988. Maternal cocaine use and genitourinary tract malformations. Teratology **37:** 201-204.
8. CHASNOFF, I. J., M. E. BUSSEY, R. SAVICH & C. M. STACK. 1986. Perinatal cerebral infarction and maternal cocaine use. J. Pediatr. **108:** 456-459.
9. BINGOL, N., M. FUCHS, V. DIAZ, R. K. STONE & D. S. GROMISH. 1987. Teratogenicity of cocaine in humans. J. Pediatr. **110:** 93-96.
10. ORO, A. S. & S. D. DIXON. 1987. Perinatal cocaine and methamphetamixe exposure: Maternal and neonatal correlates. J. Pediatr. **111:** 571-578.
11. SHIH, L., B. CONE-WESSON, B. REDDIX & P. Y. K. WU. 1988. Effects of maternal cocaine abuse on the neonatal auditory system (abstract). Pediatr. Res. **23:** 264A.
12. DIXON, S. D. & R. BEJAR. 1988. Brain lesions in cocaine and methamphetamine exposed neonates (abstract). Pediatr. Res. **23:** 405A.
13. RILEY, J. B., N. L. BRODSKY & R. PORAT. 1988. Risk for SIDS in infants with *in utero* cocaine exposure: A prospective study (abstract). Pediatr. Res. **23:** 454A.
14. BALLARD, J. L., K. KAZMAIER & M. DRIVER. 1977. A simplified assessment of gestational age (abstract). Pediatr. Res. **11:** 374.
15. BRENNER, W. E., D. A. EDELMAN & C. H. HENDRICKS. 1976. A standard of fetal growth for the United States of America. Am. J. Obstet. Gynecol. **26:** 555-564.
16. BRAZELTON, T. B. 1968. Neonatal Behavioral Assessment Scale. Spastics International. Philadelphia, PA.
17. LESTER, B. M., H. ALS & T. B. BRAZELTON. 1982. Regional obstetric anesthesia and newborn behavior. A reanalysis towards synergistic effects. Child Dev. **53:** 687-692.
18. ACKER, D., B. P. SACHS, K. J. TRACEY & W. E. WISE. 1983. Abruptio placentae associated with cocaine use. Am. J. Obstet. Gynecol. **146:** 220-221.
19. MOORE, T. R., J. SORG, L. MILLER, T. C. KEY & R. RESNIK. 1986. Hemodynamic effects of intravenous cocaine on the pregnant ewe and fetus. Am. J. Obstet. Gynecol. **155:** 883-888.
20. RITCHIE, J. M. & N. M. GREENE. 1980. Local anesthesia. *In* The Pharmacologic Basis of Therapeutics. 6th edit. A.G. Gilman, L.S. Goodman & A. Gilman, Eds.: 300-320. Macmillan. New York, NY.
21. VAN ALLEN, M. I. 1981. Fetal vascular disruption: Mechanisms and some resulting birth defects. Pediatr. Annals **10:** 219-233.
22. STEVENSON, R. E., J. C. KELLY, A. S. AYLSWORTH & M. C. PHELAN. 1987. Vascular basis for neural tube defects: A hypothesis. Pediatrics **80:** 102-106.
23. NOBIN, A. & A. BJORKLUND. 1973. Topography of the monoamine neuron systems in the human brain as revealed in fetuses. Acta Physiol. Scand. Suppl. **388:** 1-40.
24. GRIMM, V. E. 1987. Effect of teratogenic exposure on the developing brain: Research strategies and possible mechanisms. Dev. Pharmacol. Ther. **10:** 328-345.
25. CLAYTON, R. R. 1985. Cocaine use in the U.S.: In a blizzard or just being snowed. *In* Cocaine Use in America: Epidemiology and Clinical Perspectives. N. J. Kozel & E. H. Adams, Eds. NIDA Research Monograph 61: 8-34. U.S. Department of Health & Human Services. Rockville, MD.

Prenatal Cocaine Exposure to the Fetus: A Sheep Model for Cardiovascular Evaluation[a]

JAMES R. WOODS, JR., MARK A. PLESSINGER,
KIMBERLY SCOTT, AND RICHARD K. MILLER

Department of Obstetrics and Gynecology, Box 668
University of Rochester Medical Center
Strong Memorial Hospital
601 Elmwood Avenue
Rochester, New York 14642

INTRODUCTION

The abuse of cocaine as a recreational drug by women of childbearing age has increased dramatically in the past few years. A survey of over 50,000 people in 16 states and the District of Columbia indicates that women aged 18-34 constitute 15% of all regular users of recreational cocaine.[1] The widespread abuse of this drug by women who are or may become pregnant constitutes a major health issue which must be addressed by the obstetrical community.

Despite its widespread use, our understanding of the impact of prenatal cocaine exposure upon the developing fetus is incomplete. As recently as 1982, a major obstetric textbook stated, "Cocaine is not known to have direct deleterious effects on the fetus."[2] Then in 1983, Acker reported two pregnant patients who experienced abruptio placenta (separation of the placenta from the uterine wall prior to delivery) following intravenous or intranasal cocaine administration. A severely depressed newborn was delivered to one patient, while the second patient delivered a stillborn child.[3]

Clinical reports have since provided considerable evidence that cocaine administration during pregnancy may be detrimental to cardiovascular function in the mother and fetus. Chasnoff and co-workers reported an increased incidence of miscarriage in pregnant patients using cocaine when compared with those on Methadone therapy or drug-free patients.[4] Others have reported rupture of maternal intracranial aneurysm, preterm labor, abruptio placenta, and delivery of small for gestational age babies in pregnant women using cocaine.[4-7]

The increase in obstetric and perinatal complications secondary to cocaine usage in pregnant women has prompted a number of animal studies to investigate the mechanisms of cocaine action upon the developing fetus. Cocaine's effect upon the cardiovascular system are thought to be mediated primarily through its ability to block uptake and degradation of catecholamines at adrenergic nerve endings.[8] The adverse effects of cocaine upon fetal well-being may in part be explained by recent studies indicating that regional vascular beds during pregnancy may be more sensitive

[a]Supported by National Institute on Drug Abuse Grant 04415.

267

to certain vasoactive amines than those in the nonpregnant sheep. The uterine vessels are maximally dilated throughout most of pregnancy but vasoconstrict readily in response to alpha-adrenergic receptor stimulation. Greiss and Van Wilkes utilized electromagnetic flow probes to measure uterine blood flow from pregnant ewes in response to adrenergic stimulation.[9] Systemic infusion of epinephrine or norepinephrine resulted in a 40% reduction in total uterine blood flow in response to either drug. Rosenfeld and West later employed microsphere techniques to demonstrate a 39.3% reduction in total uterine blood following systemic infusion of norepinephrine, 0.24 μg/kg/min.[10] Studies in the rodent first documented the impact of cocaine upon uterine blood flow during pregnancy. Fantel and MacPhail[11] administered intraperitoneal cocaine to pregnant rats and mice on day 8 through 12. The authors observed a decrease in fetal weights in both species of animals compared with controls when animals were sacrificed on day 20 for rats and day 18 for mice. Mahalik and coworkers[12] examined the placental transport properties of sodium-22 isotope when cocaine was given to pregnant mice on days 7 through 12. Impaired placental transport of sodium-22 isotope to the fetus after cocaine administration was interpreted by the authors as evidence of cocaine-induced vasoconstriction of uteroplacental blood vessels.

During the past three years we have utilized the pregnant ewe to define more carefully the effects of maternal cocaine administration upon the fetal lamb. The sheep is ideally suited for this type of study because it exhibits a high tolerance for uterine surgery without significant risk of premature labor. Moreover, the fetal lamb is similar to a human fetus in size and is large enough to tolerate chronic arterial and venous catheterization for frequent blood sampling. For years, this model has been the subject for studies of uterine and placental blood flow, fetal cardiac function and maternal-fetal oxygen transport. It is an ideal model, therefore, for the study of cocaine during pregnancy.

In this report, we:

1. evaluate the suitability of the pregnant ewe to study the mechanisms of cocaine action upon the maternal and fetal cardiovascular systems,
2. examine the pharmacokinetics of cocaine transfer from the pregnant ewe to fetus and
3. summarize behavioral and cardiovascular complications in this model to IV cocaine administration.

METHODS AND MATERIALS

Surgical Instrumentation of the Basic Animal Model

Pregnant ewes with singleton fetuses of 116-121 days gestational age (term = 145 days) were used in these studies. Each ewe was sedated with an intravenous (IV) injection of 0.02 mg/kg of a 100:1 Ketamine hydrochloride/xylazine hydrochloride mixture prior to tracheal intubation and was maintained during surgery on Halothane/oxygen using an Air-Shield Ventimeter 2 Surgical Respirator. Through a midline abdominal approach, a small incision was made in the uterus and the left fetal leg was exposed. A small incision was made in the fetal groin and a polyvinyl catheter was placed in the femoral artery for fetal arterial blood pressure (BP), heart rate

(HR) and arterial blood gas sampling. An additional catheter was placed in the femoral vein for collecting blood samples for cocaine analysis. After catheterization of fetal vessels, the fetal incision was sutured closed, the leg was returned to the uterus and the amniotic membranes and uterine incision were sutured closed in separate layers. A polyvinyl catheter was placed in the maternal femoral artery for blood pressure and heart rate measurements. An additional catheter was placed in the femoral vein for drug administration and for the collection of samples for cocaine analysis. The fetal catheters were brought out through the abdominal incision and both maternal and fetal catheters were passed subcutaneously along the left flank and placed in a pouch secured to the ewe's side.

All studies were conducted at least five days post surgery to allow for surgical recovery. Maternal and fetal catheters were flushed daily with 1000 units/ml and 100 units/ml heparin sodium, respectively.

Dosing

Cocaine hydrochloride (Sigma Chemical Company, St. Louis, MO) doses were dissolved in 5 ml physiologic saline (0.9% NaCl). Cocaine was administered IV to the ewe at 1.0 or 2.0 mg/kg body weight as a 30-second bolus injection. Twenty-four hours were allowed to pass before each ewe received the second dose. In some animals, cocaine, in doses of 3.0 mg/kg or 5.0 mg/kg, was administered in order to evaluate its effects upon behavior and cardiopulmonary function.

Physiologic Measurements

In all experiments, cardiovascular measurements were monitored continuously over a 30-minute baseline period and for one hour after cocaine administration. Blood pressures (BP) were monitored by attaching the maternal and fetal catheters to pressure transducers (Micron MP-15D) connected to pressure amplifiers (Sensormedics 9853C). Heart rates (HR) were measured by cardiotachometers (Sensormedics 9857) connected in series with the blood pressure amplifiers. Maternal and fetal blood pressures and heart rates were continuously recorded by a Sensormedics R-611 eight-channel recorder.

Arterial Blood Gas Measurements

Baseline maternal and fetal arterial blood gas samples were obtained 25 and 5 minutes before cocaine administration. Following cocaine injection, fetal arterial blood samples for blood gas determinations were obtained at 5, 10, 15, 30, and 60 minutes after cocaine administration.

Blood samples (0.5 ml) were drawn anaerobically from the fetal catheter into a 1.0-ml heparinized glass syringe and analyzed for PO_2, pH and PCO_2 using an Instrumentations Laboratory IL-1302 blood gas analyzer, adjusted to 39°C (sheep core temperature). Before each experiment, the blood gas analyzer was calibrated with two certified gas mixtures and verified with calibrated blood samples.

Cardiovascular Measurements

Baseline maternal and fetal cardiovascular measurements were obtained 25 and 5 minutes before cocaine injection. Maternal and fetal cardiovascular measurements were obtained at 1, 2, 5, 10, 15, 30, and 60 minutes after cocaine administration.

To determine maternal and fetal cardiovascular measurements, data points at 25 and 5 minutes before, and 5, 10, 15, 30 and 60 minutes after cocaine injection each represented the mean of 4 measurements taken over a two-minute period. At 1 and 2 minutes after cocaine injection, the reported data points each represented the mean of two measurements made over a 20-second period.

Cocaine Analysis

Baseline maternal and fetal venous samples (1.5 ml) for cocaine determination were obtained 15 minutes before cocaine administration. Maternal venous blood samples for cocaine analysis were obtained at 5, 15, 30 and 60 minutes after cocaine administration. Fetal venous blood samples for cocaine analysis were obtained at 5, 15 and 60 minutes after cocaine administration. In one experiment, maternal and fetal blood samples were collected every 30 seconds to 1 minute for the first 15 minutes and then at 30 and 60 minutes to examine how quickly cocaine crosses the placenta.

Since cocaine is a methyl ester easily hydrolyzed by plasma esterases, each sample for cocaine analysis was immediately injected into a 5-ml Vacutainer 6471 containing 12.5 mg sodium fluoride and 10.0 mg potassium oxalate. Sodium fluoride inhibits plasma esterases and prevents cocaine hydrolysis. Each sample was centrifuged at 3,000 RPM for 10 minutes and the serum decanted and frozen at $-20°C$ for later analysis of cocaine levels.

Cocaine was extracted from serum samples by the use of C-18 sorbent columns. To each 1.0-ml serum sample was added mepivacaine hydrochloride 10 ng (Sterling Organics, Rensselaer, NY) as an internal standard and 1.0 ml of 0.1 M Sodium Bicarbonate ($NaHCO_3$) buffer at pH 9.0. Each Bond Elute C-18 column (Analytichem #607101, Harbor City, CA) was activated with two washes of 1.0 ml methanol followed by 1.0 ml distilled H_2O and the sample/buffer/internal standard mixture placed on top of the column. After evacuation of the column using a Baker 10SPE vacuum manifold, the columns were washed three times with 0.5 ml distilled water. Each column was dried using N_2 at 25 ml/min for 5 minutes. The mepivacaine and cocaine were eluted from the column using three washes of 100 μl each of 90:10 methanol/ether mixture. The eluate (1.0 μl) was injected onto the gas chromatograph.

Detection and quantification of mepivacaine and cocaine were made using a Hewlett Packard HP 5890A gas chromatograph with a nitrogen-phosphorous detector. Carrier gas (He) flow was 20 ml/minute into a RSL-150 polydimethylsiloxane 10-meter capillary column. The injector temperature was 225°C and the detector temperature was 270°C with H_2 flow at 3.0 ml/minute and air flow at 130 ml/minute. At injection, the oven temperature was 170°C for 0.75 minutes, increasing to 270°C (20°/minute) over the next five minutes. Retention time for mepivacaine was 2.560 ± 0.050 minutes and cocaine was 3.095 ± 0.050 minutes.

Cocaine standards of 0.5, 1.0, 2.5, 5.0, 10.0, 25.0, 50.0, 100.0 and 200.0 ng cocaine/ μl methanol were prepared and analyzed by gas chromatography prior to analysis of unknowns. In each of the standards, 10 ng mepivacaine/μl methanol was included as the internal standard, and the ratio of cocaine to mepivacaine was used to construct a standard curve for each analysis day. In addition, two controls each of 1.0, 1.5, 2.0, 2.5, 5.0, 10.0, 25.0, 50.0, 100.0 and 200.0 ng cocaine with 10 ng mepivacaine/μl methanol were extracted in the same manner as unknown samples. These samples provided a means of verifying the standard curve and as an indicator of the recovery yield by this extraction method. The overall mean recovery yield of all extracted control samples was 85.0%.

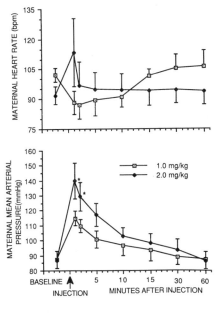

FIGURE 1. Responses of maternal HR and BP to IV injection of cocaine, 1.0 and 2.0 mg/kg in 6 animals. Data are shown as means ± SEM. (*Asterisk* indicates statistically significant differences between doses and from baseline values.)

To determine statistical significance, a two-way (factors = dose, time) repeated measures analysis of variance with a post hoc Student's Newman-Keuls test was used to determine differences between means. Statistical significance was established at *p* less than 0.05.

RESULTS

Within one minute following IV injection (FIG. 1), cocaine produced a slight decrease in maternal HR at 1.0 mg/kg but a transient tachycardia at 2.0 mg/kg when compared with basal measurements (TABLE 1). To these same two doses of cocaine, maternal BP exhibited dose-dependent increases which peaked by 1 minute. All maternal measurements had returned to baseline by 30 minutes post injection.

Maternal cocaine injection produced no significant changes in fetal pH or PCO_2. Responses of fetal HR, BP and oxygen tension (PO_2) to maternal administration of cocaine 1.0 and 2.0 mg/kg demonstrated drug-induced changes (FIG. 2). The fetal HR exhibited dose-dependent increases which were maximum by 15 minutes after maternal injection. In contrast, the fetal BP increased and the fetal PO_2 decreased to a maximum by 5 minutes, but neither change was dose dependent. All fetal values had returned to baseline by 30-45 minutes.

The concentrations of cocaine appearing in the maternal and fetal circulations following maternal administration of cocaine 1.0 and 2.0 mg/kg (TABLE 2) indicate that cocaine does not rapidly equilibrate across the placenta. By 5 minutes, fetal concentrations of cocaine were 14 and 17% of maternal concentrations. However, by 15 minutes, the fetal concentrations, although 21% of maternal concentrations for both doses, had declined significantly. By 60 minutes, no cocaine was detectable in either circulation.

In one experiment, maternal and fetal serum cocaine concentrations were determined every 30 seconds to 1 minute during the first 15 minutes and then at 30 and

TABLE 1. Baseline Cardiovascular Values prior to Maternal Adminstration of 1.0 mg/kg and 2.0 mg/kg IV Cocaine

		1.0-mg/kg Experiments	2.0-mg/kg Experiments
Maternal			
	MAP	87 ± 6	87 ± 5
	HR	102 ± 4	92 ± 4
Fetal			
	MAP	59 ± 3	60 ± 4
	HR	178 ± 7	190 ± 9
	pH	7.30 ± .02	7.31 ± .02
	PCO_2	47 ± 3	46 ± 2
	PO_2	26 ± 2	25 ± 2

60 minutes following IV injection of cocaine 2.0 mg/kg (FIG. 3). Cocaine peaked in the maternal circulation immediately following IV injection, rapidly declined in the first 2 minutes, and then declined more slowly over a 15 to 30 minute period. These data indicate that maternal cardiovascular responses coincided with peak maternal blood cocaine levels. Fetal cocaine levels increased initially to peak by 3 minutes and coincided with maximum increases in fetal mean arterial pressure (MAP). Thereafter, fetal cocaine levels fell rapidly by 4 to 6 minutes to remain at lower levels during the next 30 minutes.

In this study, maternal and fetal cardiovascular measurements in response to maternal IV cocaine injection were confined to doses of 1.0 and 2.0 mg/kg. These doses were selected since at higher doses, a number of cardiopulmonary and neurologic complications were encountered (TABLE 3). At 3.0 mg/kg, 3 of 5 animals died; one by cardiac arrhythmias (autopsy demonstrated acute myocarditis), one ruptured a pulmonary artery,[a] and one bled into the amniotic cavity (abruptio placenta).

[a] This complication, although a result of IV cocaine administration, occurred 5 days following surgical dissection of the pulmonary artery for electromagnetic flow probe placement for other ongoing studies.

TABLE 2. Maternal and Fetal Serum Cocaine Levels in ng/ml in Response to 1.0 mg/kg and 2.0 mg/kg Maternal IV Cocaine Administration

Dose mg/kg	Baseline	5 Min After	15 Min After	30 Min After	60 Min After
Maternal Levels					
1.0	0	2128 ± 446	615 ± 249	562 ± 518	0
2.0	0	2797 ± 506	751 ± 394	0.0	0
Fetal Levels					
1.0	0	327 ± 85	0	—	0
2.0	0	404 ± 95	167 ± 26	—	0

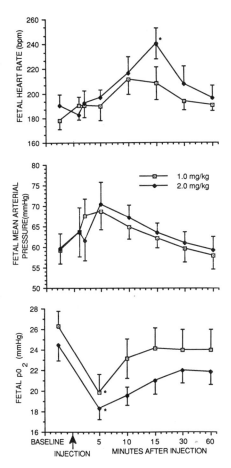

FIGURE 2. Responses of fetal HR, BP and PO_2 to maternal injection of IV cocaine, 1.0 and 2.0 mg/kg. Data are shown as means ± SEM for 6 animals. (*Asterisk* indicates statistically significant differences from baseline.)

TABLE 3. Cocaine Responses in the Pregnant Ewe

IV Dose mg/kg	N	Responses
0.5	5	no restlessness; no arrhythmias
1.0-2.0	15	increased restlessness, vocalization (15/15); increased attentiveness (15/15); mild arrhythmias
3.0	5	acute myocarditis (1); pulmonary artery rupture (1); abruptio placenta (1)
5.0	3	seizure activity and opisthotonos (3/3); death by arrhythmias (1/3); respiratory distress (3/3)

At 5.0 mg/kg, the animals uniformly exhibited cardiopulmonary distress followed by seizure (FIG. 4). Within 1 minute, each animal initially experienced increasing hypertension and tachycardia which rapidly progressed to bradyarrhythmias and collapse. By three minutes, the animals began to manifest progressive rigidity of all extremities, opisthotonos and generalized tonic seizure activity. At this time, respiratory function was extremely compromised, presumably from tonic intercostal muscle or diaphragm activity. By 5 to 8 minutes, seizure activity began to subside after which breathing became easier, cardiac rhythm stabilized and blood pressure began to decline.

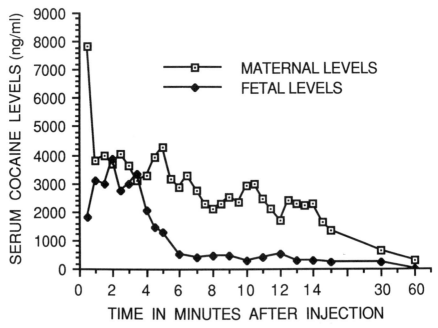

FIGURE 3. Maternal and fetal serum cocaine levels in one experiment obtained every 30 seconds to 1 minute for 15 minutes and then at 30 and 60 minutes following IV injection of cocaine 2.0 mg/kg.

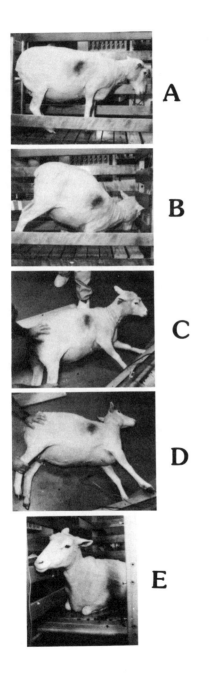

FIGURE 4. Neural-behavioral response to IV cocaine, 5.0 mg/kg. Panel (**A**) and (**B**): cocaine injection produces collapse by 1 minute: panel (**C**): animal repositioned; panel (**D**): opisthotonos, rigidity of all extremities, respiratory distress by 3 minutes; panel (**E**): resting without seizure activity or respiratory distress by 10 minutes.

By 10 minutes the animal was lying quietly and by 15 to 20 minutes each animal stood up in the cage. This pattern was observed in all 3 animals, the exception being that one animal experienced cardiopulmonary arrest midway through and failed to respond to cardiopulmonary resuscitation. Despite the complications observed at lower (3.0 mg/kg) doses, cocaine, 5.0 mg/kg, clearly produced the most significant and prolonged compromise of the cardiopulmonary and neurologic systems of the doses used in this study.

DISCUSSION

When administered to pregnant ewes, intravenous cocaine produces dose-dependent increases in maternal heart rate and blood pressure and dose-dependent decreases in uterine blood flow.[13] Fetal responses to maternal cocaine administration are characterized by fetal tachycardia and hypertension. These fetal cardiovascular responses result, in part, from fetal hypoxemia secondary to cocaine-induced uterine-artery vasoconstriction. Additionally, via maternal-placental transfer to the fetus, cocaine may increase fetal blood pressure and heart rate as a direct drug action.

Although studies have demonstrated that placental transfer of cocaine to the fetus does occur, the animal models selected and/or the methods of study employed have prevented an examination of a correlation between fetal cocaine blood levels and cardiovascular function. Shaw and co-workers observed only small amounts of Levo (3H) cocaine in fetal mice following maternal intraperitoneal injection.[14] In this study, no physiologic measurements of the fetus were made. More recently, Moore and co-workers observed that maternal injection of IV cocaine (0.5 mg/kg) produced fetal blood levels that were approximately 10-15% of maternal levels at 5 and 30 minutes, respectively.[15] These blood levels were associated with fetal mean-arterial pressure increases from 55 to 62 mmHg. A cocaine dose of 0.5 mg/kg, however, produces insufficient reductions in uterine blood flow to affect fetal PO_2 levels.[13] Moore's data would suggest, therefore, that cocaine produces direct cardiovascular actions in the fetus which are independent of fetal hypoxemia secondary to reduced uterine blood flow.

The results of the present study indicate that maternal and fetal cardiovascular changes to maternally-administered IV cocaine exhibit different patterns of response. Moreover, while maternal HR and BP responses to cocaine are dose dependent, only fetal HR responses clearly exhibit this characteristic. Maternal cardiovascular responses to cocaine are dose dependent and are a direct drug action. In contrast, fetal BP and PO_2 are both affected by IV cocaine; but neither appears to exhibit a dose-response relationship. Moreover, fetal HR and BP changes result from fetal hypoxemia secondary to reduced uterine blood flow, as well as from direct cocaine actions arising from cocaine transfer to the fetus.

Previous studies in which fetal hypoxemia was created by methods other than by cocaine injection provide insight into the fetal response to low oxygen levels. Skillman and co-workers utilized an externally-controlled constriction device around the uterine arteries in the pregnant ewe in order to evaluate the relationship of uterine blood flow reductions to fetal oxygenation.[16] A 25% reduction in uterine blood flow produced a small drop in fetal PO_2 (-2.4 mmHg), but there was no change in fetal BP. At 50% reduction in blood flow, fetal PO_2 fell by 7.9 mmHg and fetal MAP increased 5 mmHg. At 63% reduction, fetal PO_2 fell by 8.2 mmHg and MAP increased 5 mmHg. These data indicate that uterine blood-flow reductions in excess of 25% produce similar increases in fetal MAP and decreases in fetal PO_2. Cocaine at doses of 1.0 and 2.0 mg/kg previously have been shown to produce reductions in uterine blood flow of 34 and 47%, respectively.[13] In the present study, cocaine, 1.0 and 2.0 mg/kg, produced similar increases in fetal MAP (8 and 10 mmHg, respectively) and decreases in fetal PO_2 (-6 and -6.2 mmHg). The authors attribute these changes in fetal PO_2 directly to cocaine-induced uterine artery vasoconstriction.

Despite similar changes in fetal PO_2 levels, the magnitude of the fetal MAP response to maternal cocaine injection is approximately double the fetal MAP response to hypoxemia produced by mechanical uterine artery occlusion alone. These differences suggest that cocaine has direct cardiovascular actions in the fetal circulation which are not related to fetal PO_2 levels. Support for this premise is provided from a previous study, in which cocaine was injected directly into the fetal circulation.[13] When IV cocaine doses of 0.5, 1.0 and 2.0 mg/kg (estimated fetal weight for gestational age) were given directly to the fetus, no changes in fetal PO_2 were observed. Nevertheless, all three doses produced fetal hypertension by 5 minutes and fetal tachycardia by 15 minutes. The magnitude of the fetal HR and BP responses were similar at all dose levels and, therefore, were not dose dependent.

In the present study, fetal serum cocaine levels were 14 and 17% of maternal levels at 5 and 15 minutes, respectively, following IV injection of cocaine 1.0 and 2.0 mg/kg to the pregnant ewe. In a separate experiment in which more frequent fetal blood samples were taken, however, cocaine was found to cross the placenta from maternal to fetal circulations rapidly, peaking by 3 minutes. Fetal serum cocaine levels determined at 5 minutes, therefore, do not represent peak levels. Nevertheless, even these fetal concentrations of cocaine are considerably greater than would be predicted to occur in our previous study from direct fetal injection of cocaine, 0.5, 1.0 and 2.0 mg/kg (estimated fetal weight for gestational age).[13] The fetal lamb's weight is approximately 1/50 that of the pregnant ewe. Cocaine doses which were selected for direct fetal injection were, therefore, very low when compared with the maternal doses used in the current study. Yet, the fetal injections produced cardiovascular changes in the absence of fetal hypoxemia. In the current study, the levels of cocaine found in the fetal circulation following maternal administration are sufficient, therefore, to produce direct cardiovascular effects in the fetus. Of note, the distribution of cocaine at 5 minutes in maternal and fetal circulations is similar to that reported by Moore *et al.*[15] in response to a smaller dose of cocaine (0.5 mg/kg). These collective findings suggest that, unlike oxygen transport to the fetus, transport of cocaine from the maternal to the fetal compartment is not limited by cocaine-mediated uterine artery vasoconstriction.

Maternal cardiovascular and neurologic complications observed in response to IV cocaine doses of 3.0 to 5.0 mg/kg were unanticipated. These findings nevertheless coincide with cocaine-related complications observed among clinical populations.[17] Although increased restlessness and agitation were noted in all ewes following cocaine doses of 1.0 mg/kg or greater, significant cardiopulmonary complications or seizures were confined to responses following injection of 3.0 to 5.0 mg/kg. One noteworthy observation is that cocaine-induced seizures usually are described as tonic-clonic and are attributed to the neurotoxic actions of cocaine in the central nervous system.[18] In the current study, seizures following 5.0 mg/kg cocaine were identical in all three animals and also were consistent with those described following strichnine administration.[19] Strichnine seizures are characterized by stiffness of the neck and face, extension of the body and all limbs, opisthotonos, and respiratory compromise from contraction of the diaphragm, thoracic, and abdominal muscles. Strichnine-induced seizures also are characterized by hypersensitivity to sensory stimuli leading to tonic extension of the extremities. Because in this study sensory stimuli were not introduced during the cocaine-induced seizures, this component of strichnine seizure was not assessed. The lethal human dose of cocaine is estimated to be 1.4 g, or approximately 20 mg/kg for a 70 kg individual.[20] The authors' data suggest that, at least during pregnancy, the cardiovascular system of the ewe is more sensitive to such cocaine-related complications as bradyarrhythmias, seizure activity, acute respiratory distress, and death than is that of the human. Additional studies are needed to evaluate the etiology of this cardiopulmonary sensitivity to IV cocaine in the pregnant ewe.

SUMMARY

Transplacental passage of cocaine in response to maternal administration of intravenous (IV) cocaine in doses of 1.0 and 2.0 mg/kg was studied in 6 pregnant ewes and fetuses and correlated with maximum changes in maternal and fetal blood pressures (BP), heart rates (HR) and fetal arterial blood gas values. Certain animals were given larger doses (3.0 and 5.0 mg/kg) of cocaine to examine cocaine-related cardiopulmonary and neurologic sequelae. Cocaine was extracted on C-18 sorbent columns and analyzed by gas chromatography. At 1.0 and 2.0 mg/kg, cocaine produced dose-dependent increases in maternal HR and BP which were maximum by 1 minute. The fetal response was characterized by maximum increases in BP and decreases in PO_2 by 3 minutes and increases in HR by 15 minutes. Cocaine rapidly appeared in the fetal circulation, was approximately 15% of maternal concentrations by 5 minutes, and was undetectable in both circulations by 60 minutes. At cocaine doses of 3.0 and 5.0 mg/kg significant maternal cardiopulmonary and neurologic complications were encountered including bradyarrhythmias, respiratory distress, seizure and death. These data indicate that cocaine exerts direct drug actions upon maternal cardiovascular and neurologic function. In addition, cocaine affects fetal cardiovascular function directly via transplacental passage and indirectly by fetal hypoxemia from cocaine-induced uterine artery vasoconstriction. (NIDA 04415)

REFERENCES

1. EVANS, M. A. & R. D. HARBISON. 1977. Cocaine, marihuana, LSD: Pharmacologic effects in the fetus and newborn. In Drug Abuse in Pregnancy and Neonatal Effects. J. L. Rementeria, Ed.: 195-208. C. V. Mosby. New York, NY.

2. LEE, R. V. 1982. Drug abuse. In Medical Complications During Pregnancy. G. N. Burrow & T. F. Ferris, Eds. W. B. Saunders. Philadelphia, PA.

3. ACKER, D., B. P. SACHS, K. J. TRACEY & W. E. WISE. 1983. Abruptio placentae associated with cocaine use. Am. J. Obstet. Gynecol. 146: 220-221.

4. CHASNOFF, I. J., W. J. BURNS, S. H. SCHNOLL & K. A. BURNS. 1985. Cocaine use in pregnancy. N. Engl. J. Med. 313: 666-669.

5. HENDERSON, C. E. & M. TORBEY. 1988. Rupture of intracranial aneurysms associated with cocaine use during pregnancy. Am. J. Perinatol. 5: 142-143.

6. MACGREGOR, S. N., L. G. KEITH, I. J. CHASNOFF, M. A. ROSNER, G. M. CHISUM, P. SHAW & J. P. MINOGUE. 1987. Cocaine use during pregnancy: Adverse perinatal outcome. Am. J. Obstet. Gynecol. 157: 686-690.

7. ORO, A. S. & S. D. DIXON. 1987. Perinatal cocaine and methamphetamine exposure: Maternal and neonatal correlates. J. Pediatr. 111: 571-578.

8. RITCHIE, J. M. & N. M. GREENE. 1980. Local anesthetics. *In* The Pharmacological Basis of Therapeutics. 6th edit. A. G. Gilman, L. S. Goodman, T. W. Rall & F. Murad, Eds.: 307. Macmillan. New York, NY.

9. GREISS, F. C., JR. & D. VAN WILKES. 1964. Effects of sympathomimetic drugs and angiotensin on the uterine vascular bed. Obstet. Gynecol. **23:** 925-930.

10. ROSENFELD, C. R. & J. WEST. 1977. Circulatory response to systemic infusion of norepinephrine in the pregnant ewe. Am. J. Obstet. Gynecol. **157:** 376-383.

11. FANTEL, A. G. & B. J. MACPHAIL. 1982. The teratogenicity of cocaine. Teratology **26:** 17-19.

12. MAHALIK, M. P., R. F. GAUTIERI & D. E. MANN, JR.. 1984. Mechanisms of cocaine-induced teratogenesis. Res. Commun. Subst. Abuse **5:** 279-302.

13. WOODS, J. R., JR., M. A. PLESSINGER & K. E. CLARK. 1987. Effect of cocaine on uterine blood flow and fetal oxygenation. J. Am. Med. Assoc. **257:** 957-961.

14. SHAH, N. S., D. A. MAY & J. D. YATES. 1980. Disposition of Levo (^{3}H) cocaine in pregnant and nonpregnant mice. Toxicol. Appl. Pharmacol. **53:** 279-284.

15. MOORE, T. R., J. SORG, L. MILLER, T. C. KEY & R. RESNIK. 1986. Hemodynamic effects of intravenous cocaine on the pregnant ewe and fetus. Am. J. Obstet. Gynecol. **155:** 883-888.

16. SKILLMAN, C. A., M. A. PLESSINGER, J. R. WOODS, JR. & K. E. CLARK. 1985. Effect of graded reductions in uteroplacental blood flow on the fetal lamb. Am. J. Physiol. **249:** H1098-H1105.

17. ISNER, J. M., N. A. M. ESTES, P. D. THOMPSON, M. R. COSTANZO-NORDIN, R. SUBRAMANIAN, G. MILLER, G. KATSAD, K. SWEENEY & W. Q. STURNER. 1986. Acute cardiac events temporally related to cocaine abuse. N. Engl. J. Med. **315:** 1438-1443.

18. RICHIE, J. M. & N. M. GREENE. 1985. Central nervous system stimulants. *In* The Pharmacologic Basis of Therapeutics. 6th edit. A. G. Gilman, L. S. Goodman, T. W. Ralls & F. Murad, Eds.: 304. Macmillan. New York, NY.

19. FRANZ, D. N. 1985. Central nerous system stimulants. *In* The Pharmacologic Basis of Therapeutics. 6th edit. A. G. Gilman, L. S. Goodman, T. W. Ralls & F. Murad, Eds.: 584. Macmillan. New York, NY.

20. SMART, R. G. & L. ANGLIN. 1987. Do we know the lethal dose of cocaine? J. Forensic Sci. **32:** 303-312.

Long-Term Neurochemical and Neurobehavioral Consequences of Cocaine Use during Pregnancy[a]

DIANA L. DOW-EDWARDS

Department of Neurosurgery
Laboratory of Cerebral Metabolism
State University of New York
Health Science Center
450 Clarkson Avenue, Box 1189
Brooklyn, New York 11203-2098

With the increase in cocaine use among the general population in recent years,[1] ill effects of the drug have occurred in all social strata and age groups, including pregnant women. For example, over 300 babies were born at the Kings County Hospital (Brooklyn) during 1986 from women admitting to frequent cocaine use during pregnancy.[2] These babies were more frequently delivered at 37 weeks or earlier, were 3.6 times more likely to have intrauterine growth retardation, and 2.8 times more likely to have a head circumference below the tenth percentile for gestational age than were cohort-matched babies. Other clinical reports have also appeared associating cocaine use during pregnancy with serious physical abnormalities in the newborn.[3,4] In a large, well-controlled series, Chasnoff *et al.*[5] were able to identify cocaine-exposed infants as being jittery, irritable, and exhibiting decreased interactive behavior and poor organizational responses. There is ample clinical evidence then, that intrauterine exposure to cocaine can result in neurobehavioral and developmental abnormalities in the infant.

Maternal Cocaine Administration

Animal studies pertaining to the developmental toxicity of cocaine appeared as early as 1980 (see REF. 6 for review). Together, the animal data indicate that cocaine use during pregnancy is associated with decreased maternal weight gain, intrauterine growth retardation, and neurobehavioral abnormalities. The strength of the animal data is that it shows with certainty that the changes are the effects of cocaine exposure per se and are not merely the result of polydrug interactions, which are so difficult to control in clinical populations. The limitation of the animal studies rests on whether the rat is an appropriate model for the effects of cocaine on human development.

[a] Supported in part by National Institute on Drug Abuse Grant DA04118, National Institute of Neurological and Communicative Disorders and Stroke Grant NS22766, and the State University of New York.

Our first published report examining the neurobehavioral effects of prenatal cocaine exposure[7] shows that the drug significantly alters activity levels at a time around the day of weaning (21 days). In this series of studies, two doses of cocaine, 30 and 60 mg/kg were administered by gastric intubation each day between gestation day 8 and 22 of the rat. A pair-fed, pair-watered, vehicle-intubated control group and a control group receiving no treatment were maintained. All litters were fostered at birth to eliminate the possible residual effects of cocaine or the pair-feeding procedures on postnatal development of the pups. While these doses had minimal effects on fetal development as determined by litter size, birth weight, etc. (TABLE 1), activity levels

TABLE 1. Maternal and Offspring Effects (Mean ± SEM)

	Nontreated	Pair-Fed	30 mg/kg	60 mg/kg
Litters	13	9	9	11
Mean maternal wt gain (g)	202.8 ± 7.0	165.5 ± 5.3[a]	170.8 ± 5.1[a]	169.2 ± 5.1[a]
Mean implantation sites	15.1 ± 0.8	14.9 ± 0.8	14.6 ± 0.3	16.7 ± 0.6
% resorptions	1.36%	4.46%	3.77%	1.77%
% perinatal mortality	0.47%	3.21%	0.00%	1.01%
Total offspring mortality	1.87%	7.66%	3.77%	2.78%
Number born live				
Male	105 (55%)	68 (56%)	57 (45%)	91 (51%)
Female	86 (45%)	56 (44%)	69 (55%)	88 (49%)
Mean litter size	14.7 ± 0.7	13.8 ± 0.7	14.0 ± 0.4	16.3 ± 0.6[b]
Mean birthweight (g)				
Male	7.26 ± 0.15	6.83 ± 0.23	7.16 ± 0.10	6.34 ± 0.14[c]
Female	6.63 ± 0.15	6.36 ± 0.18	6.82 ± 0.15	5.98 ± 0.15[c]

[a] $p < 0.001$, univariate F test, significantly different from nontreated group.
[b] $p < 0.02$, univariate F test, significantly different from pair-fed and 30 mg/kg cocaine groups.
[c] By ANOVA significant effect of treatment but not by ANCOVA.

determined in intact litters were significantly *elevated* on postnatal days 20 and 23 in the high-dose cocaine group (FIG. 1). Since this is a time when the central neurons regulating activity are rapidly undergoing synaptogenesis,[8] it is possible that prenatal cocaine exposure alters the normal developmental sequence in these important central neuronal pathways.

Spear et al.[9,10] have also reported that prenatal cocaine exposure at a dose too small to produce obvious malformations nevertheless does induce abnormal behavioral development which persists at least until the time of weaning. These results, discussed by Spear et al. in this volume, emphasize that prenatal cocaine alters the development of central pathways regulating activity levels as well as cognitive abilities. The majority of these neurobehavioral changes occur at a time in the rat equivalent to the last trimester of pregnancy and the early postnatal period in human development. Several other groups have now found that prenatal cocaine exposure induces long-term neurobehavioral changes including altered startle responses[11] and altered male sexual behavior.[12]

The possible mechanisms whereby cocaine induces these neurobehavioral effects has also been the subject of much interest recently. Woods in this volume presents impressive evidence that cocaine lowers fetal oxygen tension and raises fetal heart rate and blood pressure in a dose-dependent manner when administered iv to a pregnant

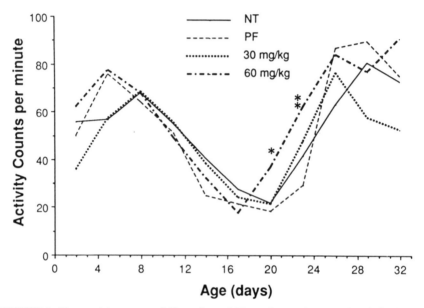

FIGURE 1. Mean activity counts of 60 mg/kg and 30 mg/kg cocaine-treated, pair-fed (PF), and nontreated (NT) litters. Dam is removed and whole litter activity levels are recorded for 1 hour on a Stoelting Activity Monitor between days 2 and 32 of life. * $p < 0.001$, univariate F test, significantly different from all other groups. ** $p < 0.006$, univariate F test, significantly different from PF group.

ewe. The possibility of chronic hypoxia as well as the likelihood of chronic undernutrition (which are both associated with cocaine use) together would be expected to have significant effects on growth of the fetus and neurochemistry of the brain. Since clinical studies have documented that cocaine is present in the urine of exposed newborns, cocaine must be present in the fetal circulation. Thereafter, due to its high lipid solubility, cocaine has direct access to all developing tissues, including the brain.

Direct Effects of Cocaine on Brain Development

The presence of psychoactive drugs affecting any of several neurotransmitter systems can result in long-term alterations in the structure and function of these systems and their associated behaviors.[13-16] In the case of cocaine, altered activity at the dopaminergic, noradrenergic, and serotonergic synapses might be expected. Since the developing brain responds to drugs affecting these systems, we hypothesized that cocaine administration during the transition between the day-1 dopamine receptor pattern and the day-21 pattern (see below, FIG. 3) would alter the structure and function of these highly dopaminergic forebrain regions. Our first experimental approach was to administer cocaine at a time approximately equivalent to the third trimester in utero for humans: during the early postnatal period of the rat, a time when synaptogenesis is occurring in the forebrain (see FIG. 3).[8,17-20] This period is characterized by rapid axonal and dendritic expansion, and is highly sensitive to environmental influences.[21] Others have found that drug administration during this period alters the function of these synapses both immediately and perhaps permanently (see above). The results of our experiments with cocaine correlate with these findings.[22,23]

In the first study, we administered 50 mg/kg cocaine HCl (sc) to half of the pups in a litter and the vehicle (water) to the other half. On days 1 and 2 (day of birth = 1) the dose was divided into two portions and administered 8 hours apart. On days 3 through 10, the injections were administered only once a day in the morning. Reflex ontogeny was assessed on a small sample of pups throughout this early period and was found not to be affected. Growth of the pups before and after day of weaning (day 21) was also not affected (FIG. 2). At 60 days of age, there were no statistically significant differences between groups in mean arterial blood pressure, arterial blood gases or pH, hematocrit, or plasma glucose concentration (TABLE 2).

Brain glucose metabolism, an index of functional activity, was determined using the deoxyglucose method[24] as previously described.[25] The female rats were all examined during diestrus to minimize differences in brain metabolism which occur across days of the estrus cycle.[26] The female treated rats showed significantly increased rates of brain functional activity with specific highly dopaminergic regions showing the greatest percentage changes compared to the control females (TABLE 3). Two structures associated with the mesocortical dopaminergic system, the cingulate cortex and the ventral tegmental area, were very significantly stimulated with p values < 0.002 (FIG. 4). Most of the regions examined in the female rats were 10 to 15% more metabolically active in the treated female animals (TABLE 3). This is in sharp contrast to the findings with the male rats (FIG. 4, TABLE 3). Here, neonatal cocaine treatment had little effect on brain glucose metabolism (TABLE 3). Therefore, one might conclude that cocaine administration at 50 mg/kg during the first 10 postnatal days has no long-term effect on brain glucose metabolism in male rats, but a large stimulatory effect in females.

The increased sensitivity to cocaine in female rats has often been described by others. Cocaine induces a greater amount of turning in females than in males while behavioral sensitization to cocaine has a lower threshold and is longer lasting in females than in males.[27-29] We have also now repeated our experiments by injecting the developing rats between postnatal days 11 and 20 and have found very similar results (TABLE 4). Many highly dopaminergic brain regions were metabolically stimulated in the female treated rats while others, such as the sensory cortex, were not. Again, there were no long-term changes in brain functional activity in the males.

In order to determine whether changes in glucose metabolic activity reflected changes in activity of the dopamine system, per se, patterns of tritiated dopamine-specific ligand binding were determined. Brain sections from animals undergoing identical treatments to those used in the deoxyglucose experiments were incubated with either ^{3}H SCH 23390 for marking the D_1 receptor or ^{3}H sulpiride for marking the D_2 receptor. FIGURE 5 shows the altered pattern of D_1 receptors in adult females exposed between postnatal days 11 and 20. The caudal portions of the caudate nucleus showed the greatest percentage increase in D_1 binding ($+72\%$). At this time we do not know whether the increase in binding represents an increase in affinity of the ligand for the receptor or whether there is an increase in the B_{max}. However, it appears that the presence of cocaine in the brain during the time of synaptogenesis can result in long-term changes in the neurochemistry of the dopaminergic system.

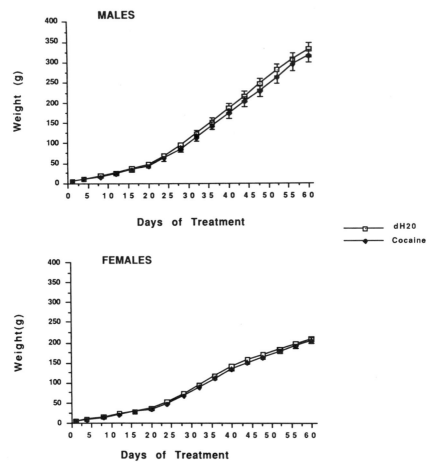

FIGURE 2. Growth curves of both male (*top*) and female (*bottom*) treated and control Sprague-Dawley rats. The treatment consisted of 50 mg/kg cocaine sc between days 1 and 10 of life. Each point represents approximately 8 observations. There were no statistically significant differences between treated and control values.

Due to the importance of the dopaminergic system in determining activity levels, we wanted to examine several behaviors in the exposed adults. Therefore, we prepared another group of rats by injecting half with cocaine at 50 mg/kg and the other half with the vehicle (water), following the same injection schedules and treatments as we had previously. Again, at 60-65 days of age, the rats (with females all in diestrus)

TABLE 2. Physiologic Parameters of Rats Treated Postnatally (Days 1-10) with Cocaine[a]

	Female		Male	
	Water (N = 6)	Cocaine (N = 6)	Water (N = 6)	Cocaine (N = 7)
Weight (g)	197 ± 3	204 ± 7	347 ± 16	343 ± 13
Glucose (mg/ml)	1.22 ± .02	1.22 ± .07	1.19 ± .05	1.20 ± .06
Temperature (°C)	37.9 ± .18	37.7 ± .07	37.4 ± .08	37.4 ± .13
Pressure (mmHg)	127 ± 3	121 ± 2	120 ± 3	117 ± 2
Hematocrit (%)	48.6 ± 2.1	49.2 ± 1.4	45.7 ± 1.5	47.3 ± 0.9
Arterial blood gases				
PO_2 (mmHg)	89.8 ± 11.5	94.3 ± 6.6	85.0 ± 5.3	86.3 ± 5.9
PCO_2 (mmHg)	24.6 ± 2.1	23.4 ± 2.9	29.0 ± 2.1	30.9 ± 2.9
pH	7.36 ± .04	7.38 ± .05	7.41 ± .05	7.40 ± .05
Estrus cycle	diestrus	diestrus		

[a] Values are means ± SEM for the number of animals indicated.

were examined for baseline activity for 15 minutes in a Digiscan Activity Monitor (Omnitech Equipment Corp). The monitor has 8 photosensors on each side, a second row of sensors placed 16 cm above the floor, a sound-insulated wood enclosure with two 5-watt lights, and a Par ventilator fan. The behaviors occurring during fifteen one-minute intervals were automatically recorded and grouped into three 5-minute intervals.

As shown in FIGURE 6, neonatal cocaine exposure in female rats significantly decreased the distance traveled per minute during the fifteen minutes of baseline recording. In fact, overall scores in all behaviors except rest time were significantly lower in the treated females compared to the controls. Male rats, however, did not

TABLE 3. Percent Change in Brain Glucose Metabolism in Selected Regions from Rats Treated with Cocaine between Postnatal Days 1 and 10[a]

	Female Rats	Male Rats
CORTEX:		
cingulate	+19[b]	− 4
primary motor	+14	− 1
primary sensory	+12	+ 1
Caudate n	+14[b]	+ 4
N. accumbens	+14	0
Globus pallidus	+ 4	0
Substantia nigra	+ 9	+ 2
Ventral tegmental area	+16[b]	− 2
Interpeduncular n	+20[b]	− 6
Hippocampus		
CA1	+15[b]	− 4

[a] Calculated from mean rate of glucose utilization in μMol/100g tissue/min for 6 control and 6 treated females and 5 control and 6 treated males.
[b] Means are significantly different with p values ≤ 0.05 by t test.

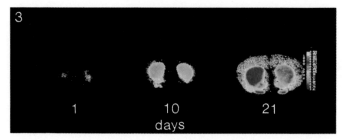

FIGURE 3. Computer-generated images of ³H SCH 23390 binding in rat forebrain during the first 21 days of life. All sections taken through the caudate nucleus including the nucleus accumbens and olfactory tubercle where possible. Sections depict concentrations of dopamine (D₁) receptors which attain adult levels by postnatal day 30. The presence of dopamine fluorescence from the terminals in these regions generally precedes the appearance of the receptors. System from Amersham Corp. (Chicago, IL) with the software from Loats Associates (MD). (× 1.4).

appear to demonstrate any change in baseline behaviors of any kind. Again, female rats appear to be more sensitive to the effects of cocaine exposure during development than male rats. These studies should not be taken to mean that cocaine-exposed infants will be less active because extrapolation of behavior from rat to man is quite difficult. The most prudent conclusion is that cocaine exposure induces long-term alterations in animal behavior implicating long-term changes in the central pathways regulating these complex actions.

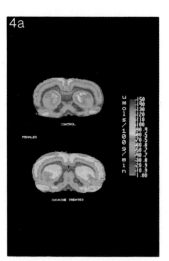
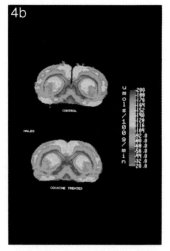

FIGURE 4. Computer-generated images of coronal sections of rat brain comparing rates of glucose metabolism in adult rats receiving either vehicle or cocaine injections during the pre-weaning period. (**4a**) Female control (*top*) and cocaine-treated (*bottom*). (**4b**) Male control (*top*) and cocaine-treated (*bottom*). (Amersham/Loats imaging system.) Values in μMol/100g/min. (× 1.4).

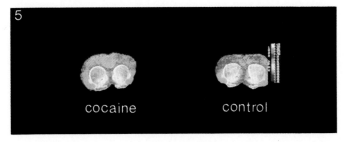

FIGURE 5. Computer-generated images of ³H SCH 23390 binding in coronal sections of the brains of adult female rats which had received either vehicle or cocaine injections during the preweaning period. (Amersham/Loats imaging system.) ($\times$ 1.3).

CONCLUSION

Exposure to cocaine during critical periods of development has been shown to produce lasting neurochemical changes in brain of the rat coupled with both early and late behavioral alterations. Females appear to be more sensitive than males. Brain effects occur at a dose where little general toxicity is seen. If the rat is a suitable model to study the effects of cocaine on development of the human nervous system, our data would suggest that cocaine may place exposed children at risk for neurochemical and neurobehavioral abnormalities which may last into adulthood.

ACKNOWLEDGMENTS

The contributions of T. H. Milhorat, L. A. Freed, G. Pringle, R. J. Wolintz, A. Fingesten, Z. Gamagaris, and D. Segal are greatly appreciated.

TABLE 4. Percent Change in Brain Glucose Metabolism in Selected Regions from Rats Treated with Cocaine between Postnatal Days 11 and 20[a]

	Female Rats	Male Rats
CORTEX:		
cingulate	+18[b]	− 7
primary motor	+20[b]	− 7
primary sensory	+13	− 2
Caudate n	+22[b]	+ 4
N. accumbens	+22[b]	− 2
Globus pallidus	+28[b]	− 7
Substantia nigra	+21[b]	− 5
Ventral tegmental area	+30[b]	− 1
Interpeduncular n	+24[b]	+ 5
Hippocampus		
CA1	+33[b]	− 9

[a] Calculated from mean rate of glucose utilization in μMol/100g tissue/min for 4 control and 5 treated females and 5 control and 5 treated males.

[b] Means are significantly different with p values ≤ 0.05 by t test.

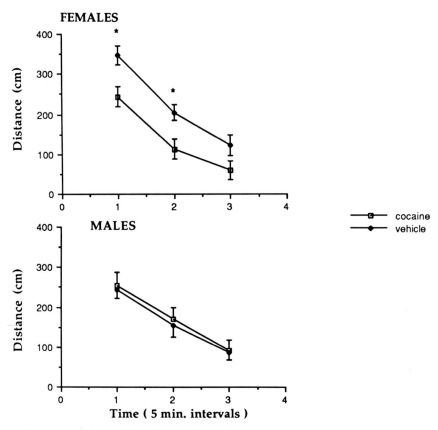

FIGURE 6. Baseline activity collected with a Digiscan Activity Monitor with vertical sensors 16 cm from the base of the floor. Values represent average distance traveled (cm/min) in 5 one-minute intervals (mean ± SEM) of data obtained from 46 adult rats receiving vehicle or 50 mg/kg cocaine between days 11 and 20 of life. * represents a statistically significant difference from control by t test. Overall difference in distance travelled for females significant at $p = 0.004$. All females were in diestrus at the time of the behavioral observation.

REFERENCES

1. ADAMS, E. H. & D. DURELL. 1984. Cocaine: A growing public health problem. In Cocaine: Pharmacology, Effects and Treatment of Abuse. J. Grabowski, Ed.: 9-14. NIDA Research Monograph 50. DHHS Pub. #(ADM) 84-1326. National Institute on Drug Abuse. Rockville, MD.

2. CHERUKURI, R., H. MINKOFF, J. FELDMAN, A. PAREKH & L. A. GLASS. 1988. Cohort study of alkaloidal cocaine ("crack") in pregnancy. Obstet. Gynecol. **72:** 147-151.

3. BINGOL, H., M. FUCHS, V. DIAZ, R. K. STONE & D. S. GROMISH. 1987. Teratogenicity of cocaine in humans. J. Pediatr. **110:** 93-96.

4. CHASNOFF, I. J., G. M. CHISUM & W. E KAPLAN. 1988. Maternal cocaine use and genitourinary tract malformations. Teratology **37:** 201-204.

5. CHASNOFF, I. J., W. J. BURNS, S. H. SCHOLL & K. A. BURNS. 1985. Cocaine use in pregnancy. New Engl. J. Med. **313:** 666-669.

6. DOW-EDWARDS, D. L. 1988. Developmental effects of cocaine. In Mechanisms of Cocaine

Abuse and Toxicity. K. Ashgar, R. Brown & D. Clouet, Eds.: 290-303. NIDA Research Monograph 88. National Institute on Drug Abuse. Rockville, MD.

7. HUTCHINGS, D. E., T. A. FICO & D. L. DOW-EDWARDS. Prenatal cocaine: Maternal toxicity, fetal effects, and motor activity in rat offspring. Neurotoxicol. Teratol. In press.

8. HARTLEY, E. J. & P. SEEMAN. 1983. Development of receptors for dopamine and noradrenaline in rat brain. Eur. J. Pharmacol. **91:** 391-397.

9. SPEAR, L. P., C. KIRSTEIN, J. BELL, R. GREENBAUM, J. O'SHEA, V. YOOTTANASUMPUN, H. HOFFMAN & N. E. SPEAR. 1987. Effects of prenatal cocaine on behavior during the early postnatal period in rats (abstract). Teratology **35:** 8B.

10. SPEAR, L. P., N. FRAMBES, C. KIRSTEIN, J. BELL, L. ROGERS, V. YOOTTANASUMPUN & N. E. SPEAR. 1988. Neurobehavioral teratogenic effects of prenatal exposure to cocaine (abstract). Teratology **37:** 517.

11. FOSS, J. A. & E. P. RILEY. 1988. Behavioral evaluation of animals exposed prenatally to cocaine (abstract). Teratology **37:** 517.

12. McGIVERN, R. F., W. J. RAIM, R. Z. SOKOL & P. PETERSON. 1988. Long-term effects of prenatal cocaine exposure on scent marking and the HPG axis in male rats (abstract). Teratology **37:** 518.

13. LOIZOU, A. L. 1972. The postnatal ontogeny of monoamine-containing neurons in the CNS of albino rats. Brain Res. **40:** 395-418.

14. COYLE, J. T. & D. HENRY. 1973. Catecholamines in fetal and newborn rat brain. J. Neurochem. **21:** 61-67.

15. ROSENGARTEN, H. & A. J. FRIEDHOFF. 1979. Enduring changes in dopamine receptor cells of pups from drug administration to pregnant and nursing rats. Science **203:** 1133-1135.

16. FRIEDHOFF, A. J. & J. C. MILLER. 1983. Prenatal psychotrophic drug exposure and the development of central dopaminergic and cholinergic neurotransmitter systems. Monogr. Neural Sci. **9:** 91-98.

17. LEVITT, P. & R. Y. MOORE. 1979. Development of the noradrenergic innervation of neocortex. Brain Res. **162:** 243-259.

18. FILLION, G. & C. BAUGUEN. 1984. Postnatal development of ^{3}H-5-HT binding in the presence of GTP in rat brain cortex. Dev. Pharmacol. Ther. 7(Suppl.): 1-5.

19. MOON-EDLEY, S. & M. HERKENHAM. 1984. Comparative development of striatal opiate receptors and dopamine revealed by autoradiography and histofluorescence. Brain Res. **305:** 27-42.

20. MURRIN, L. C., D. L. GIBBENS & J. R. FERRER. 1985. Ontogeny of dopamine, serotonin and spirodecanone receptors in rat forebrain—an autoradiographic study. Dev. Brain Res. **23:** 91-109.

21. DOBBING J. 1968. Vulnerable periods in developing brain. *In* Applied Neurochemistry. A. Davison & J. Dobbing, Eds.: 287-316. Davis, Co. Philadelphia, PA.

22. DOW-EDWARDS, D. L., L. A. FREED & T. H. MILHORAT. 1986. The effects of cocaine on development. Soc. Neurosci. Abstr. **12:** 59.12.

23. DOW-EDWARDS, D. L., L. A. FREED & T. H. MILHORAT. 1988. Stimulation of brain metabolism by perinatal cocaine exposure. Dev. Brain Res. **42:** 137-141.

24. SOKOLOFF, L., M. REIVICH, C. KENNEDY, M. H. DES ROSIERS, C. S. PATLAK, K. D. PETTIGREW, O. SAKURADA & M. SHINOHARA. 1977. The [^{14}C] deoxyglucose method for measurement of local cerebral glucose utilization: Theory, procedure and normal values in the conscious and anesthetized albino rat. J. Neurochem. **28:** 897-916.

25. VINGAN, R. D., D. L. DOW-EDWARDS & E. P. RILEY. 1986. Effects of prenatal exposure to ethanol on local cerebral glucose utilization. Alcohol. Clin. Exp. Res. **10:** 22-26.

26. NEHLIG, A., L. PORRINO, A. CRANE & L. SOKOLOFF. 1985. Local cerebral glucose utilization in normal female rats: Variations during the estrus cycle and comparison with males. J. Cereb. Blood Flow Metab. **5:** 393-400.

27. GLICK, S. D., P. A. HINDS & R. M. SHAPIRO. 1983. Cocaine-induced rotation: Sex-dependent differences between left- and right-sided rats. Science **221:** 775-777.

28. GLICK, S. D. & P. A. HINDS. 1984. Sex differences in sensitization to cocaine-induced rotation. Eur. J. Pharmacol. **99:** 119-123.

29. POST, R. M. 1981. Central stimulants: Clinical and experimental evidence on tolerance and sensitization. *In* Research Advances in Alcohol and Drug Problems. Y. Israel, F. Glaser, H. Kalant, R. E. Dopham, W. Schmidt & R. Smart, Eds. Vol. 6: 1-65. Plenum Press. New York, NY.

Cocaine Effects on the Developing Central Nervous System: Behavioral, Psychopharmacological, and Neurochemical Studies

LINDA PATIA SPEAR, CHERYL L. KIRSTEIN, AND
NANCY A. FRAMBES

Department of Psychology
Center for Developmental Psychobiology
Center for Neurobehavioral Sciences
State University of New York at Binghamton
Binghamton, New York 13901

There is an escalating number of human offspring born to mothers who have used cocaine during pregnancy (see, for example, REF. 1). As neonates, these offspring have been reported to exhibit a depression of interactive behavior, poor state organization, abnormal sleep patterns, feeding deficits, visual dysfunctions, excitement, irritability, and tremulousness, along with EEG abnormalities and an increased incidence of Sudden Infant Death Syndrome.[1-5] Although there is a need to establish animal models for further systematic assessment of potential neurobehavioral consequences of early cocaine exposure, published laboratory studies are limited in this area and have focused largely on maternal toxicity and fetal teratogenicity following gestational cocaine exposure.[6-9] Recently, a number of researchers have begun to examine the neurobehavioral consequences of early cocaine exposure in rodent populations, including the laboratories of Drs. Dow-Edwards,[10-12] Riley and Foss,[13] McGivern,[14] and R. F. Smith[15] in addition to our laboratory. It is likely that knowledge of the effects of early cocaine exposure on brain function and behavior will escalate rapidly due to the diversity of approaches being used across different laboratories in this research.

Establishment of a Rodent Model System for Gestational Cocaine Exposure: Issues of Dose and Route of Administration

At this early stage in the investigation of the consequences of gestational cocaine exposure, it is important to verify the appropriateness of the animal model chosen for investigation. Important considerations include issues of dose and route of administration used for the substance, as well as dose-dependency of effects. It has been suggested that doses used in animal experiments should not be merely based on equivalency of administered doses on a mg/kg basis, due to species differences in pharmacokinetics (see, for example, REF. 16). Ideally, use of drug doses that produce equivalent fetal brain or plasma levels between laboratory animals and exposed human offspring would be desired; yet, there are no data on cocaine levels in human fetuses to provide a standard for use in animal studies. Based on the clinical information available, equivalent maternal blood levels across species would appear to be the best available index of the appropriateness of the doses chosen for use in the establishment of animal models for gestational cocaine exposure (see REF. 16). In developmental toxicology studies, it is also important to establish dose-response relationships, an issue which may be particularly critical with cocaine given that the vasoconstrictor actions of cocaine may potentially retard cocaine uptake differentially across dose with certain routes of administration.

For these reasons, we felt that it was important to document the appropriateness of the doses and the subcutaneous (sc) route that we had chosen for our initial work. This route has been frequently used to administer drugs during gestation, although its utility as a means of administering cocaine to pregnant rodents has not been previously examined. A number of studies, however, have investigated the distribution and pharmacokinetics of cocaine administered acutely or chronically via this route in nonpregnant adult rodents.[17-21] In spite of the localized vasoconstriction and necrosis induced by sc cocaine, absorption of cocaine from the sc injection site has been reported to be relatively rapid and complete,[17] although slower and more sustained than that observed after intraperitoneal (ip) injection (see REF. 20). Peak plasma and brain levels of cocaine in rats have been reported to be reached about 4 hr following acute sc injection and approximately 2 hr following chronic daily sc cocaine administration (see, for example, REF. 18).

To address issues of appropriate plasma levels and dose-dependency across the chosen range given sc to gravid rat dams, we conducted two investigations. In both studies, pregnant Sprague-Dawley rats were injected daily with cocaine from the time of neural tube closure (gestational day 8 = E8) until shortly before term (E20). The doses chosen for investigation were 10 mg/kg, a dose sufficient to produce self-administration in rats,[22,23] 20 mg/kg, and 40 mg/kg, a dose slightly below that reported to cause increased fetal mortality upon chronic sc administration to gravid rat dams.[9] In the first study, the behavior of the dams was observed in the home cage at 0.5, 1, 2, and 4 hr following drug injection in order to determine whether there were dose-dependent behavioral effects in the dams across the chosen drug range. Dams were examined on E8, 12, 16 and 20 using a time-sampling procedure. Behaviors measured included sniffing and an index of total activity which included both vertical movements (rearing) and horizontal movements (exploration and locomotor activity). These data averaged over test day are represented in FIGURE 1. At 0.5, 1 and 2 hr postinjection, all doses produced similar increases in sniffing and activity. At 4 hr postinjection, there were significant differences only between the 10 and 40 mg/kg dose groups on both measures. Thus, these behavioral data do not provide convincing evidence for dose-dependency across the doses examined. One possible explanation of these data is that there may be a "ceiling effect" with respect to cocaine-induced stereotyped sniffing behavior and activity. Indeed, the data of Ellinwood and colleagues[24,25] suggest that there are minimal differences in the amount of stereotyped behavior elicited by 15-20 mg/kg versus 40 mg/kg cocaine in adult animals following either acute or chronic cocaine exposure. Another possible explanation of these results, however, is that drug-induced vasoconstriction may have retarded cocaine uptake differentially across dose, with the result that there were not reliable dose-related differences in brain cocaine levels across the test doses utilized. This does not appear to be the case, based on the results of our next study.

In our second study, we examined brain and plasma levels of cocaine and the

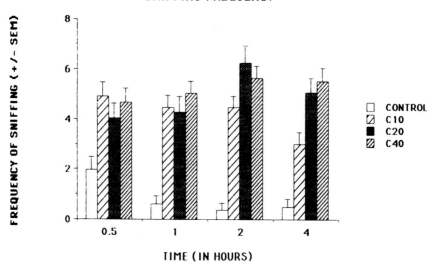

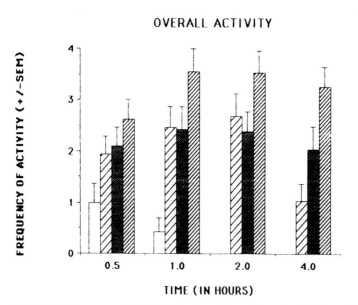

FIGURE 1. Frequency of sniffing behavior and overall activity (both vertical and horizontal movements) exhibited by gravid dams in their home cages at 0.5, 1, 2 and 4 hr following treatment with either saline (CONTROL), 10 mg/kg (C10), 20 mg/kg (C20) or 40 mg/kg (C40) cocaine HCl.

cocaine metabolite benzoylecgonine (BE) in dams and fetuses sacrificed either 0.5 or 2 hr following drug administration on E20. These results are illustrated in FIGURE 2, which presents maternal and fetal data from the 2-hr sacrifice interval for both cocaine (*top panel*) and BE (*bottom panel*). Dose-dependent increases in both plasma and brain levels of cocaine were observed, an effect seen in both the dams and fetuses. It should also be noted that maternal levels of cocaine in plasma were observed to be in the range of, or to exceed, those reported in human cocaine users (reported to range from approximately 200-240 ng/ml with intranasal cocaine use[26] to around 800-900 ng/ml for free base smoking[27]). Fetal concentrations of cocaine in brain and plasma were approximately 2-fold less than those of the dams, suggesting that the placenta may somewhat restrict cocaine entry into fetal circulation. These data are similar to those reported after ip administration of cocaine to pregnant mice[28] and somewhat greater than those reported following intravenous administration of cocaine to pregnant ewes.[29] In addition to numerous other factors that may influence the pharmacokinetics of drug distribution to the fetus, it is possible that the vasoconstrictor actions of cocaine may reduce vascular flow in the placenta, thereby influencing the penetration of cocaine itself across the placenta (see REF. 28). Given that brain/plasma cocaine ratios were similar between the dams and fetuses, with ratios averaging 2.35 (± 0.10 SE), it appears that once cocaine enters circulation, however, its affinity for brain tissue is similar in the fetus and dam.

Whereas plasma levels of the cocaine metabolite BE, like cocaine levels per se, were greater in the dams than fetuses, BE concentrations in fetal brain were greater than those observed in maternal brain (see FIG. 2). This polar metabolite, which is formed by hydrolysis predominantly in periphery, only poorly penetrates the blood-brain barrier in adult animals (see, for example, REF. 20). It is likely that the immaturity of this barrier system in fetuses (see, for example, REF. 30) may be a major contributing factor to the high concentrations of BE observed in fetal brain. In adult animals, BE has been shown to have potent stimulatory effects upon central administration[31,32] which may be in part related to the ability of this active metabolite to form molecular complexes with calcium ions.[33] Given the multiplicity of neuronal functions that have been shown to be calcium regulated in adult as well as developing brain (see, for example, REFS. 34,35), it is possible that potential neuroteratogenic effects of gestational cocaine exposure may be in part related to a disruption in calcium regulation induced by substantial brain levels of this cocaine metabolite.

Taken together, the results of these studies suggest that the sc route may be an appropriate means for administering cocaine to gravid rat dams. In spite of a lack of convincing dose-dependency in behavioral testing of dams in the home cage, dose-dependent increases in brain and plasma cocaine levels in both the dams and fetuses were observed. Clinically-relevant plasma levels of cocaine were reached in the dams, with significant amounts of both cocaine and the active, calcium-binding metabolite BE being observed in fetal brain during a time of rapid neural development.

Neurobehavioral Teratogenic Experiments

In our investigations of the neurobehavioral consequences of gestational cocaine exposure, we have focused initially on assessment during the early postnatal period. Given that the available clinical population of exposed offspring is still quite young, correlations between human and animal data might be expected to be closer when analogously examining laboratory animal populations early in life. Assessment of

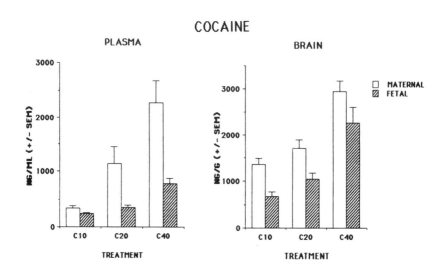

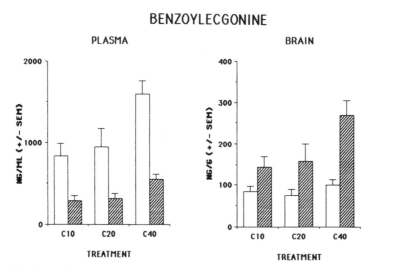

FIGURE 2. Plasma and brain levels of cocaine and the cocaine metabolite benzoylecgonine in gravid dams and their fetuses at 2 hr postinjection on gestational day 20 (E20) following daily sc injection of 10 mg/kg (C10), 20 mg/kg (C20) or 40 mg/kg (C40) cocaine from E8 to E20. Samples were assayed via gas chromatography/mass spectrometry in the laboratory of Dr. Roger Foltz at the University of Utah.

potential teratogenic effects of test compounds in developing animals may also provide more direct indices regarding the underlying primary alterations induced by teratogens that testing conducted in adulthood.[36,37] In these early assessments, we assessed not only the maturation of reflexes and physical landmarks which are often included in developmental toxicology studies, but also examinations of cognitive function early in life, and behavioral, psychopharmacological and neurochemical measures designed to assess potential alterations in dopaminergic function.

At present, we have completed two experimental series examining the neurobehavioral consequences of gestational cocaine exposure in Sprague-Dawley rats. In both experiments, cocaine was administered sc from E8-E20 as in the studies presented above. In Experiment 1, offspring from 3 groups of dams were assessed: dams given 40 mg/kg/3cc cocaine HCl daily; dams pair-fed to the cocaine-treated dams and injected sc daily with 3cc/kg of a 0.9% saline solution; and nontreated dams allowed ad lib access to lab chow. In Experiment 2, offspring of dams given 10, 20 or 40 mg/kg cocaine in addition to saline-injected dams pair-fed to the high dose cocaine group and nontreated ad lib dams were assessed. In this second experiment, all offspring were surrogate-fostered on the day after birth (*i.e.*, on postnatal day 1 (P1)). In both experiments, offspring from a given litter were partitioned into a variety of different test procedures, with only one pup from any litter being placed into a given testing condition unless otherwise specified.

Maternal/Litter Data

There were no significant differences among treatment groups in the number of offspring born per litter, the ratio of male/female offspring, number of implantation sites (examined in Experiment 2 only), or offspring body weights on P1 or P21. In Experiment 2, we observed a slight attenuation in weight gain during pregnancy among dams in the 40 mg/kg cocaine group, an effect not observed in Experiment 1 where the dams were approximately 50-70 g heavier at the onset of mating than in Experiment 2. Whether this initial weight difference is the causal factor leading to a reduction in weight gain during pregnancy in the high dose cocaine group still remains to be determined. It should be noted, however, that in Experiment 2 there were no notable differences between offspring of dams pair-fed to the high dose group and dams given ad lib access to lab chow, suggesting that the consequences of exposure to the 40 mg/kg dose of cocaine during gestation may not be related merely to potential nutritional alterations during fetal development.

Reflex/Physical Maturation

In Experiment 1, one male and one female pup per litter were used to examine the maturation of reflexes and physical landmarks (day of eye opening and upper and lower incisor eruption). The reflex test battery included: righting reflex, cliff aversion, horizontal screen, vertical screen and negative geotaxis. Cocaine-exposed offspring were not observed to differ reliably from control offspring in these tests.

Cognitive Function

Although normal patterns of physical maturation and reflex development were observed in cocaine-exposed offspring, these offspring did exhibit cognitive deficits in some but not all conditioning situations. Data from an appetitive conditioning test conducted at P7-8 in Experiment 1 are shown in FIGURE 3. In this task, paired pups were exposed to a CS+ odor in the presence of milk and a CS− odor in the absence of milk. Unpaired animals received milk exposure separate from odor exposure. On both the immediate (*top panel* of FIG. 3) and 24-hr (*bottom panel*) retention tests, prenatally exposed offspring exhibited impaired performance on the task. Paired pups from the pair-fed and nontreated groups exhibited an increase in preference for the CS+ odor (*i.e.,* positive (CS+)-(CS−) difference scores) relative to nonpaired pups. In contrast, there were no significant differences between paired and unpaired pups in the prenatal cocaine treatment group on either the immediate or 24-hr retention test. It should be realized, of course, that the impaired performance observed in cocaine-treated offspring at 24 hr after conditioning may not reflect retention deficits per se, but may rather reflect a lack of significant conditioning (as indexed by impaired performance on the immediate retention test).

We have preliminary data to suggest that offspring prenatally exposed to cocaine also exhibit impaired performance in an aversive conditioning task at P17-18 (work conducted in conjunction with Drs. James Miller and N. E. Spear). For this study, offspring of dams exposed to 40 mg/kg cocaine as well as pair-fed and ad lib dams were examined. These offspring were littermates of pups examined in Experiment 2. As can be seen in FIGURE 4, control offspring (collapsed across the pair-fed and ad lib groups) exposed to footshock in the presence of the CS+ odor spent significantly less time in the presence of that odor on the immediate (*top panel*) and 60-min (*bottom panel*) retention test than control animals receiving unpaired exposures of the odor and footshock. This effect was attenuated in offspring of dams given 40 mg/kg cocaine chronically during gestation. On the 60-min retention test, only the control animals exhibited significant retention.

Pups exposed gestationally to cocaine, however, do not display cognitive deficits in all conditioning situations. In Experiment 2, no differences among the treatment groups were observed on immediate or 24-hr retention tests following aversive (odor/footshock) conditioning on P7. The training parameters used in this task resulted in excellent conditioning and retention in all groups of animals. In future work, we plan to investigate more carefully the types of circumstances under which cocaine-exposed offspring exhibit learning/retention deficits. Given that such offspring were observed to exhibit learning deficits in two of three testing situations, all of which involved simple classical conditioning, it would be expected that they might show even more pronounced deficits in tasks that are more challenging cognitively, such as those requiring the integration or organization of various stimuli.

Behavioral and Psychopharmacological Assessments of Dopaminergic Function

Wall climbing, a behavior characterized by alternate forelimb treading against a vertical surface with the body positioned in a near vertical plane, is elicited predominately during the second postnatal week, and not thereafter, by a variety of aversive

IMMEDIATE TEST

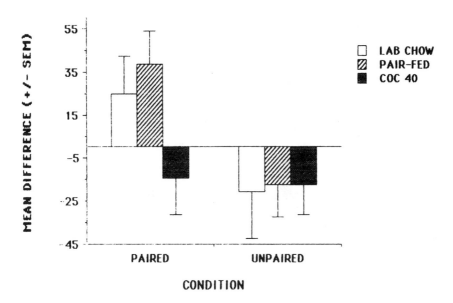

CONDITION

24 HR RETENTION TEST

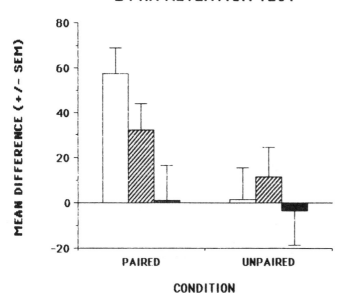

CONDITION

FIGURE 3. Mean (± SEM) odor preference difference scores [(CS+) - (CS−)] on the immediate and 24-hr appetitive conditioning retention test for paired and unpaired offspring of nontreated dams allowed ad lib access to lab chow (LAB CHOW), pair-fed dams (PAIR-FED) and dams injected sc daily with 40 mg/kg cocaine from E8 to E20 (COC 40).

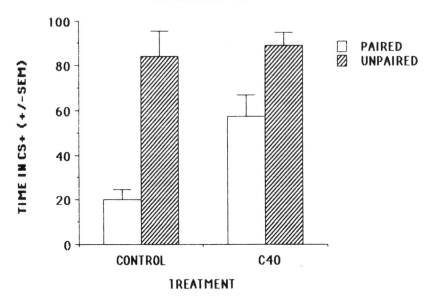

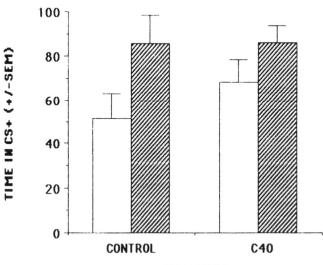

FIGURE 4. Mean amount of time spent in the presence of the CS+ (in sec) on the immediate and 24-hr aversive conditioning retention test for paired and unpaired offspring of control dams (CONTROL) and of dams injected sc daily with 40 mg/kg cocaine from E8 to E20 (C40).

environmental stimuli including high temperature[38] and footshock.[39] This behavior appears to be dependent upon levels of catecholaminergic activity during the second postnatal week (see REF. 37 for review and references). In Experiment 1, the incidence of shock-precipitated wall climbing was assessed on postnatal days 8, 10, 12, 14 and 16. On each test day pups received two 3-min test sessions during which they were exposed to a 0.5 sec, 0.6 mA footshock intermittently on a FI 30-sec schedule. As can be seen in the *top panel* of FIGURE 5, pups exposed gestationally to cocaine exhibited a significant reduction in shock-precipitated wall climbing on P12. There were, however, no significant differences among the treatment groups in their footshock sensitivity thresholds at this age; thus, it is unlikely that the observed reduction in wall climbing is associated with any alterations in sensitivity to the footshock. At this age, offspring exposed gestationally to cocaine also exhibited an increase in locomotor activity in this test situation (FIG. 5, *bottom panel*). The reduction in wall climbing does not appear to be related to this increase in matrix crossing as the correlation between amount of wall climbing and the number of quadrants entered was not significant. It should be noted that, although the cocaine-exposed offspring exhibited increased locomotor activity in this test situation in which they were exposed intermittently to footshock, it does not appear that they are hyperactive under less stressful testing situations. In Experiment 2, no alterations in baseline activity levels were seen among the treatment groups at P7-8 or P11-12 in testing situations that involved exposure to a novel, but otherwise unstressful test apparatus.

The reduction in wall climbing observed in offspring that were prenatally exposed to cocaine suggests the possibility that there may be an attenuation in catecholaminergic (dopaminergic and/or noradrenergic) activity in these offspring. In contrast, no treatment-induced alterations were observed in the amount of milk-induced mouthing behavior elicited at P7-8 (Experiments 1 and 2), or in the normal ontogenetic decline in wall climbing which diminishes rapidly following 14 days or so postnatally (Experiment 1). This is notable because these behaviors have been shown to be related to serotonergic and cholinergic activity, respectively, at the test ages (see REF. 37 for further discussion and references). These data support the suggestion that functional alterations induced by prenatal cocaine exposure may be at least somewhat specific to the catecholaminergic system. This working hypothesis, based on testing conducted during the preweaning period, needs to be examined in more detail in developing as well as mature offspring.

The results of the psychopharmacological studies conducted as a part of Experiment 2 support the suggestion that there may be an attenuation in dopamine (DA) activity in offspring that were exposed gestationally to cocaine. Psychopharmacologically, an attenuation in DA activity would typically be characterized by a reduced sensitivity to DA agonists along with a converse increased sensitivity to DA antagonists. We tested this by assessing offspring following exposure to 0, 0.1 or 3.0 mg/kg apomorphine on P12, or to 0, 0.1 and 0.5 mg/kg haloperidol in testing conducted both in the presence and absence of milk on P8. As can be seen in TABLE 1, offspring of dams given 20 and 40 mg/kg cocaine exhibited an attenuated sensitivity to the dopamine agonist apomorphine. Conversely, offspring of dams given 40 mg/kg, and to some extent 20 mg/kg, cocaine exhibited an increased sensitivity to the relatively low test doses of the DA antagonist haloperidol that had minimal effects on the behavior of control animals (see TABLE 2). These psychopharmacological data, together with the wall climbing data, are consistent with the hypothesis that gestational cocaine exposure may result in an attenuation in DA activity evident during the preweanling period.

Cocaine is an indirect DA agonist, blocking DA uptake into the presynaptic terminal region. Our data thus far support the suggestion that chronic treatment with

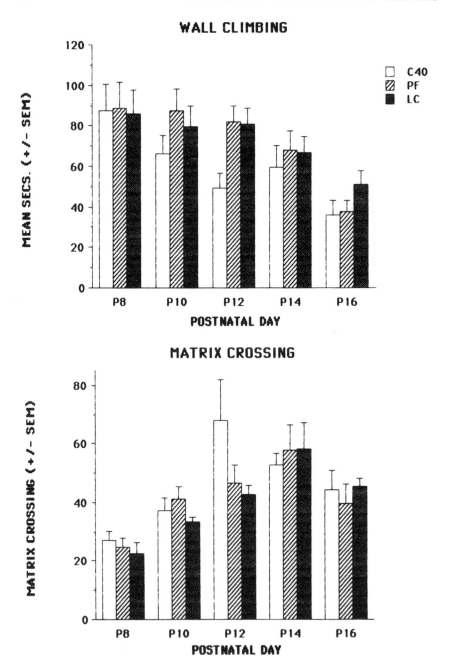

FIGURE 5. Mean duration of shock-precipitated wall climbing and number of matrix crossings for offspring of nontreated dams allowed ad lib access to lab chow (LAB CHOW), pair-fed dams (PAIR-FED) and dams injected sc daily with 40 mg/kg cocaine from E8 to E20 (COC 40).

TABLE 1. Response of Offspring of the Various Treatment Groups to 0.1 and 3 mg/kg (Respectively) Apomorphine on P12

Behavior	LC	PF	C10	C20	C40
BA*	↑↑	↑↑	↑↑	↑↑	−↑
Probe	−↑	−↑	↑↑	−−	−−
MC**	↑↑	↑↑	↑↑	↑↑	−↑
Lie still	↓↓	↓↓	↓↓	−−	−↓

− = no significant difference when compared with saline control.
↑ = significant increase over saline control.
↓ = significant decrease over saline control.
*BA = behavioral activation (forward locomotion, forelimb paddle, hindlimb tread, and roll/curl).
**MC = matrix crossing.

this DA agonist during gestation may result in a down regulation of the DA system. It is interesting that early chronic treatment with DA antagonists such as haloperidol has also been reported to result in DA down regulation,[40–43] an effect apparently related at least in part to a decrease in the number of DA receptors with no alteration in their affinity.[40,42] If further research supports the suggestion of an attenuation in DA activity following gestational cocaine exposure, future work could be profitably directed towards comparing the neural mechanisms underlying the observed down regulation in the DA system following early exposure to DA antagonists in comparison with those induced by the DA agonist cocaine.

Neurochemical Investigations

An attenuation in DA activity induced by gestational cocaine exposure could reflect drug-induced compensations evident presynaptically (reflected by alterations in DA turnover) and/or postsynaptically (evident in alterations in DA receptor binding). To assess potential alterations in postsynaptic DA activity, we are currently collaborating with Dr. Ron Hammer of the University of Hawaii who is conducting

TABLE 2. Response of Offspring of the Various Treatment Groups to 0.1 and 0.5 mg/kg (Respectively) Haloperidol on P6

Behavior	LC	PF	C10	C20	C40
BA*	−−	−−	−−	−↓	−−
Probe	−↓	−−	−−	−−	↓↓
Mouth	−−	−−	−−	−−	−↓
Lie still	−−	−−	−−	−−	−↑

− = no significant difference when compared with saline control.
↑ = significant increase over saline control.
↓ = significant decrease over saline control.
*BA = behavioral activation (forward locomotion, forelimb paddle, hindlimb tread, roll/curl).

autoradiographic examinations of dopamine and opiate receptor binding in P1 and P21 littermates of pups tested in Experiment 2. With regard to presynaptic function, we have examined DA turnover at P21 in animals from Experiment 2 using the alpha-methyl-para-tyrosine (ampt) technique for estimating turnover of DA (see REF. 44). In this study, high pressure liquid chromatography (HPLC) was used to measure forebrain DA levels at 0, 1, 2 and 4 hr following treatment with the tyrosine hydroxylase inhibitor ampt. In FIGURE 6 the log of forebrain DA concentrations is graphed over time following ampt treatment. No differences were observed among the groups in the slope of the regression lines, suggesting that the turnover rates of DA were similar across the different treatment groups. There were also no differences observed at this age across groups in forebrain or hindbrain levels of serotonin (5HT), 5-hydroxyindoleacetic acid (5HIAA) or the ratio of 5HIAA/5HT (used as an index of 5HT turnover).

In Experiment 2, we also assessed whole brain levels of DA, 5HT and 5HIAA in culled animals from the various treatment groups, analyzing the data using litter means. Although the number of litters represented is low (ranging from 4-6/treatment group) due to the use of only culled pups, there was a trend in this data for DA levels to be increased in P1 neonates exposed gestationally to cocaine (see FIG. 7). These preliminary findings will be examined in more detail in future work.

SUMMARY

Implications and Future Directions

The data we have collected thus far support the following conclusions:

1. Subcutaneous administration of cocaine results in dose-dependent increases in brain and plasma cocaine in both dams and fetuses, and maternal plasma levels in the range of or above those observed in human cocaine users. Fetal levels are lower than those of the dam, suggesting that the placenta may partially restrict cocaine entry into the fetus. Concentrations of the active cocaine metabolite benzoylecgonine, however, are greater in fetal than in maternal brain; this may have important implications for brain development given the calcium-binding properties of this metabolite.

2. Chronic subcutaneous administration of 10, 20 or 40 mg/kg cocaine from E8-E20 does not alter litter size, body weights at birth or weaning, or development of reflexes or physical landmarks in the offspring.

3. Offspring exposed gestationally to cocaine exhibit learning and/or retention deficits in some but not all conditioning situations.

4. Behaviorally and psychopharmacologically, there is evidence for a potential attenuation in DA activity in preweanling pups exposed gestationally to cocaine. There is, however, no sign of any alteration in DA turnover in treated offspring sacrificed at weaning, although preliminary data suggest that DA levels may be increased in exposed pups during the neonatal period. Possible alterations in DA receptor function are currently being assessed.

We are still at the initial stages of our work, and the data we have collected thus far have raised as many questions as they have answered. We plan to assess further the cognitive deficits observed in cocaine-exposed offspring. Under what contingencies are these learning and/or retention deficits observed, and are they permanent deficits

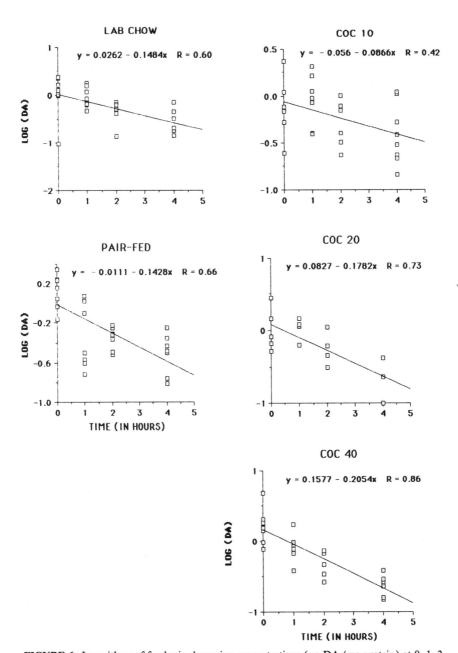

FIGURE 6. Logarithms of forebrain dopamine concentrations (ng DA/mg protein) at 0, 1, 2 and 4 hr following injection with the tyrosine hydroxylase inhibitor alpha-methyl-para-tyrosine among offspring from the various treatment groups. The least-squares linear regression line and correlation coefficient for each group is indicated.

or does recovery eventually occur? Is there actually an attenuation in DA activity in treated offspring? If so, is this attenuation related to compensations at the presynaptic and/or postsynaptic level, and what is the time course for this effect on the DA system? What are the critical periods for the production of these alterations; is cocaine exposure during the second or third trimester alone sufficient? How do our results compare with those of other laboratories that are using other methods for administering cocaine during gestation? At some point in the future we also hope to examine potential therapeutic approaches to reduce the cognitive deficits observed in exposed offspring. It is clear that there are still many questions to be answered concerning the neuro-behavioral consequences of gestational cocaine exposure as manifested during different stages of ontogeny.

We believe that our findings may eventually have implications for clinicians working with offspring born to cocaine-using females. Although obvious species differences between rodents and humans require careful assessment of the relevance of such animal models, at least in the case of the Fetal Alcohol Syndrome "striking similarities between the results of . . . animal studies and the related clinical and epidemiological

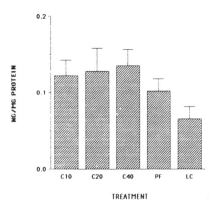

FIGURE 7. Litter means of whole brain dopamine concentrations in offspring from the various treatment groups sacrificed on postnatal day 1 (P1).

literature" (REF. 45, p. 184) have been observed. From our results thus far, it would appear that careful analysis of learning and retention processes in human infants exposed gestationally to cocaine may be warranted. It would seem to be critical to determine whether these infants exhibit cognitive deficits early in life that could have pronounced consequences on subsequent behavioral and social functioning. Recent advances in methods to analyze learning and retention capabilities in human infants (*e.g.,* REF. 46) could potentially be profitably utilized in such work.

Another possible clinical implication is with regard to our initial findings that cocaine-exposed offspring may exhibit an attenuation in DA activity. Given evidence that reduced activity in the DA system may be related to hyperactivity and attentional deficits (*e.g.,* see REF. 47 for review and references), it is possible that offspring of cocaine-using females may be at risk for the development of Attentional Deficit Disorder (ADD). Whereas clinical studies of cocaine-exposed offspring have necessarily focused to date on infants, as these offspring mature it may be important to include assessments of potential attentional deficits, learning problems, impulsivity and hyperactivity that are characteristic signs of ADD.

At this early stage in both clinical and laboratory animal studies of the neuro-behavioral consequences of early cocaine exposure, there is but a limited data base from which to assess the clinical relevance of potential animal models of early cocaine exposure. Yet, establishment of appropriate animal models is crucial for detailed examination of the consequences of early cocaine exposure, given the greater degree of control of variables, increased options for assessing physiological function, and shorter time frame for lifespan studies than is possible in clinical investigations alone. Research efforts at both the clinical and basic science level would appear to be ultimately necessary to determine the prognosis for future development of human offspring exposed gestationally to cocaine.

ACKNOWLEDGMENTS

The authors would like to acknowledge the assistance of K. Monti and C. Sakashita at the University of Utah, and Drs. N. E. Spear and J. Miller along with J. Bell, R. Greenbaum, H. Hoffmann, J. O'Shea, L. Rogers and V. Yoottanasumpun for their active contribution to the work presented in this paper.

[a] Supported in part by National Institute on Drug Abuse (NIDA) Grant R01 DA04478. The assays of plasma and brain cocaine and benzoylecgonine were conducted under NIDA contract to Dr. R. Foltz at the University of Utah.

REFERENCES

1. CHASNOFF, I. J., K. A. BURNS & W. J. BURNS. 1987. Cocaine use in pregnancy: Perinatal morbidity and mortality. Neurotox. Teratol. **9:** 291-293.
2. CHASNOFF, I. J., W. J. BURNS, S. H. SCHNOLL & K. A. BURNS. 1985. Cocaine use in pregnancy. N. Engl. J. Med. **313:** 666-669.
3. DIXON, S. D., R. W. COEN & S. CRUTCHFIELD. 1987. Visual dysfunction in cocaine-exposed infants. Pediatr. Res. **21:** 359A.
4. DOBERCZAK, T. M., S. SHANZER & S. R. KANDALL. 1987. Neonatal effects of cocaine abuse in pregnancy. Pediatr. Res. **21:** 359A.
5. ORO, A. S. & S. D. DIXON. 1987. Perinatal cocaine and methamphetamine exposure: Maternal and neonatal correlates. J. Pediatr. **111:** 571-578.
6. FANTEL, A. G. & B. J. MACPHAIL. 1982. The teratogenicity of cocaine. Teratology **26:** 17-19.
7. MAHALIK, M. P., R. F. GAUTIERI & D. E. MANN, JR. 1980. Teratogenic potential of cocaine hydrochloride in CS-1 mice. J. Pharmaceut. Sci. **69:** 703-706.
8. MAHALIK, M. P., R. F. GAUTIERI & D. E. MANN, JR. 1984. Mechanisms of cocaine-induced teratogenesis. Res. Commun. Subst. Abuse **5:** 279-302.
9. CHURCH, M. W., B. A. DINCHEFF & P. K. GESSNER. 1988. Dose-dependent consequences of cocaine on pregnancy outcome in the Long-Evans rat. Neurotox. Teratol. **10:** 51-58.
10. DOW-EDWARDS, D. L., L. A. FREED & T. H. MILORAT. 1986. The effects of cocaine on development. Soc. Neurosci. Abstr. **12:** 59.12.
11. DOW-EDWARDS, D. L., T. A. FICO & D. E. HUTCHINGS. 1988. Functional effects of cocaine given during critical periods of development. Teratology **37:** 518.
12. DOW-EDWARDS, D. L. 1988. Cocaine effects on the developing CNS: Studies of brain function. This volume.
13. FOSS, J. A. & E. A. RILEY. 1988. Behavioral evaluation of animals exposed prenatally to cocaine. Teratology **37:** 517.
14. MCGIVERN, R. F., W. J. RAUM, R. Z. SOKOL & P. PETERSON. 1988. Long-term effects

of prenatal cocaine exposure on scent marking and the HPG axis in male rats. Teratology 37: 518.

15. SMITH, R. F., K. M. MATTRAN, M. F. KURKJIAN & S. L. KURTZ. 1989. Alterations in offspring behavior induced by chronic prenatal cocaine dosing. Neurotox. Teratol. In press.

16. KUTSCHER, C. L. & B. K. NELSON. 1985. Dosing considerations in behavioral teratology testing. Neurobehav. Toxicol. Teratol. 7: 663-664.

17. MISRA, A. S. 1976. Disposition and biotransformation of cocaine. In Cocaine: Chemical, Biological, Clinical, Social and Treatment Aspects. S. J. Mule, Ed.: 73-90. CRC Press. Cleveland, OH.

18. NAYAK, P. K., A. L. MISRA & S. J. MULE. 1976. Physiological disposition and biotransformation of [³H]cocaine in acutely and chronically treated rats. J. Pharmacol. Exp. Ther. 196: 556-569.

19. MULE, S. J. & A. L. MISRA. 1977. Cocaine: Distribution and metabolism in animals. In Cocaine and Other Stimulants. E. H. Ellinwood, Jr. & M. M. Kilbey, Eds.: 215-228. Plenum Press. New York, NY.

20. BENUCK, M., A. LAJTHA & M. E. A. REITH. 1987. Pharmacokinetics of systemically administered cocaine and locomotor stimulation in mice. J. Pharmacol. Exp. Ther. 243: 144-149.

21. REITH, M. E. A., M. BENUCK & A. LAJTHA. 1987. Cocaine disposition in the brain after continuous or intermittent treatment and locomotor stimulation in mice. J. Pharmacol. Exp. Ther. 243: 281-287.

22. DOUGHERTY, J. & R. PICKENS. 1976. Pharmacokinetics of intravenous cocaine self-injection. In Cocaine: Chemical, Biological, Clinical, Social and Treatment Aspects. S. J. Mule, Ed.: 105-120. CRC Press. Cleveland, OH.

23. PICKENS, R. & T. THOMPSON. 1968. Cocaine-reinforced behavior in rats: Effects of reinforcement magnitude and fixed-ratio size. J. Pharmacol. Exp. Ther. 161: 122-129.

24. KILBEY, M. M. & E. H. ELLINWOOD, JR. 1977. Chronic administration of stimulant drugs: Response modification. In Cocaine and Other Stimulants. E. H. Ellinwood, Jr. & M. M. Kilbey, Eds.: 409-429. Plenum Press. New York, NY.

25. STRIPLING, J. S. & E. H. ELLINWOOD, JR. 1977. Sensitization to cocaine following chronic administration in the rat. In Cocaine and Other Stimulants. E. H. Ellinwood, Jr. & M. M. Kilbey, Eds.: 327-351. Plenum Press. New York, NY.

26. JAVAID, J. I., M. W. FISCHMAN, C. R. SCHUSTER, H. DEKIRMENJIAN & J. M. DAVIS. 1978. Cocaine plasma concentration: Relation to physiological and subjective effects in humans. Science 202: 227-228.

27. SEIGEL, R. K. 1982. Cocaine smoking. J. Psychoactive Drugs 14: 271-359.

28. SHAH, N. S., D. A. MAY & J. D. YATES. 1980. Disposition of levo-[³H]cocaine in pregnant and nonpregnant mice. Toxicol. Appl. Pharmacol. 53: 279-284.

29. MOORE, T. R., J. SORG, L. MILLER, T. C. KEY & R. RESNIK. 1986. Hemodynamic effects of intravenous cocaine on the pregnant ewe and fetus. Am. J. Obstet. Gynecol. 155: 883-888.

30. REINIS, S. & J. M. GOLDMAN. 1980. The Development of the Brain: Biological and Functional Perspectives. C. C. Thomas. Springfield, IL.

31. MISRA, A. L., P. K. NAYAK, R. BLOCH & S. J. MULE. 1975. Estimation and disposition of [³H]benzoylecgonine and pharmacological activity of some cocaine metabolites. J. Pharm. Pharmacol. 27: 784-786.

32. WILLIAMS, N., D. H. CLOUET, A. L. MISRA & S. MULE. 1977. Cocaine and metabolites: Relationship between pharmacological activity and inhibitory action on dopamine uptake into striatal synaptosomes. Prog. Neuro-Psychopharmacol. 1: 265-269.

33. MISRA, A. L. & S. J. MULE. 1975. Calcium-binding property of cocaine and some of its active metabolites—Formation of molecular complexes. Res. Commun. Chem. Pathol. Pharmacol. 11: 663-666.

34. CARAFOLI, E. & J. T. PENNISTON. 1985. The calcium signal. Sci. Am. 253: 70-78.

35. BARNES, D. M. 1986. Neurotransmitters regulate growth cones. Science 234: 1325-1326.

36. RILEY, E. P., J. H. HANNIGAN & M. A. BALAZ-HANNIGAN. 1985. Behavioral teratology as the study of early brain damage: Considerations for the assessment of neonates. Neurobehav. Toxicol. Teratol. 7: 635-638.

37. SPEAR, L. P., E. K. ENTERS & D. G. LINVILLE. 1975. Age-specific behaviors as tools for examining teratogen-induced neural alterations. Neurobehav. Toxicol. Teratol. **7:** 691-695.
38. JOHANSON, I. B. & W. G. HALL. 1980. The ontogeny of feeding in rats: III. Thermal determinants of early ingestive responding. J. Comp. Physiol. Psych. **94:** 977-992.
39. BARRETT, B. A., P. CAZA, N. E. SPEAR & L. P. SPEAR. 1982. Wall climbing, odors from the home nest and catecholaminergic activity in rat pups. Physiol. Behav. **29:** 501-507.
40. ROSENGARTEN, H. & A. J. FRIEDHOFF. 1979. Enduring changes in dopamine receptor cells of pups from drug administration to pregnant and nursing rats. Science **203:** 1133-1135.
41. SPEAR, L. P., I. A. SHALABY & J. BRICK. 1980. Chronic administration of haloperidol during development: Behavioral and psychopharmacological effects. Psychopharmacology **70:** 47-58.
42. ROSENGARTEN, H., E. FRIEDMAN & A. J. FRIEDHOFF. 1983. Sensitive period for the effect of haloperidol on development of striatal dopamine receptors. *In* Nervous System Regeneration. Birth Defects: Original Article Series. B. Haber, S. R. Perez-Polo, F. A. Hashim, A. M. G. Stella & N. W. Paul, Eds. Vol. 19, No. 4. Allan R. Liss. New York, NY.
43. SPEAR, L. P. & F. M. SCALZO. 1986. Behavioral, psychopharmacological and neurochemical effects of chronic neuroleptic treatment during development. *In* Handbook of Behavioral Teratology. E. P. Riley & C. V. Vorhees, Eds.: 173-184. Plenum Press. New York, NY.
44. BRODIE, B., E. COSTA, A. DLABAC, N. NEFF & H. SMOOKLER. 1977. Application of steady-state kinetics to the estimation of synthesis rate and turnover time of tissue catecholamines. J. Pharmacol. Exp. Ther. **154:** 493-498.
45. ABEL, E. L. 1984. Fetal alcohol syndrome and fetal alcohol effects. Plenum Press. New York, NY.
46. ROVEE-COLLIER, C. 1984. The ontogeny of learning and memory in human infancy. *In* Comparative Perspectives on the Development of Memory. R. Kail & N. E. Spear, Eds.: 103-134. Lawrence Erlbaum Associates. Hillsdale, NJ.
47. BROWN, R. M. & R. H. B. FISHMAN. 1984. An overview and summary of the behavioral and neural consequences of perinatal exposure to psychotropic drugs. *In* Neurobehavioral Teratology. J. Yanai, Ed.: 3-54. Elsevier. New York, NY.

Prenatal Amphetamine Effects on Behavior: Possible Mediation by Brain Monoamines

LAWRENCE D. MIDDAUGH

Medical University of South Carolina
Department of Psychiatry and Behavioral Sciences
Room 803 Research Building
171 Ashley Avenue
Charleston, South Carolina 29425-0742

INTRODUCTION

Amphetamines were used and abused extensively in the 1960s and early 1970s, including use during pregnancy.[1,2] More recent surveys indicate that amphetamine use has declined over the past several years.[3] Based on requests for information regarding the possibility of adverse effects of prenatal amphetamine exposure, however, some community interest continues. Unfortunately, the current literature is too incomplete to provide very sound advice. Perhaps more important than the community interest is the potential contribution amphetamine studies might provide toward understanding possible mechanisms for some of the behavioral effects of prenatal drug exposure. The amphetamines have several well documented short- and long-term effects on the nervous and endocrine systems of adults. Exposing these systems to amphetamines during early stages of development might have long-lasting or permanent consequences. Since many effects of amphetamines and cocaine are similar, it might be advantageous to compare the effects of prenatal exposure to the two compounds as data become available.

Evidence that prenatal exposure to amphetamines might be detrimental to the offspring was first published in 1965. First, Bell, Drucker, and Woodruff[4] reported that single injections of *d*-amphetamine sulfate on either Gestation Days (GD) 6-9 or 12-15 caused a reduction in motor activity of 45-day-old offspring. In the same year, Nora, Trasler, and Fraser[5] reported that a single intraperitoneal injection of *d*-amphetamine sulfate (50 mg/Kg) into A/Jax mice on GD 8 significantly increased the number of resorptions and malformations in fetuses two days prior to term.

Although the first published evidence that prenatal amphetamine exposure affected offspring was over 20 years ago, the literature on the topic remains sparse. This literature was recently reviewed by two authors[6,7] and all of the published studies on the topic are tabulated in one or the other review. Each author noted several studies indicating that prenatal amphetamine exposure had both behavioral and neurochemical effects on the offspring; however, some inconsistency in the literature was also noted. Rather than duplicating these reviews, the present paper is concerned with a rationale for anticipating detrimental effects of prenatal amphetamine exposure based on information about the drug's effects on adults and on information about particular aspects of development. The studies included in the above-noted reviews are discussed to help identify empirical support for the detrimental consequences of prenatal amphetamine exposure, and hopefully to resolve some of the apparent inconsistency in the literature as well as to identify areas which need further research. The results of this analysis indicate that the literature is currently too limited to draw anything but very tentative conclusions about whether amphetamine during pregnancy is detrimental to the offspring. However, that exposure to either amphetamine or methamphetamine throughout pregnancy can have long-term consequences for rodent offspring appears to be supported by the literature, and is logically consistent with known effects of amphetamines and related drugs on adult and developing systems.

RATIONALE

The rationale for anticipating that exposure to amphetamines will be detrimental to the developing fetus is based on the well documented effects of amphetamines on neuronal and/or endocrine systems of adults, on the assumption and limited empirical evidence that the drug produces similar effects on the developing fetus, and on some evidence that these effects are detrimental and long-lasting.

Work from our laboratory resulted in one of the early published effects of prenatal amphetamine exposure;[8] and the present discussion will be organized according to the general framework used to guide our prenatal drug research. The emphasis of our work and this discussion is on whether prenatal exposure to the drug can produce functional deficits in fully mature offspring and on possible mediating mechanisms for the deficits. It is felt that the emphasis on long-term effects of prenatal drug exposure is particularly appropriate for animal research because the long intervening interval between birth and maturity in humans is likely to prevent relating an abnormality in a mature person to an event occurring prior to birth. In addition, only by establishing differences in the fully mature offspring can we be sure that in utero drug exposure produces more than a transient effect that may or may not have long-term consequences. Since laboratory animals mature much more rapidly than humans, studying long-term effects is feasible. By characterizing the long-term behavioral effects of prenatal drug exposure and providing possible mediating mechanisms, the results of animal studies might then direct research on humans.

The hypothesis that has guided our work and is applicable to the present discussion is that exposure to psychoactive drugs during pregnancy can alter the development of specific neural systems utilizing one of the monoamines as a transmitter and/or of the pituitary-adrenal system; that the changes in either of these systems will be long-lasting, and that the altered systems will be reflected in behavioral changes.

The hypothesis requires that either the maternally administered drug, one of its metabolites, or a product of the drug's effect on the mother must cross the placenta and access the fetus. Both the amphetamines[9] and corticosterone,[10] which is released by amphetamine, most likely cross the placenta and are available to exert effects on the developing neural or endocrine systems. Because of evidence that psychoactive drugs have similar influences on fetal and adult brains, it is instructive to consider the wealth of information about effects of these compounds on adult animals.

Amphetamine Effects on Adult Animals

Amphetamines produce many of their behavioral effects in adults by their action on neural systems utilizing one of the monoamines, dopamine (DA), norepinephrine (NE) or serotonin (5-HT), as a neurotransmitter.[11] Amphetamines stimulate the release, inhibit monoamine oxidase and thus transmitter degradation, and block re-uptake of DA, NE and 5-HT. Like cocaine, although possibly by a slightly different mechanism,[12] the net effect of amphetamine is to increase the availability of monoamine to the postsynaptic receptor.

Very high doses of amphetamine or methamphetamine (16 mg/kg/day) given continuously to rats over a three-day period via osmotic minipumps cause degeneration of DA neurons which begins at the terminals[13] and then extends retrograde to the cell bodies.[14] The exact mechanism for these degenerative effects is currently unknown but seems to depend on the DA synthetic mechanism, since pretreatment with the tyrosine hydroxylase inhibitor, alpha-methyltyrosine, prevents the degeneration. In addition to degeneration of DA neurons, high doses of methamphetamine, but not *d*-amphetamine, cause degeneration of 5-HT neurons. Methamphetamine also produces long-term DA and 5-HT depletion in neonatal rats; however, the latter appear to be less sensitive than adult animals to these effects.[15] Since young animals are more sensitive than adults to the neurotoxin, 6-hydroxy dopamine, the reduced sensitivity to methamphetamine appears to be related to some aspect of the drug rather than to a reduced vulnerability of the monoamine systems. Neonates might be less sensitive to the neurotoxic effects of methamphetamine because of their limited capacity to metabolize the drug to an active metabolite. This mechanism for a reduction in neurotoxicity would not be available to the fetus, however, since the drug could be metabolized by the mother and then transferred to the fetus. Currently it is not known whether prenatal amphetamine exposure produces similar neural degeneration in the fetus.

Somewhat lower doses of amphetamine (2-5 mg/kg) injected into adult rats stimulate motor activity, with stimulation depending upon an intact nigrostriatal tract. Chronic administration of the upper limits of this dose range depletes catecholamine stores and reduces motor activity. These results and the finding that similar amphetamine doses increase DA turnover strongly implicate the DA system in the mediation of amphetamine-induced motor stimulation. Very low doses of amphetamine (0.01-0.10 mg/kg) reduce motor activity presumably via its action on 5-HT neurons.[16] On the basis of the different effects produced by different doses and lengths of exposure to amphetamine in adults, it is reasonable to expect that the effects of the compound on the developing fetus might well depend upon the amount of drug reaching the fetus and the duration of exposure.

In addition to its effects on monoamine systems, there is evidence that amphetamine[17] and other dopamine agonists[18] elevate serum levels of corticosterone. The increased corticosterone levels produced by DA agonists appear to be the result of DA-stimulated release of ACTH, since the release could be blocked by pretreatment with haloperidol.[19] Transplacentally derived amphetamine might produce a similar release of ACTH in the developing fetus. Alternatively, transplacentally derived corticosterone released by amphetamine in the dam could also provide a mechanism by which fetal development could be altered.

Development of Monoaminergic and Pituitary-Adrenal Systems

The hypothesis regarding the long-term effects of prenatal drugs also depends on Dobbing's identification of rapidly developing systems as being particularly susceptible to external insult.[20] Considering periods of rapid development as sensitive periods to external insult extends the time of concern for drug exposure considerably beyond neurogenesis (GD 12-15), and can include some early neonatal periods. It is possible that some drugs will have a greater impact on subsequent behavior by disrupting these later periods of "neural organization" than by altering neurogenesis. Because its primary action is on monoaminergic nerve terminals which are limited during neurogenesis, amphetamine may be such a drug. In rodents, the monoamine tracts and the pituitary-adrenal system are developing rapidly during the last third of gestation and early neonatal period; hence, these time periods should be sensitive to the drugs affecting them. A very large literature has established many relationships between the three monoamines[21] or the pituitary-adrenal system[22] and the behavior of adult animals; hence, a change in either system produced by prenatal drug exposure might well be reflected in altered behavior.

Several studies confirm that the monoamine systems are developing rapidly during the perinatal period. Utilizing histofluorescence techniques, Golden[23] detected DA in mouse brain beginning on GD 13. By GD 16, the entire nigrostriatal tract could be visualized and the adult fluorescence pattern was noted by GD 18. NE was visible in the locus coeruleus on GD 14 and terminals were first seen in hypothalamus on GD 19. 5-HT cells were visualized in pontine and mesencephalic raphe areas on GD 13. No 5-HT terminals were evident in the fetus suggesting slower maturation of the serotonergic system. In rats, the peak times for cell differentiation are GD 12 for NE (in locus coeruleus); GD 13 for DA (in substantia nigra); and GD 13-14 for 5-HT (in raphe nuclei).[24] In rats, DA and NE are detectable on GD 15 (13.2 and 10.5 pg/mg tissue) and the concentrations increase to 193 and 156 pg/mg tissue by birth.[25] In light of these data indicating that monoaminergic systems are developing very rapidly during gestation, they should be sensitive to amphetamine. It is interesting to note that the enzymes for synthesis and degradation, the uptake mechanism, and the storage vesicles for catecholamines are available by Gestation Day 18 and the regulatory processes at this time are under controls similar to those previously established for adult animals.[25]

The organization of the interaction between the hypothalamus, pituitary, and adrenals is also beginning to develop during the later stages of gestation and continues into the early neonatal period. It has been recognized for a number of years that the full development and functional activity of the fetal adrenal cortex depends on ACTH. Excess or reduced availability of ACTH, respectively, results in hypertrophy and atrophy of the fetal adrenal cortex.[26] Pituitary control of the developing fetal adrenals in rats occurs around GD 16-17 and the fetal adrenals increase from less than 0.5 mg on GD 16.5 to more than 2.5 mg on GD 20.5. Plasma corticosterone in fetus increases from 16.5 μg% on GD 17.5 to 42.1 μg% on GD 20.5.[27] In addition, hypothalamic control of the pituitary is thought to develop during GD 18-22.[28] Thus, it is apparent that the hypothalamic-pituitary-adrenal axis is developing rapidly during the latter stages of gestation.

Prenatal Drug Effects on Monoaminergic and Pituitary-Adrenal Systems

Since monoaminergic systems in the developing fetus appear to be under controls similar to the adult, amphetamine given to a pregnant animal should also influence the monoamine systems of the developing fetus. Early studies indicated that catecholamines can be depleted in the brains of newly hatched chicks injected with reserpine[29] or alpha-methyltyrosine[30] prior to hatching. Work from our laboratory indicated that NE was reduced in brains of newborn mice exposed to d-amphetamine sulfate *in utero*.[8] Altered levels of transmitters at critical stages of development could, through repression or derepression, transiently or permanently alter the synthesis of regulatory enzymes[31] which in turn could alter neurotransmitter synthesis. This possibility is supported by reports indicating that catecholamine levels were elevated in brains of 30-day-old chicks depleted of the amines with reserpine prior to hatching,[29] and of 30-day-old mice depleted of the amines with amphetamine prior to birth.[8] These reports, and a report that maternal injections of haloperidol increased the number of DA receptors in rat offspring for at least 60 days, indicate that the developing MA systems can be manipulated with psychoactive drugs given to the mother and that the effects can be long-lasting.

Drugs given during pregnancy could also alter development of the pituitary-adrenal system either directly by affecting the fetal system or indirectly by a product of the drug effect on the dam. In either case, the effect might be due to the dependence of the fetal adrenals on fetal ACTH for proper development. Most psychoactive drugs act on the mature pituitary-adrenal system to either elevate or reduce corticosteroids. Since corticosteroids can cross the placenta,[10] changes in their concentration in the mother could, via placental transfer, alter their availability to the developing fetus.[10] The change in availability of steroid could, in turn, alter secretion of fetal ACTH and thus alter adrenal development. Alternatively, drugs crossing the placenta could directly influence ACTH release with increases and decreases producing hypertrophy and atrophy of the adrenal cortex. In either case, these prenatal effects could cause long-term changes in pituitary-adrenal function by altering the homeostatic mechanism which is set at an early age.

Several early reports suggest that hypothalamic-pituitary-adrenal activity in early life has long-term consequences for the system.[32] For example, stressing neonatal rats via handling was reported to increase the secretion of corticosterone,[33] and to cause increased exploratory activity accompanied by a decrease in plasma corticosterone after maturity.[34] In addition, neonatal injections or implants of corticosterone have been shown to produce long-term alterations in behavior and physiological systems associated with pituitary-adrenal function.[35-37] Finally, it has been demonstrated that maternal exposure to either phenobarbital[38] or ethanol[39] can alter this system in offspring at birth, and the effects appear to be long-lasting.

EFFECTS OF PRENATAL AMPHETAMINE EXPOSURE

The above discussion suggests that monoaminergic and pituitary-adrenal systems of the developing fetus can be affected by maternally administered drugs. Clearly, amphetamines affect monoaminergic neurons and pituitary-adrenal function in adult animals, and some of these effects appear to be long-lasting. Thus, it is reasonable to anticipate that amphetamines will exert these effects on the developing fetus and that such changes will be reflected in altered behavior.

The reported behavioral effects of prenatal amphetamine exposure include altered motor activity which is either increased or decreased depending upon several factors;[4,8,40-44] better performance on active avoidance,[45,46] poor performance on passive avoidance[47] and poor performance on a Lashley-III maze.[44] Not surprisingly, motor activity was the most frequently studied behavior. The literature on prenatal amphetamine effects on motor activity appears to lack consistency. The apparent contradictions in this literature, however, might be related to differences in the drug dose, to the duration and gestation time of drug exposure, as well as to the age at which the offspring were tested.[48] When the drug was given throughout gestation, and activity was tested on weanling or adult offspring, the literature consistently indicates that prenatal amphetamine exposure increased activity whether measured in the open-field or in activity wheels.[41,43,44,46] The literature is less clear when the duration of amphetamine exposure was for a restricted period during gestation or when animals were tested at an earlier age.

Elevated activity has been reported for prenatal-amphetamine-exposed adult mice[8] (5 mg/Kg d-amphetamine on GD 12-19) and adult rats[42] (5 mg or 10 mg/Kg d-amphetamine on GD 5-9 or 12-16). These reports of elevated motor activity in animals exposed to amphetamine contrast sharply with several reports in which exposure was limited to GD 12-15 and doses were 3 mg/Kg or less. Although, some of these experiments indicated that motor activity of prenatal-amphetamine-exposed animals was altered,[48,49] the results were inconsistent, and several of the studies indicated that prenatally exposed rats were not different from control animals.[48,50-52] These studies suggest that amphetamine at doses of 3 mg/Kg or less when restricted to GD 12-15, i.e., the period of neurogenesis, has little influence on activity of relatively young (45-50 days) offspring. Holson, et al.[48] on the basis of a thorough experimental analysis, concluded that the effects of prenatal amphetamine exposure on activity were complex and subtle depending on such factors as age of testing, sex, dose, and type of test. In general, amphetamine-related differences in motor activity occurred in older offspring (120 days or older) tested in a novel environment. It should be noted, however, that an earlier study[42] indicated that motor activity was elevated in 54-day-old offspring exposed to a 10-mg but not a 5-mg/Kg dose of amphetamine on GD 12-16 and to both doses given on GD 5-9. These studies suggest that, in contrast to many drugs, neurogenesis might not be the most sensitive period for the effects of amphetamine. Current information, however, does not establish whether the stage of development or the duration of drug exposure accounts for the different results obtained in the above studies.

When animals were tested prior to weaning, prenatal amphetamine exposure has been reported to either reduce[40] or to have no influence on motor activity when given throughout[53] or for restricted periods of gestation.[8,52] Although there is insufficient information for any firm conclusion on the basis of these results, it is possible that prenatal amphetamine exposure may have less effect or a different effect on young than on mature offspring.

Prenatal amphetamine exposure has also been reported to alter catecholaminergic systems which can be observed in mature offspring. There are few studies on the topic, however, and the reported changes provide no consistent pattern. An early study indicated that methamphetamine (dose unspecified, but behaviorally active) given to rats via drinking water throughout gestation and lactation altered catecholamines in brains of adult (9 mo) offspring.[54] Concentrations of both DA and NE were elevated in cortical and reduced in thalamic tissues. In addition, NE was elevated in tissue from hippocampus, hypothalamus, and corpora quadrigemini. In another study,[42] d-amphetamine (3 mg/Kg) was injected subcutaneously into rats during Gestation Days 5-21. NE and DA were lower in the brainstem and NE was lower in the diencephalon of adult offspring (84 days). In contrast to the above study, catecholamines were not elevated in the cortex or other brain regions. This study also indicated that whole brain concentrations of NE were reduced in 35-day-old offspring. Neither DA nor 5-HT differed from controls at either age except as noted for the adult brain. In two additional studies on rats, d,l-amphetamine (0.5 mg/Kg) injected throughout pregnancy altered several monoamine measures in adult (90-120 day) animals. Although catecholamine levels were unchanged in whole brain, tissue from animals prenatally exposed to amphetamine had higher tyrosine hydroxylase activity and increased rates of incorporation of [^{3}H]-tyrosine into either DA or NE suggesting increased turnover rates.[55] In addition, tissue from brains of adult rats prenatally exposed to amphetamine had reduced binding of alpha, but not beta adrenergic receptor ligands.[56] Finally, in a single study on mice, d-amphetamine (5 mg/Kg) injected IP for the last third of pregnancy reduced whole brain concentration of NE at birth.[8] Both DA and NE were elevated at 21 and 30 days of age but did not differ from controls at 75-days of age.

The effects of amphetamine on monoaminergic systems of adults certainly depend on the dose and the duration of exposure. Future studies on the prenatal effects of amphetamine should include in their design a relatively long duration of exposure, different stages of gestation than GD 12-15, and doses higher than 3 mg/Kg. It might also be important to consider the relative effects of periodic higher peak levels of the drug compared to more sustained exposure to lower doses. Recent work indicates that high peak levels of ethanol are more detrimental to developing rats than exposure to similar amounts of the drug distributed over longer time periods.[57] Unpublished work from our laboratory indicated that when injected subcutaneously, prenatal amphetamine did not produce the effects on offspring observed when the drug was injected intraperitoneally. Although alternative explanations are possible, the more rapid drug absorption and higher peak levels resulting from IP than SC injections might account for the different effects. Although the IP route of administration should be avoided in prenatal drug studies for a number of good reasons, more attention should be given to the effects of short exposure to higher doses of the drug.

The effects of amphetamines during pregnancy on the development of the pituitary-adrenal system have not been reported; however, as discussed above, there is a reasonable rationale for anticipating an effect. It should also be noted that increased exploratory activity and reduced passive avoidance performance which have been reported in offspring prenatally exposed to amphetamine are also reported for early exposure to corticosterone.[35-37] Thus, an altered pituitary-adrenal system is a logical and testable mechanism for the long-term behavioral effects of prenatal amphetamine exposure.

SUMMARY AND CONCLUSIONS

The present analysis indicates that the literature is currently too limited to draw anything but very tentative conclusions about whether amphetamine during pregnancy is detrimental to the offspring. However, exposure to very high doses of the drug appears to be teratogenic; and studies in which animals were exposed to lower doses of either amphetamine or methamphetamine throughout pregnancy indicate that this class of drugs can have long-term neurochemical and behavioral consequences for rodent offspring. The commonly reported behavioral effects include abnormal responding on aversively motivated tasks, and heightened motor activity which might be associated with slower habituation. Neurochemical studies have focused on various aspects of the monoamine neurotransmitter systems and suggest that prenatal amphetamine exposure can increase the synthesis and turnover of DA and NE and reduce the number of adrenergic receptors in adult offspring. In addition, concentrations of NE appear to be reduced at birth suggesting prenatal depletion and are sometimes found to be altered at later times. Although these studies are provocative, the absence of pair-fed controls and cross-fostering prevent ruling out the possible confounding effects of undernutrition and altered maternal care.

In addition to the above limited empirical support, the effects of amphetamines on adult brain provide a logical rationale for anticipating that prenatal exposure to the drug could be detrimental. This rationale is essentially that amphetamine can have long-term effects of monoaminergic systems in the brains of adults, including neural degeneration; and, since the drug can cross the placenta, it should also have long-lasting consequences for the developing fetus. It is proposed that the later stages of gestation might be particularly sensitive to the long-term behavioral effects of amphetamine. Although there are no systematic studies on critical periods for the effects of prenatal amphetamine exposure, several reports indicate that exposure restricted to GD 12-15 has little effect. Since amphetamine predominantly affects the neuron terminals and terminals develop later than GD 15, it is proposed that amphetamine exposure later in gestation, after the monoaminergic systems are more mature, will have a greater effect. The rationale for the long-term behavioral effects of prenatal amphetamine is based on studies indicating that 1) rapidly developing systems are very sensitive to insult from external agents; 2) the monoaminergic systems and pituitary-adrenal organization are developing rapidly during the later gestation and early neonatal periods; 3) amphetamine influences each of these systems in adults and the monoamine systems in fetuses; and, 4) alterations in the systems cause predictable behavioral changes. It is thus proposed that prenatal amphetamine exposure during the later stages of gestation will have long-lasting effects on behavior which are mediated via its effects on the monoamines and/or the pituitary-adrenal system.

REFERENCES

1. HILL, R. M. 1973. Drugs ingested by pregnant women. Clin. Pharmacol. Ther. **14:** 654-659.
2. FORFAR, J. O. & M. M. NELSON. 1973. Epidemiology of drugs taken by pregnant women: Drugs that may affect the fetus adversely. Clin. Pharmacol. Ther. **14:** 632-642.
3. MORGAN, J. P. 1981. Amphetamine. *In* Substance Abuse: Clinical Problems and Perspectives. J. H. Lowinson & P. Ruiz, Eds.: 167-184. Williams & Wilkins. Baltimore, MD.
4. BELL, R. W., R. R. DRUCKER & A. B. WOODRUFF. 1965. The effects of prenatal injections of adrenaline chloride and *d*-amphetamine sulfate on subsequent emotionality and ulcer proneness of offspring. Psychonomic Science **2:** 269-270.
5. NORA, J. J., D. G. TRASLER & F. C. FRASER. 1965. Malformations in mice induced by dexamphetamine sulphate. Lancet **2:** 1021-1022.
6. BUELKE-SAM, J. 1986. Postnatal functional assessment following central nervous system stimulant exposure. Amphetamine and caffeine. *In* Handbook of Behavioral Teratology. E. P. Riley & C. V. Vorhees, Eds.: 161-172. Plenum Press. New York, NY.
7. MARTIN, J. 1986. Irreversible changes in mature and aging animals following intrauterine drug exposure. Neurobehav. Toxicol. Teratol. **8:** 335-343.
8. MIDDAUGH, L. D., L. A. BLACKWELL, C. A. SANTOS III & J. W. ZEMP. 1974. Effects of *d*-amphetamine sulfate given to pregnant mice on activity and on catecholamines in the brains of offspring. Dev. Psychobiol. **7:** 429-438.
9. PINDER, R. & H. KOPERA. 1984. Stimulants of the central nervous system. *In* Clinical Pharmacology in Pregnancy. H. P. Keummerle & K. Brendel, Eds.: 339-341. Thieme-Stratton. New York, NY.
10. MILKOVIC, K., J. PAUNOVIC, Z. KNIEWALD & S. MILKOVIC. 1973. Maintenance of the plasma corticosterone concentration of adrenalectomized rat by the fetal adrenal glands. Endocrinology **93:** 115-118.

11. MOORE, K. E. 1978. Amphetamines: Biochemical and behavioral actions in animals. *In* Handbook of Psychopharmacology, Vol. II. Stimulants. L. L. Iverson, S. D. Iverson & S. H. Snyder, Eds.: 41-98. Plenum Press. New York, NY.

12. RITZ, M. C., R. J. LAMB, S. R. GOLDBERG & M. J. KUHAR. 1987. Cocaine receptors on dopamine transporters are related to self-administration of cocaine. Science **237:** 1219-1223.

13. RICAURTE, G. A., L. S. SEIDEN & C. R. SCHUSTER. 1984. Further evidence that amphetamines produce long-lasting dopamine neurochemical deficits by destroying dopamine nerve fibers. Brain Res. **303:** 359-364.

14. COMMING, D. L. & L. S. SEIDEN. 1986. *a*-Methyltyrosine blocks methylamphetamine-induced degeneration in the rat somatosensory cortex. Brain Res. **365:** 15-20.

15. LUCOT, J. B., G. C. WAGNER, C. R. SCHUSTER & L. S. SEIDEN. 1982. Decreased sensitivity of rat pups to long-lasting dopamine and serotonin depletions produced by methylamphetamine. Brain Res. **247:** 181-183.

16. BRADBURY, A. J., B. COSTALL, R. J. NAYLOR & E. S. ONAIVI. 1987. 5-Hydroxytryptamine involvement in the locomotor activity suppressant effects of amphetamine in the mouse. Psychopharmacology **93:** 457-465.

17. PINTER, E. J. & C. J. PATTEE. 1970. Fat-mobilizing action of amphetamine. *In* Amphetamines and Related Compounds. E. Costa & S. Garattini, Eds.: 653-672. Raven Press. New York, NY.

18. FULLER, R. W., H. D. SNODDY, N. R. MASON, J. A. CLEMENS & K. G. BEMIS. 1983. Elevation of serum corticosterone in rats by dopamine agonists related in structure to pergolide. Neuroendocrinology **36:** 285-290.

19. JEZOVA, D., J. JURCOVICOVA, M. VIGAS, K. MURGAS & F. LABRIE. 1985. Increase in plasma ACTH after dopaminergic stimulation in rats. Psychopharmacology **85:** 201-203.

20. DOBBING, J. 1968. Vulnerable periods in developing brain. *In* Applied Neurochemistry. A. Davison & J. Dobbing, Eds.: 278-316. Davis. Philadelphia, PA.

21. IVERSON, S. D. & L. L. IVERSON. 1975. Central neurotransmitters and the regulation of behavior. *In* Handbook of Psychobiology. M. S. Gazzaniga & C. Blakemore, Eds.: 153-200. Academic Press. New York, NY.

22. WIEGANT, V. M. & D. DE WIED. 1981. Behavioral effects of pituitary hormones, *In* Neuroendocrine regulation and altered behaviour. P. D. Hrdina & R. L. Singhal, Eds.: 31-49. Plenum Press. New York, NY.

23. GOLDEN, G. S. 1973. Prenatal development of the biogenic amine system of the mouse brain. Dev. Biol. **33:** 300-311.

24. LAUDER, J. M. & F. E. BLOOM. 1974. Ontogeny of monoamine neurones in the locus coeruleus, raphe nuclei and substantia nigra of the rat. I. Cell differentiation. J. Comp. Neurol. **155:** 469-482.

25. COYLE, J. T. & D. HENRY. 1973. Catecholamines in fetal and newborn rat brain. J. Neurochem. **21:** 61-67.

26. JOST, A. 1966. Problems in fetal endocrinology: The adrenal glands. Recent Prog. Horm. Res. **22:** 541-574.

27. COHEN, A. 1977. Plasma corticosterone concentration in the foetal rat. Horm. Metab. Res. **5:** 66.

28. EGUCHI, Y., O. HIRAI, Y. MORIKAWA & Y. HASHIMOTO. 1973. Critical time in the hypothalamic control of the pituitary-adrenal system in fetal rats: Observations in fetuses subjected to hypervitaminosis A and hypothalamic destruction. Endocrinology **93:** 1-11.

29. SPARBER, S. B. 1972. Effects of drugs on the biochemical and behavioral responses of developing organisms. Fed. Proc. **31:** 74-80.

30. LYDIARD, R. B. & S. B. SPARBER. 1977. Postnatal behavioral alterations resulting from prenatal administration of dl-alphamethylparatyrosine. Dev. Psychobiol. **10:** 305-314.

31. EIDUSON, S. 1966. 5-hydroxytryptamine in the developing chick brain: Its normal and altered development and possible control by end-product repression. J. Neurochem. **13:** 923-932.

32. LEVINE, S. & R. J. MULLINS, JR. 1966. Hormonal influences on brain organization in infant rats. Science **152:** 1585-1592.

33. DENENBERG, V. H., J. T. BRUMAGHIM, G. C. HALTMEYER & M. X. ZARROW. 1967.

Increased adrenocortical activity in the neonatal rat following handling. Endocrinology **81:** 1047-1052.

34. LEVINE, S., G. C. HALTMEYER, G. KARAS & V. H. DENENBERG. 1967. Physiological and behavioral effects of infantile stimulation. Physiol. Behav. **2:** 55-59.

35. HOWARD, E. 1973. Increased reactivity and impaired adaptability in operant behavior of adult mice given corticosterone in infancy. J. Comp. Physiol. Psychol. **85:** 211-220.

36. HOWARD, E., D. S. OLTON & M. H. TAYLOR. 1974. Polydipsia in adult mice and rats given corticosterone in infancy: Accentuation by variable interval food reinforcement. J. Comp. Physiol. Psychol. **87:** 120-125.

37. OLTON, D. S., C. T. JOHNSON & E. HOWARD. 1974. Impairment of conditioned active avoidance in adult rats given corticosterone in infancy. Dev. Psychobiol. **8:** 55-61.

38. MIDDAUGH, L. D., W. O. BOGGAN, C. WILSON-BURROWS & J. W. ZEMP. 1979. Prenatal maternal phenobarbital alters plasma concentrations of corticosterone in developing offspring. Life Sci. **24:** 999-1002.

39. TAYLOR, A. N., B. J. BRANCH, S. H. LIU, A. F. WIECHMANN, M. A. HILL & N. KOKKA. 1981. Fetal exposure to ethanol enhances pituitary-adrenal and temperature responses to ethanol in adult rats. Alcohol. Clin. Exp. Res. **5:** 237-246.

40. CLARK, C. V. H., D. GORMAN & A. VERNADAKIS. 1970. Effects of prenatal administration of psychotropic drugs on behavior of developing rats. Dev. Psychobiol. **3:** 225-235.

41. SELIGER, D. L. 1973. Effect of prenatal maternal administration of d-amphetamine on rat offspring activity and passive avoidance learning. Physiol. Psychol. **1:** 273-280.

42. HITZEMANN, B. A., R. J. HITZEMANN, D. A. BRASE & H. H. LOH. 1976. Influence of prenatal d-amphetamine administration of development and behavior of rats. Life Sci. **18:** 605-612.

43. MARTIN, J. C. & D. C. MARTIN. 1981. Voluntary activity in the aging rat as a function of maternal drug exposure. Neurobehav. Toxicol. Teratol. **3:** 261-264.

44. NASELLO, A. G. & O. A. RAMIREZ. 1978. Open-field and Lashley III maze behaviour of the offspring of amphetamine-treated rats. Psychopharmacology **58:** 171-173.

45. NASELLO, A. G., C. A. ASTRADA & O. A. RAMIREZ. 1974. Effects on the acquisition of conditioned avoidance responses and seizure threshold in offspring of amphetamine-treated gravid rats. Psychopharmacologia **40:** 25-31.

46. MARTIN, J. C. 1975. Effects on offspring of chronic maternal methamphetamine exposure. Dev. Psychobiol. **8:** 397-404.

47. SELIGER, D. L. 1975. Prenatal maternal d-amphetamine effects on emotionality and audiogenic seizure susceptibility of rat offspring. Dev. Psychobiol. **8:** 261-268.

48. HOLSON, R., J. ADAMS, J. BUELKE-SAM, B. GOUGH & C. A. KIMMEL. 1985. d-amphetamine as a behavioral teratogen: Effects depend on dose, sex, age and task. Neurobehav. Toxicol. Teratol. **7:** 753-758.

49. BUELKE-SAM, J., C. A. KIMMEL, J. ADAMS, D. R. MILLER & C. J. NELSON. 1982. Behavioral assessment of rats treated prenatally with low doses of d-amphetamine: II. Activity and pharmacological challenge testing. Teratology **25:** 30A-31A.

50. ADAMS, J., J. BUELKE-SAM, C. A. KIMMEL & J. B. LABORDE. 1982. Behavioral alterations in rats prenatally exposed to low doses of d-amphetamine. Neurobehav. Toxicol. Teratol. **4:** 63-70.

51. BUELKE-SAM, J., C. A. KIMMEL, J. ADAMS, C. J. NELSON, C. V. VORHEES, D. C. WRIGHT, V. ST. OMER, B. A. KOROL, R. E. BUTCHER, M. A. GEYER, J. F. HOLSON, C. L. KUTSCHER & M. J. WAYNER. 1985. Collaborative behavioral teratology study: Results. Neurobehav. Toxicol. Teratol. **7:** 591-624.

52. VORHEES, C. V. 1985. Behavioral effects of prenatal d-amphetamine in rats: A parallel trial to the collaborative behavioral teratology study. Neurobehav. Toxicol. Teratol. **7:** 709-716.

53. MONDER, H. 1981. Effects of prenatal amphetamine exposure on the development of behavior in rats. Psychopharmacology **75:** 75-78.

54. TONGE, S. R. 1973. Permanent alterations in catecholamine concentrations in discrete areas of brain in the offspring of rats treated with methylamphetamine and chlorpromazine. Br. J. Pharmacol. **47:** 425-427.

55. NASELLO, A. G. & O. A. RAMIREZ. 1978. Brain catecholamines metabolism in offspring of amphetamine treated rats. Pharmacol. Biochem. Behav. **9:** 17-20.

56. RAMIREZ, O. A., E. A. KELLER & O. A. ORSINGHER. 1983. Prenatal amphetamine reduces alpha but not beta adrenergic receptor binding in brain of adult rats. Life Sci. **32:** 1835-1838.

57. BONTHIUS, D. J., C. R. GOODLETT & J. R. WEST. 1988. Blood alcohol concentration and severity of microencephaly in neonatal rats depend on the pattern of alcohol administration. Alcohol **5:** 209-214.

Phencyclidine during Pregnancy: Behavioral and Neurochemical Effects in the Offspring

THERESA A. FICO AND
CHRISTINA VANDERWENDE [a]

New York State Psychiatric Institute
722 West 168th Street
Box 40
New York, New York 10032
and
[a] *Rutgers, The State University of New Jersey*
P.O. Box 789
Piscataway, New Jersey 08854

INTRODUCTION

Phencyclidine (PCP, angel dust) was developed by the Parke-Davis pharmaceutical company in the 1950s as an anesthetic agent. PCP is a dissociative anesthetic with minimal cardiovascular and respiratory depression. However, its medical use was discontinued following reports of adverse side effects which include postanesthetic confusion, agitation, delirium and persistent hallucinations.[1,2] Presently, the only legal use for PCP is as a veterinary anesthetic.

PCP first emerged as a popular drug of abuse in the early 1970s. PCP usage peaked in 1979, remained relatively constant and by 1981 began to decline. Since then, however, the Drug Abuse Warning Network and National Institute on Drug Abuse National Drug Surveys have indicated PCP abuse is on the rise. The popularity of PCP is thought to be due in part to an uncomplicated synthesis from readily available precursors,[3] low cost and the ability of the drug to elicit hallucinations, excitation, euphoria and feelings of tranquillity.

The drug is not without untoward side effects. PCP can also produce feelings of paranoia, impending death, outbursts of bizarre, agitated or violent behavior and a psychosis which mimics schizophrenia.[4-6] In the early 1980s, when I entered the laboratory of C. VanderWende, Wilmot and VanderWende[7,8] had just reported that in a pathological model of aggressive behavior—isolation-induced aggressive behavior—PCP intensified fighting in male mice.

With the increased use of PCP by women of reproductive age, physicians were beginning to identify and report on the effects of prenatal exposure to phencyclidine. Golden *et al.*[9] were the first to describe the appearance and neurobehavioral development of an infant prenatally exposed to PCP. Three case studies reported neonates born to women who abuse PCP during their pregnancy to be jittery, hyperreactive to stimuli and irritable, alternating with periods of lethargy and blank staring.[9-11] There were a limited number of animal studies of the developmental toxicity of PCP.

Placental transfer of PCP was reported to occur in the pig,[12,13] rabbit, mouse[14] and human.[15] Tonge[16,17] administered PCP to rats throughout gestation and lactation and reported permanent increases in the concentrations of dopamine and serotonin in discrete brain areas of the male offspring. However, behavioral assessment of these offspring was not carried out so that the functional significance of these neurochemical alterations was not clear. PCP administered prenatally to the mouse[18] and rat[19] was found to produce a variety of gross structural defects but only at doses that were highly toxic to the dam. Low doses of PCP administered throughout gestation to mice delayed the development of behavioral reflexes[14] but had no effect on locomotor activity.[20]

In 1980, Hutchings[21] published a commentary on phencyclidine abuse noting that PCP had emerged as one of the most dangerous and widespread drugs of abuse. Hutchings reasoned that given the psychoactive potency of the drug in the adult it would not be surprising that it would produce deleterious effects in the developing central nervous system and suggested further animal and clinical studies.

The studies summarized here developed out of several major issues of concern related to prenatal drug abuse in the early 1980s. These include problems of long-term tolerance, addiction liability, abstinence and the assumption that adult toxicity may be predictive of developmental toxicity.

Experiment 1

All of the results reported here are part of a larger study; the pharmacokinetic and aggression studies are in press,[22] while the postnatal sensitivity and binding experiments are in preparation.[23] Throughout these studies, adult female CF-1 mice were time-mated to male mice and randomly assigned to a dosage group and treatment period. Three subteratogenic doses (i.e., below those reported to produce dysmorphogenesis) were administered during two different but overlapping critical periods. The first spanned organogenesis (gestation day (G) 6-15) and the second, the period of central nervous system PCP receptor ontogeny (G12-18).[24] Because Misra and co-workers[25] reported that PCP persisted in tissues for more than 14 days after a single injection, we were concerned that persistence of pharmacologically active concentrations PCP in the offspring of treated mothers could disturb maternal pup interactions and confound behavioral measures. The half-life of PCP in fetal brain was determined on the last day of drug administration (G15 and 18). Other groups of treated and control offspring were fostered, growth determined and ontogeny of isolation-induced aggressive behavior examined. As a measure of tolerance, sensitivity to postnatal PCP-induced motor activity and ataxia and ontogeny of 3H-PCP binding in discrete brain areas were examined. Details of the methods have been provided elsewhere.[22]

Maternal Effects

There were no maternal deaths among the more than 400 PCP-treated and control dams in either period of treatment. Among the mid-gestation-treated dams, there was a significant effect of PCP on maternal weight gain from G6 to 15. The dams treated with 20 mg/kg PCP gained approximately 20% less than all other treated groups.

Among the late-gestation-treated dams, there was no significant effect of phencyclidine on maternal weight gain from G12 to 18, although the 20-mg/kg group gained less weight than all other treatment groups.

Pharmacokinetics

In a separate study, dams were bred and administered 20 mg/kg PCP as previously described. On the last day of injections (G15 or 18) the dams received the injection of PCP to which a known quantity of 3H-PCP had been added. The method of Martin et al.[26] was employed to quantitate PCP in fetal brain tissue at various times after the dams' last injection. PCP appears rapidly in brain and is already present as early as 15 min (FIG. 1). The time course of PCP on G15 and 18 is virtually identical,

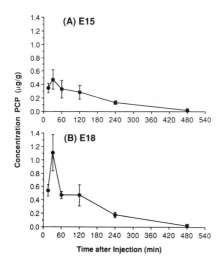

FIGURE 1. Time course of PCP in fetal brain on (A) E15 and (B) E18. Concentration of PCP in μg per g wet weight of tissue after a subcutaneous injection of 20 mg/kg PCP with the addition of 3H-PCP. Each value is the mean $\pm$ SEM of 3-6 litter determinations.

however, on G15 the concentration of PCP was half that of G18 at all time points. Thirty minutes after sc injection of PCP to the dams peak concentrations of 0.473 and 1.108 μg/g fetal brain on G15 and 18, respectively, were reached. The two major metabolites of PCP, 4-phenyl-4-piperidinocyclohexanol (PPC) and 1-(1-phencyclohexyl)-4-hydroxypiperidine (PCHP) followed a similar time course (data not shown). PCP, PPC and PCHP were not detectable after 24 hours in fetal brain tissue.

Offspring Effects

As seen in TABLE 1, prenatal exposure to PCP in either treatment period had no effect on mean litter size. There was a significant dose response effect of PCP on the number of males and females: as dose increased, there was a corresponding decrease in the number of live males and increase in the number of live females at birth. The data suggests that PCP increases prenatal male mortality, however, without implantation site data, number of stillborns and number of resorptions, this observation remain tentative.

Birthweight of the males was greater than the females in all groups. There was a significant effect of prenatal PCP on birth weight of both male and female offspring. The offspring of the 10- and 20-mg/kg groups weighed significantly less at birth than all other treatment groups (TABLE 1); however, this is a modest reduction of approximately 7%. Male weights were recorded at weaning, postnatal day (P) 21 and 35; female growth was not recorded as females were not included in postnatal testing. Although there was a significant effect of prenatal treatment on male birthweight, the difference was not present on P21 and 35.

PCP had no effect on the percentage of animals that exhibited aggressive behavior, ontogeny of aggressive behavior or fighting intensity. Surprisingly, the timing of the prenatal handling and injection did significantly affect the intensity of the fighting behavior, an effect we attributed to prenatal maternal stress.

TABLE 1. Offspring Effects[a]

| | | | PCP (mg/kg) | | |
	UTC	Saline	5	10	20
Number of litters	200	55	43	48	57
Number of born live					
males[b]	1097 (55%)	310 (58%)	236 (56%)	246 (49%)	273 (51%)
females	910 (45%)	228 (42%)	188 (44%)	255 (51%)	266 (49%)
Mean litter size	10	10	10	10	9
Mean birthweight (g)					
Males[b]	1.61 ± 0.01	1.59 ± 0.02	1.58 ± 0.02	1.54 ± 0.02^c	1.52 ± 0.02^c
Females	1.58 ± 0.01	1.54 ± 0.02	1.54 ± 0.02	1.48 ± 0.02^c	1.48 ± 0.02^c

[a] Data for mid and late gestation period of treatments were pooled within each treatment group. Birthweights are mean ± SEM.

[b] $p < 0.05$, Duncan's multiple range test, significantly different from females.

[c] $p < 0.05$, Duncan's multiple range test, significantly different from UTC, saline and 5-mg/kg PCP groups of the same sex.

Experiment 2

On P34-36, four male offspring from each litter were randomly chosen and each received either 0, 2.5, 5.0, or 7.5 mg/kg PCP-HCl, sc. Immediately following the injection, the mice were placed on an activity meter and activity counts were recorded for one hour. Using the rating scale of Castellani and Adams[27] ataxia was scored by the investigator in 15-sec observation periods at 5-min intervals for 50 min.

Neurobehavioral Effects

Neither PCP administration nor treatment period had any effect on the total motor activity score; however, postnatal challenge had a significant effect on the total score.

A repeated measure analysis was conducted on the 10 6-min intervals comprising the total score. This analysis confirmed the significant dose-dependent effect of postnatal challenge on motor activity but revealed no effect of prenatal treatment on the temporal pattern of motor activity. Similarly, there was no significant effect of prenatal PCP on ataxia. However, within each period of treatment, the highest scores were demonstrated by those animals which were prenatally exposed to PCP as compared to saline. Ataxia score was increased in a dose-dependent manner by postnatal challenge of PCP.

Receptor Binding

Since the PCP receptor is present in brain membranes from developing rats as early as embryonic day 13,[24] we investigated whether prenatal administration of PCP could alter the development of the PCP receptor. Modification of the receptor could explain any postnatal changes in responsivity to PCP. On P21 and 35 males were decapitated an the striatum, cortex and hippocampus were dissected out. For each assay the tissue was pooled from five to six males of a litter. Membranes were prepared and 3H-PCP binding assay of Zukin et al.[28] was employed.

On P21, the number of 3H-PCP binding sites was increased in the cortex and striatum of the late-gestation offspring. There was no effect of prenatal PCP on the Bmax in the three brain regions. On P35, there were no differences in the binding affinity or number of receptors among the treatment groups.

DISCUSSION

The low doses (5 to 20 mg/kg) of PCP used in this study, produce mild maternal toxicity, selective male embryolethal effect and reduced bodyweights at birth but not effects on postnatal growth. PCP and its monohydroxylated metabolites, PPC and PCHP, rapidly enter fetal brain, but do not appear to persist for more than 24 hr after administration. Prenatal PCP did not effect the ontogeny or intensity of isolation-induced aggressive behavior, postnatal sensitivity to PCP-induced motor activity and ataxia or 3H-PCP binding to brain membranes on P21 and 35.

PCP has been reported to produce embryolethality and dysmorphogenesis in both the mouse[18] and rat,[19] but only at doses that approximated the maternal LD40. Results of the present experiments support other reports[14,20,29] that subteratogenic doses of PCP produce mild maternal toxicity but no significant neurobehavioral deficits in the offspring. Recently, Nebeshima et al.[30] reported that prenatal administration of 10 mg/kg/day PCP to rats resulted in mild maternal toxicity, a modest reduction in birthweights, decreased male/female ratio but no gross morphological abnormalities, findings in agreement with the existing literature. They also reported transient sex-dependent effects on neurobehavioral development, but since fostering was not employed, these effects may have been produced by drug-induced alterations of maternal behavior and not prenatal drug exposure.

Because the persistence of pharmacologically active concentrations of PCP in the offspring could alter postnatal development, we were concerned about the reports of accumulation and persistence of PCP and metabolites after acute or multiple dosing.

Misra and co-workers[25] reported that when PCP is behaviorally active, the concentration in the brain is 5000-8000 ng/g tissue; After 24 hr the concentration of PCP is less than 150 ng/g tissue. Martin et al. reported that 24 hr after receiving PCP, less than 24 ng/g brain of PCP and metabolites were detected. More recently, Ahmad and co-workers[31] investigated PCP persistence in fetal brain after multiple dosing and reported that 24 hr after the last dose there was 17.2 ng/g PCP in fetal brain. We were not able to detect the presence of PCP or its metabolites in the brains of fetuses 24 hr after the last injection; if PCP was present the concentration was less than the 50 ng/g limit of detection. The functional significance of the persistence of such trace concentrations is unknown but adult data do not support the notion that these low concentrations are pharmacologically active.

Unlike alcohol, a syndrome associated with prenatal exposure to phencyclidine has not been established. In 1980, Golden et al.[9] first described an infant that was extremely jittery, was hyperresponsive to stimuli and had increased muscular tone. The mother admitted to smoking approximately 6 marijuana cigarettes contaminated with PCP each day throughout her pregnancy; however, no drug screen was done on the infant or mother. Based solely on the mother's history, the infant's symptoms were attributed to PCP but, curiously, neither to a direct effect of marijuana nor to a possible interaction of marijuana and PCP. Furthermore, the symptoms shown by this infant are not unique to PCP but common to many prenatal abuse compounds.[32] In a follow-up prospective study, Golden et al.[33] using a urine toxicology screen of over 2000 women, found 188 that used PCP during their pregnancy. The infants of these women had more nonspecific abnormal neurological and behavioral findings at birth than did control infants. However, many of the PCP users were polydrug abusers and the authors could not discount interactions with other drugs.

Chasnoff[34] reported on nine infants whose mothers primarily abused PCP throughout pregnancy. PCP offspring were more difficult to console than drug-free controls, exhibited rapid state changes but did not show signs of withdrawal. The rapid changes in state, increased responsivity to stimuli and coarse flapping movements are consistent with PCP intoxication of the neonate. PCP-exposed infants had a smaller head circumference and showed neurobehavioral deficits in the neonatal period.[35] Subsequent follow-up studies through two years of age, however, failed to reveal any differences in mental or psychomotor development between PCP-exposed infants and controls.[34]

In the eight years since the case report of a neonate prenatally exposed to PCP appeared, there have been only three individual case reports—two brief reports each on approximately seven neonates and a larger study of 188 PCP-exposed offspring—totaling 206 children. Polydrug exposure occurred in virtually all of the reports. PCP-exposed offspring were uniformly described as difficult to console and as showing rapid changes in state. No congenital defects were reported. Furthermore, follow-up studies by Chasnoff[34] suggested that the infant's environment contributed more to developmental outcome by age two than did maternal drug use during pregnancy.

If PCP is, indeed, developmentally toxic in humans and produces either dysmorphogenesis or chronic neurobehavioral deficits in the offspring, one would expect corroborating epidemiological data from information networks such as the Center for Disease Control; to the best of our knowledge, such information has not been reported. Perhaps PCP-exposed offspring are underreported because women that abuse PCP during their pregnancy are less likely to admit to PCP use compared with other drugs of abuse. Even if this were true, it would be reasonable to expect that programs such as Chasnoff's[34] or Golden's,[33] in which toxicology drug screens are routinely done during pregnancy, would identify nonreporters. Alternatively, the action of PCP in the immature organism may simply be pharmacologic and not toxic; though PCP receptors first appear during organogenesis, they may either be nonfunctional or produce an immature response. On the other hand, as in the adult, PCP may interact with its receptors to produce a pharmacological response and is metabolized and eliminated but without producing any long-term effects. Of course, one cannot rule out the possibility that PCP produces effects in the offspring that are extremely subtle and currently undetectable with state-of-the-art techniques.

REFERENCES

1. GREIFENSTEIN, F. E., M. DEVAULT, J. YOSHITAKE & J. E. GAIEWSKI. 1958. 1-Aryl cyclo hexyl amine for anesthesia. Anesth. Anal. **37:** 283-294.
2. JOHNSTON, M., V. EVANS & S. BAIGEL. 1959. Br. J. Anaesth. **31:** 433-439.
3. SHULGIN, A. T. & D. E. MACLEAN. 1976. Illicit synthesis of phencyclidine and several of its analogs. Clin. Toxicol. **9:** 553-560.
4. FAUMAN, M. A. & B. J. FAUMAN. 1979. Violence associated with phencyclidine abuse. Am. J. Psychiatry **136:** 1584-1586.
5. MCCARRON, M. M., B. W. SCHULZE, G. A. THOMPSON, M. C. CONDER & W. A. GOETZ. 1981. Acute phencyclidine intoxication: Incidence of clinical findings in 1,000 cases. Ann. Emerg. Med. **10:** 237-242.
6. STILLMAN, R. & R. C. PETERSEN. 1979. Paradox of phencyclidine abuse. Ann. Intern. Med. **90:** 428-430.
7. WILMOT, C. A. & C. VANDERWENDE. 1981. Phencyclidine increases the intensity and spontaneity of fighting in isolated mice. Soc. Neurosci. Abstr. **7:** 261.
8. WILMOT, C. A. & C. VANDERWENDE. 1987. The effects of phencyclidine on the fighting of differentially housed mice. Pharmacol. Biochem. Behav. **28:** 341-346.
9. GOLDEN, N. L., R. J. SOKOL & I. L. RUBIN. 1980. Angel dust: Possible effects on the fetus. Pediatrics **65:** 18-20.
10. STRAUSS, A. A., D. MODANLOU & S. K. BOSU. 1981. Neonatal manifestations of maternal phencyclidine (PCP) abuse. Pediatrics **68:** 550-552.
11. PETRUCHA, R. A., K. R. KAUFMAN & F. N. PITTS. 1982. Phencyclidine in pregnancy: A case report. J. Reprod. Med. **27:** 301-303.
12. CUMMINGS, A. J. 1979. Transplacental disposition of phencyclidine in the pig. Xenobiotica **9:** 447-452.
13. COOPER, J. E., A. J. CUMMINGS & H. JONES. 1977. The placental transfer of phencyclidine in the pig, plasma levels in the sow and its piglets. J. Physiol. **267:** 17P-18P.
14. NICHOLAS, J. M. & E. C. SCHREIBER. 1983. Phencyclidine exposure and the developing mouse: Behavioral teratological implications. Teratology **28:** 319-326.
15. KAUFMAN, K. R., R. A. PETRUCHA & F. N. PITTS. 1983. Phencyclidine in amniotic fluid and breast milk: A case report. J. Clin. Psychiatry **44:** 269-270.
16. TONGE, S. R. 1973. Neurochemical teratology: 5-hydroxyindole concentrations in discrete areas of rat brain during the pre- and neonatal administration of phencyclidine and imipramine. Life Sci. **12:** 481-486.
17. TONGE, S. R. 1973. Catecholamine concentrations in discrete areas of rat brain after the pre- and neonatal administration of phencyclidine and imipramine. J. Pharm. Pharmacol. **25:** 164-166.
18. MARKS, T. A., W. C. WORTHY & R. E. STAPLES. 1980. Teratogenic potential of phencyclidine in the mouse. Teratology **21:** 241-246.
19. JORDAN, R. L., T. R. YOUNG, S. H. DINWIDDIE & G. J. HARRY. 1979. Phencyclidine-induced morphological and behavioral alterations in the neonatal rat. Pharmacol. Biochem. Behav. **11(S):** 39-45.
20. GOODWIN, P. J. 1980. Phencyclidine: Effects of chronic administration in the mouse on gestation, maternal behavior and the neonate. Psychopharmacology **69:** 63-67.
21. HUTCHINGS, D. E. 1980. Falling angels: Hazards of PCP abuse. Neurobehav. Toxicol. **2:** 287.

22. FICO, T. A. & C. VANDERWENDE. 1988. Phencyclidine during pregnancy: Fetal brain levels and neurobehavioral effects. Neurotoxicol. Teratol. **10:** 349-354.
23. FICO, T. A. & C. VANDERWENDE. Phencyclidine during pregnancy: Effects on 3H-PCP binding and PCP-induced motor activity and ataxia. Neurotox. Teratol. In press.
24. SIRCAR, R. & S. R. ZUKIN. 1983. Ontogeny of sigma opiate/PCP binding sites in rat brain. Life Sci. **33:** 255-257.
25. MISRA, A. L., R. B. PONTANI & J. BARTOLOMEO. 1979. Persistence of phencyclidine (PCP) and metabolites in brain and adipose tissue and implications for long-lasting behavioral effects. Res. Commun. Chem. Pathol. Pharmacol. **24:** 431-445.
26. MARTIN, B. R., W. C. VINCEK & R. L. BALSTER. 1980. Studies on the disposition of phencyclidine in mice. Drug Metab. Dispos. **8:** 49-54.
27. CASTELLANI, S. & P. M. ADAMS. 1981. Acute and chronic phencyclidine effects on locomotor activity, stereotypy and ataxia in rats. Eur. J. Pharmacol. **73:** 143-154.
28. ZUKIN, S. R., M. L. FITZ-SAYAGE, R. NICHTENHOUSER & R. S. ZUKIN. 1983. Specific binding of 3H-PCP in rat central nervous tissue: Further characterization and technical considerations. Brain Res. **258:** 277-284.
29. HUTCHINGS, D. E., S. R. BODNARENKO & R. DIAZ-DELEON. 1984. Phencyclidine during pregnancy in the rat: Effects on locomotor activity in the offspring. Pharmacol. Biochem. Behav. **20:** 251-254.
30. NABESHIMA, T., K. YAMAGUCHI, M. HIRAMATSU, K. ISHIKAWA, H. FURUKAWA & T. KAMEYAMA. 1987. Effects of prenatal and perinatal administration of phencyclidine on the behavioral development of rat offspring. Pharmacol. Biochem. Behav. **28:** 411-418.
31. AHMAD, G., L. C. HALSALL & S. C. BONDY. 1987. Persistence of phencyclidine in fetal brain. Brain Res. **415:** 194-196.
32. HUTCHINGS, D. E. 1987. Drug abuse during pregnancy: Embryopathic and neurobehavioral effects. *In* Genetic and Perinatal Effects of Abused Substances. M. C. Braude & A. M. Zimmerman, Eds.: 131-151. Academic Press. New York, NY.
33. GOLDEN, N. L., B. R. KUHNERT, R. J. SOKOL, S. MARTIER & T. WILLIAMS. 1987. Neonatal manifestations of maternal phencyclidine exposure. J. Perinat. Med. **15:** 185-191.
34. CHASNOFF, I. J., K. A. BURNS, W. J. BURNS & S. H. SCHNOLL. 1986. Prenatal drug exposure: Effects on neonatal and infant growth and development. Neurobehav. Toxicol. Teratol. **8:** 357-362.
35. CHASNOFF, I. J., W. J. BURNS, R. P. HATCHER & K. A. BURNS. 1983. Phencyclidine: Effects on the fetus and neonate. Dev. Pharmacol. Ther. **6:** 404-408.

Neurobehavioral Effects of Prenatal Caffeine

THOMAS J. SOBOTKA

Division of Toxicological Studies
Food and Drug Administration
Center for Food Safety and Applied Nutrition
200 C Street, S.W.
Washington, DC 20204

INTRODUCTION

Caffeine is a unique chemical in that it is a constituent of both drug preparations and commonly used foods and beverages. The widespread presence of this pharmacologically and behaviorally active compound[1] raises obvious questions about the health consequences of continuous exposure to excessive levels of this chemical. The consequences to the development of the immature organism are of particular interest, given the fact that caffeine can cross the placenta and reach the fetus.[2-4] This paper gives an overview and summary of the experimental information pertaining to the neurodevelopmental effects of prenatal exposure to caffeine and highlights areas in which additional information is needed.

Sources and Estimated Intakes of Caffeine

Some of the more common sources of caffeine include coffee, tea, soft drinks, chocolate, and prescription and nonprescription medication. The general average content of caffeine for each of these sources and their approximate ranges[5,6] are listed in TABLE 1. Note that the content of caffeine listed in the table is based on 5 ounces of coffee, tea, or cocoa, 12 ounces of soft drink, and 1 ounce of chocolate. The variability in caffeine content is due to a number of factors, including the specific products involved and the particular method of preparation (strong or weak coffee or tea). The average daily intakes of caffeine from all sources across various age groups[1,5,7-9] are presented in TABLE 2. Human exposure to caffeine appears to occur primarily through its availability in beverages, *i.e.,* coffee, tea, and soft drinks.[1,7] Across all age groups, the average daily dose of caffeine ranges from less than 1 mg/kg in infants to approximately 3 mg/kg in adults. Approximately 10% of the population takes in more than 5 mg/kg/day and 1% consumes more than 9 mg/kg/day.

TABLE 1. Common Sources of Caffeine[a]

Type of Product	Average mg. caffeine	Range
Coffee (5 oz)		
Brewed	98	40-180
Instant	65	30-120
Decaffeinated	3	1-5
Tea (5 oz)		
Brewed	50	20-110
Instant/Iced	30	25-76
Cocoa beverage (5 oz)	4	2-26
Chocolate (1 oz)	14	1-35
Soft drink (12 oz)	40	1-59
Prescription drugs	51	32-100
Nonprescription drugs		
Weight-control aids	170	100-200
Alertness tablets	150	100-200
Analgesic/pain relief	41	32-65
Diuretics	167	100-200
Cold/allergy remedies	27	16-30

[a] Adapted from Lecos.[6]

TABLE 2. Estimated Daily Intakes of Caffeine and Representative Plasma Half-Lives $(T\frac{1}{2})$[a]

Group	Intakes, mg/kg/day			$T\frac{1}{2}$ (Hours)
	Mean	Highest 10%	Highest 1%	
0-5 months	0.07	0	3.3	98
6-23 months	0.86	2.6	12.0	4
2-17 years	1.45	5.1	12.3	2-3
18+ years	2.7	5.7	9.3	5-6
Pregnant	2.3	5.2	11.0	
1st trimester				6
2nd trimester				10
3rd trimester				18
1 week postpartum				6
Oral contraceptive use				12
Smokers				3.5

[a] Adapted from SCOGS-89[5] and Lecos.[6]

Caffeine Rate of Metabolism

The half-life of caffeine, which reflects its rate of metabolism, is generally less than 5-6 h in adult humans, although this varies somewhat among individuals.[10–12] Comparable half-lives are found in many species of adult animals.[5,8,13] Factors that influence the rate of caffeine metabolism include age, pregnancy, and concurrent drug use (TABLE 2). The influence of age on caffeine metabolism is most apparent in the newborn or preterm infant.[11,14] At birth, the half-life of caffeine is 3-4 days, which is approximately 16-fold longer than in adults. Within 6 to 7 months, the half-life reverts to normal adult levels. Pregnancy also appears to slow the metabolism of caffeine.[11,15,16] During pregnancy, the half-life of caffeine increases steadily from the typical adult level to about 18 h in the third trimester; then it returns rapidly to normal by the first week postpartum. A somewhat smaller increase in caffeine's half-life results from the use of oral contraceptives. Smoking appears to have the opposite effect, lowering the half-life to about 3 h. The difference in the rate of elimination from the body is important in assessing the potential impact of caffeine on biological systems. In a representative sample of adult men and women the typical plasma levels of caffeine were less than 6.5 mg/1 in 97% of those surveyed.[8] Levels in the remaining 3% reached approximately 13 mg/1.

Is Excessive Use of Caffeine "Substance Abuse"?

The question of what constitutes "caffeine abuse" is particularly difficult to answer.[10] Clearly, caffeine is a pharmacologically active substance that can exert mild stimulant effects on human performance at doses of 2-4 mg/kg,[1,17,18] which approximates the adult average daily intake. The ingestion of caffeine in doses greater than 5-10 mg/kg, which represents moderate to excessive levels of caffeine consumption,[4] has been associated with adverse effects such as anxiety, tension, headache, disturbed sleep, irritability, and a decrease in hand steadiness.[10,18] Contrary to popular belief, related differences in sensitivity to caffeine are not discernible between children and adults.[17] A similar absence of age-related differences has been reported in animals.[19] Interestingly, adverse reactions to caffeine occur most notably in those who typically abstain from caffeine or normally consume small amounts (abstainers); habitual "users" typically exhibit few of these adverse symptoms.[10,17,20,21] Although the repeated exposure to caffeine results in tolerance to at least some of the pharmacological and toxic effects,[1,10,22] some factor(s) other than tolerance may be involved in the differential response of users versus abstainers. For example, it is still unclear whether individuals who normally abstain from caffeine may have an inordinate sensitivity to its adverse effects. Because of such uncertainty, the "normal" consumption of caffeine has been a problematic confound in the design and interpretation of many epidemiological and clinical studies.

The habitual use of caffeine at levels in excess of 5 mg/kg is also associated with a mild form of withdrawal.[1,23] User withdrawal from caffeine precipitates an array of symptoms remarkably similar to the adverse effects induced by caffeine administration in abstainers. These symptoms include irritability, nervousness, restlessness, and headache. Although signs of dependency, *i.e.,* tolerance and withdrawal, are associated with the habitual use of moderate to high levels of caffeine, there is no evidence of compulsive drug-seeking behavior or adverse social consequences, which are key elements in the functional criteria upon which most definitions of substance abuse are based.[1,24] Therefore, it seems inappropriate to refer to excessive use of caffeine as "substance abuse" in the commonly accepted sense. This distinction, however, should not trivialize the potential biological consequences of the excessive use of caffeine.

Reproduction and Teratogenesis

Caffeine has been shown to affect animal reproduction and to be an animal teratogen.[25] However, these effects may be influenced by several experimental variables. Exposure of the pregnant rat throughout gestation to daily doses of caffeine by intubation, at approximately 80 mg/kg or above, results in signs of maternal toxicity, increased resorptions, decreased fetal weight and size, teratogenic effects involving limbs, and skeletal ossification deficiencies.[26] Peak plasma levels of caffeine in rat dams intubated with similar dose levels approximate 63 mg/l.[27] At intubated doses as low as 6 mg/kg/day, there is little evidence of maternal or fetal toxicity,[26] although the offspring display delayed skeletal ossification, a condition which is reversible.[3] The dosing method is important in the production of teratogenesis and other effects. Administration of caffeine in the drinking water to pregnant rats at total daily doses as high as 204 mg/kg results in no teratogenic effects; however, signs of maternal and fetal toxicity occur at doses of 87 mg/kg/day.[28] The latter two dose levels have resulted in dam plasma caffeine levels ranging from approximately 5 to 18 mg/l.[2,27] Species differences also appear to play a significant role in the developmental effects of caffeine. Resorptions and stillbirths have been reported in primates given caffeine during gestation in the drinking water at doses as low as 10-20 mg/kg/day.[29]

Although, as mentioned above, caffeine is a demonstrated animal teratogen, there is no supportable evidence that it is teratogenic in humans.[8] Some epidemiological studies have associated high levels of intake of caffeine in pregnant women with a higher than normal incidence of prematurity, lower birth weights, and reduced head circumference.[30,31] Other studies, however, have not shown the same positive association.[32,33] Such inconsistencies point out the difficulties in conducting and interpreting epidemiological studies. A variety of potential confounders, such as smoking, alcohol consumption, maternal age, level of prenatal care, and amount and duration of caffeine exposure from all sources, must be addressed and considered. The failure to adjust for such confounders makes valid inferences from the results difficult or impossible.

ASSESSMENT OF CAFFEINE'S NEURODEVELOPMENTAL EFFECTS

Over the last decade, a number of experimental animal studies have investigated the neurodevelopmental consequences of in utero exposure to caffeine. Unfortunately, there have been no comparable epidemiological studies. TABLE 3 lists a representative number of the animal studies and outlines the principal elements of their experimental designs. To maintain relevance to the mode of human exposure, only those studies that administered caffeine via an oral route, *i.e.*, in the drinking water, in the food, or by intubation, have been included. Other neurodevelopmental studies of caffeine have been carried out using parenteral routes.[34–36]

Overview of Experimental Designs

The rodent, primarily the rat, has been the experimental species of choice. Most investigators used multiple dose groups, with caffeine usually being administered daily for a specified period of time. Across studies the median low dose was 24 mg/kg/day, ranging from 5 to 60, and the median high dose was 83 mg/kg/day, ranging from 35 to 180. Unfortunately, since few investigators reported the plasma levels of caffeine in either the dams or pups,[2,12] it is not possible to assess accurately the actual physiological exposures to caffeine. It is interesting, however, that the two groups that reported blood levels found caffeine in the dams at 5-18 mg/l. This is not very dissimilar from the range reported in a sample population of humans, *i.e.*, 6.5 to 13 mg/l.[8] Because the availability of this type of information would enable a more accurate interpretation of study results, it is recommended that future investigations include blood and tissue levels of caffeine and its primary metabolites. In terms of the treatment period, all studies exposed animals to caffeine during gestation; many extended the exposure to include the lactational period;[2,37–43] and a few also included a premating period of exposure.[2,12,44] Cross-fostering was not a common practice in these studies, although several investigators placed the experimental pups with control mothers.[44–46] In the absence of cross-fostering it is difficult to determine whether any treatment-related effects were due to the prior in utero exposure, to a direct exposure of the pups to caffeine in the milk, to some influence of caffeine on maternal behavior, or to some combination of these events. In the few studies that fostered the experimental pups to control dams, positive caffeine effects were found in the offspring, suggesting that in utero exposure is involved in at least some of caffeine's effects. One interesting facet of habitual caffeine exposure in humans, which has received very limited attention in animal studies, is the effect of caffeine withdrawal. There is no specific information as to whether abruptly stopping exposure to caffeine, for example by restricting exposure to the gestational period or by cross-fostering caffeine pups to control dams, affects either the dams or the developing offspring.

A majority of investigators attempted to assess the extent of maternal toxicity, but only a few included actual measurements of maternal behavior.[46,48] The experimental offspring were tested using a variety of multiple behavioral and neurochemical endpoints to assess the functional development of the nervous system. However, there were no apparent attempts to standardize the testing protocols for any of the behavioral or neurochemical measures.

Most studies included testing during the 3-week postnatal period of development. Several included testing of the 30- to 60-day-old adolescent, and others, specifically focusing on the long-term consequences of prenatal caffeine exposure, tested the adult offspring. One study even included testing of an F_2 generation to assess the possibility of transgenerational effects.[49]

Despite the fact that caffeine is known to interact with other chemical substances,[8,50] virtually no experiments have investigated the consequences of such interactions on the neurofunctional development of the immature organism.

TABLE 3. Experimental Designs of Neurodevelopmental Studies

Reference (Type of Study)	Species	Route of Administration	%	Dose (mg/kg/day)	Dam Blood Levels[a] (mg/l)	Premate	Gestation	Lactation	X-Foster	Dam	Pups	Adolesc.	Adult
Sobotka et al., 1979[37] (behavior; neurochemistry)	rat	drinking water	0.0125 0.025 0.05	30 62 115	ND	c	b	w	no	0 0 0	+ 0 +	+ + +	0 0 +
Enslen et al., 1980[49] (behavior; neurochemistry)	rat	food	0.0125 0.025 0.1	11 22 83	ND	c	b		no	+ + 0	+ 0		0 + +
Sinton et al., 1981[44] (behavior)	mouse	drinking water	0.03/0.04	60 80 100	ND	c	b		partial group				+ + +
Holloway, 1982[48] (behavior)	rat	drinking water	0.0125 0.05	25 93	ND	c	b		no	0 +	+ +		
Concannon et al., 1983[38] (behavior; neurochemistry)	rat	drinking water	0.05	32	ND	c	b	w	no	0	+	+	
Peruzzi et al., 1983[39] (behavior; neurochemistry)	rat	drinking water	0.02 0.04 0.08	38 81 148	ND	c	b	w	no	0 0 +	+ + +		+ + +
Tanaka et al., 1983[12] (neurochemistry)	rat	drinking water	0.04	70	5.75	c	b		no	+	+		

Reference	Species	Route	Dose	N	g/day	Exposure period (c–b–w)	Cross-fostered	Effects
Lombardelli et al., 1984[40] (behavior)	rat	drinking water	0.08	180	ND	c — b — w	no	+
Marangos et al., 1984[41] (neurochemistry)	mouse	food	0.4	50	ND	c — b — w	no	+ + +
Butcher et al., 1984[2] (behavior)	rat	drinking water	0.014 / 0.056	25 / 90	5 / 18	c — b — w	no	+/+ +/+ +/+
Peruzzi et al., 1985[42] (behavior; neurochemistry)	rat	drinking water	0.02 / 0.04 / 0.08	38 / 81 / 148	ND	c — b — w	no	+/+/+ + +
Glavin and Krueger, 1985[45] (behavior)	rat	drinking water	0.017 / 0.034 / 0.05	13 / 25 / 35	ND	c — b	yes	0/0/0 0/0/+ 0/0/0 0/+/+
West et al., 1986[47] (behavior)	rat	gavage		5 / 25 / 50 / 75	ND	c — b	no	+/+/+/+ 0/0/+/+ +/+/+
Nakamoto et al., 1986[43] (neurochemistry)	rat	food	—	10	ND	c — b — w	no	+
Hughes and Beveridge, 1987[46] (behavior)	rat	drinking water	0.015 / 0.03	24 / 44	ND	c — b	yes	+/+ +/+ 0/+

[a] ND = not determined.
[b] c = conception, b = birth, w = weaning.

NEURODEVELOPMENTAL EFFECTS OF PRENATAL EXPOSURE TO CAFFEINE

Maternal Effects

In agreement with the teratology and reproduction literature, the developmental neurobehavioral studies indicated that only minor maternal toxicity occurs across the range of oral doses used. Typically, the types of effects reported involved small transient changes in weight gain and/or food or water intake.[2,12,37-39,45-49] Even though there were few signs of maternal toxicity, there was clear evidence that the doses were behaviorally effective. For example, the motor activity of the dams was significantly elevated following exposure to caffeine in either the drinking water (24 mg/kg/day)[46] or via intubation (5 mg/kg/day).[47] However, even higher doses appeared to have no effect on more specific maternally relevant behaviors, such as nursing, nesting, or pup retrieval.[47,48]

Effects in Preweanling Offspring

TABLE 4 summarizes the predominant effects in the exposed preweaned offspring and approximates the lower range of doses at which each effect was found. As a general index of consistency of effect, the table also shows the proportion of studies reporting a treatment-related effect out of the total number of studies measuring a similar endpoint (testing protocols were not standardized across studies). In general, the exposed offspring tended to exhibit signs suggesting delayed development, including slight transient decreases in body weight,[2,37,47,48] delayed appearance of physical landmarks such as eye opening[37,39,42,47] and incisor eruption,[2,47] and depressed neuromotor development.[2,38,39,42,48,51] Concomitant with these developmental delays, the exposed neonates also exhibited altered sensitivity, predominantly decreased, to acute challenge with caffeine.[48] This latter effect was specific for caffeine, since the response to theophylline was unaffected. Because caffeine's acute behavioral effects are associated with adenosine receptor antagonism,[1,10,52] the altered sensitivity to caffeine challenge in the exposed offspring is consistent with the fact that perinatal caffeine also up-regulates neuronal adenosine receptors in the neonates.[41] Furthermore, since adenosine may be involved in the modulation of arousal,[53] it would be interesting to determine whether alterations to the adenosine system are specifically related to the delayed neuromotor development in the caffeine-exposed offspring.

Effects in Adolescent/Adult Offspring

The neurofunctional consequences of prenatal exposure to caffeine were not restricted to the neonatal period but also appeared to occur in the adolescent/adult offspring (TABLE 5). For the most part, the growth of the exposed offspring seemed to normalize in the older animals with only scattered reports of persistent minor reductions in body weights.[2,47]

TABLE 4. Summary of Treatment-Related Effects in Preweanling Offspring

Effect (No. Positive Studies/No. Studies)	Effective Dietary Dose (mg/kg/day)
↓ Body weight (4/11)	≥ 30
↓ Incisor eruption (2/3)	≥ 90 (≥ 50 via intubation)
↓ Eye opening (4/6)	≥ 30
— Vaginal opening (0/2)	≤ 90
— Testicular descent (0/2)	≤ 90
↓ Swimming (1/2)	≥ 35
↓ Righting (2/5)	≥ 35
↓ Climbing (1/1)	≥ 35
↓ Balance (1/1)	≥ 35
↓ Activity (4/6)	≥ 25
— Negative geotaxis (0/1)	≤ 90
— Homing (0/1)	≤ 90
↓↑ Caffeine sensitivity (1/1)	≥ 25
— Theophylline sensitivity (0/1)	≤ 93
↑ Adenosine receptors (1/1)	≥ 50
— Benzodiazepine receptors (0/1)	≤ 50

The treatment-related effects on neuromotor development noted in the neonatal period persisted in the adolescent/adult exposed offspring at dietary dose levels of caffeine in excess of 25 mg/kg/day. However, in contrast to the depressed neuromotor function in the neonate, the older offspring exhibited elevated motor activity,[2,37,39,40,44] although decreases and no effects in postweaning motor activity were reported.[45-47]

Several investigators reported alterations in tests of learning and memory in the adolescent/adult offspring.[2,37,39,44,47] However, these effects were quite variable and generally associated with rather high doses of caffeine, suggesting that perinatal caffeine has only nominal, if any, effects on the development of cognitive function.

TABLE 5. Summary of Treatment-Related Effects in Postweanling Offspring (Adolescent/Adult)

Effect (No. Positive Studies/No. Studies)	Effective Dietary Dose (mg/kg/day)
↓ Body weight (2/10)	≥ 90 (≥ 50 via intubation)
↑ Activity (5/8)	≥ 25
↓↑ Passive avoidance (2/5)	≥ 148 (≥ 5 via intubation)
— ↓ Active avoidance (1/2)	≤ 115 (↓ at ≥ 5 via intubation)
↓ Position discrimination (1/1)	≥ 30
↓ Extinction (2/2)	≥ 60
↑ Scheduled behavior (1/2)	≥ 115
↑ Paradoxical sleep (1/1)	≥ 20
↑ GI ulcer sensitivity (1/1)	≥ 25
↓ Caffeine sensitivity (1/2)	≥ 180
↑ Adenosine sensitivity (1/1)	≥ 38
↓ Dopamine (locus coeruleus) (1/2)	≥ 20
— Norepinephrine (0/3)	≤ 115
↓ CAMP (2/3)	≥ 140

Increases in paradoxical sleep were reported by Enslen et al.[49] in exposed adult offspring at in utero exposure levels in excess of 20 mg/kg/day. This was associated with a selective decrease of dopamine in the locus coeruleus. Regional brain levels of norepinephrine were unaffected. Other investigators found no changes in whole brain levels of either dopamine or norepinephrine.[37,38] However, the analysis of whole brain samples is comparatively less sensitive than the analysis of discrete brain regions. What is particularly notable about the study of Enslen et al.[49] is that the altered sleep patterns were found not only in the F_1 generation adult offspring, but also in the subsequent F_2 adult offspring without additional exposure to caffeine. The F_2 effect, however, occurred only at a higher exposure level of 83 mg/kg/day and no dopamine changes were evident in the F_2 animals. Further investigation should be carried out to confirm and explore the finding of altered regional brain levels of dopamine and the suggestion of a transgenerational effect on sleep functions.

Prenatal caffeine at exposure levels in excess of 25 mg/kg/day has also been reported to increase, in dose-related fashion, the susceptibility to stress-induced ulcer formation in adult offspring.[45] Confirmation of this observation is certainly warranted.

Adult offspring exposed in utero to doses of caffeine in excess of approximately 40 mg/kg/day exhibited increased sensitivity to adenosine.[39] In contrast to the neonate, the sensitivity of the exposed adult offspring to caffeine challenge was unaffected except in those groups exposed in utero to very high levels of caffeine. The altered adenosine sensitivity in the adult, together with the report of up-regulation of adenosine receptors in the exposed neonates,[41] suggests a persistent effect of in utero caffeine on the functional development of this neurochemical system. Because both adenosine and caffeine have been associated as factors in stress responding, a promising area of investigation would be to examine more closely the possible interaction between perinatal caffeine exposure, the development of adenosine function, and sensitivity to stress-induced ulcer formation in the offspring.

Finally, several investigators reported changes in brain levels of cyclic adenosine monophosphate.[38,39,42] The fact that this generally involved in utero exposure to rather high dose levels of caffeine is consistent with the current opinion that phosphodiesterase activity is no longer considered to be a significant factor in caffeine's biological effects.[1,10]

CONCLUSION

The preponderance of evidence indicates that rodent offspring exposed in utero to pharmacologically active doses of caffeine in excess of 20-30 mg/kg/day exhibit a range of subtle alteration in their physical, behavioral, or neurochemical development. Some of the postnatal effects appear to persist in some fashion in the adolescent/adult offspring long after the actual exposure to caffeine. For the most part, these effects are neither very dramatic, nor consistently evident across doses or studies.[51] The nature of these effects indicates that caffeine is not acting as a neurotoxicant to disrupt the development of primary neuronal systems but may be subtly modifying the course of development of discrete neuronal subsystems, such as adenosine and possibly dopamine, which may function to modulate the organism's response to environmental stimuli.[46]

REFERENCES

1. HIRSH, K. 1984. Central nervous system pharmacology of the dietary methylxanthines. *In* The Methylxanthine Beverages and Foods: Chemistry, Consumption, and Health Effects. Alan R. Liss. New York, NY.
2. BUTCHER, R., C. VORHEES & V. WOOTTEN. 1984. Behavioral and physical development of rats chronically exposed to caffeinated fluids. Fundam. Appl. Toxicol. **4:** 1-13.
3. COLLINS, T., J. WELSH, T. BLACK, K. WHITBY & M. O'DONNELL. 1987. Potential reversibility of skeletal effects in rats exposed *in utero* to caffeine. Food Chem. Toxicol. **25:** 647-662.
4. WATKINSON, B. & P. FRIED. 1985. Maternal caffeine use before, during and after pregnancy and effects upon offspring. Neurobehav. Toxicol. Teratol. **7:** 9-17.
5. SCOGS-89. Select Committee on GRAS Substances (1978). Evaluation of the health aspects of caffeine as a food ingredient. FASEB. National Technical Information Service, PB-283-441/AS. Springfield, VA.
6. LECOS, C. 1984. The latest caffeine scorecard. FDA Consumer **18**(2): 14.
7. Committee on GRAS List Survey, Phase III. 1977. Estimating distribution of daily intakes of caffeine. National Academy of Sciences. Washington, DC.
8. BERGMAN, J. & P. DEWS. 1987. Dietary caffeine and its toxicity. *In* Nutritional Toxicology. Vol. 11. Chapt. 8. Academic Press. New York, NY.
9. BARONE, J. & H. ROBERTS. 1984. Human consumption of caffeine. *In* Caffeine. P. Dews, Ed. Springer-Verlag. Berlin/Heidelberg.
10. ABBOTT, P. 1986. Caffeine: A toxicological overview. Med. J. Aust. **145:** 518-521.
11. MILLER, S. & J. HARRIS. 1983. Drugs in our food supply: Caffeine and other substances in beverages. *In* Nutrition and Drugs. M. Winick, Ed. John Wiley. New York, NY.
12. TANAKA, H., K. NAKARAWA & M. ARIMA. 1983. Adverse effect of maternal caffeine ingestion on fetal cerebrum in rat. Brain Dev. **5:** 397-406.
13. ARNAUD, M. 1984. Products of metabolism of caffeine. *In* Caffeine: Perspectives from Recent Research. International Life Sciences Institute. P. Dews, Ed. Springer-Verlag. Berlin.
14. ALDRIDGE, A., J. ARANDA & A. NIEMS. 1979. Caffeine metabolism in the newborn. Clin. Pharmacol. Ther. **25:** 447-453.
15. GULLBERG, E., F. FERRELL & H. CHRISTENSEN. 1986. Effects of postnatal caffeine exposure through dam's milk upon weanling rats. Pharmacol. Biochem. Behav. **24:** 1695-1701.
16. BRAZIER, J., J. RITTER, M. BERLAND, D. KHENFER & G. FAUCON. 1983. Pharmacokinetics of caffeine during and after pregnancy. Dev. Pharmacol. Ther. **6:** 315-322.
17. RAPOPORT, J., M. JENSVOLD, R. ELKINS, M. BUCHSBAUM, H. WEINGARTNER, C. LUDLOW, T. ZAHN, C. BERG & A. NEIMS. 1981. Behavioral and cognitive effects of caffeine in boys and adult males. J. Nerv. Ment. Dis. **169:** 726-731.
18. WEISS, B. & V. LATIES. 1962. Enhancement of human performance by caffeine and the amphetamines. Pharmacol. Rev. **14:** 1-36.
19. HOLLOWAY, W. & D. THOR. 1982. Caffeine sensitivity in the neonatal rat. Neurobehav. Toxicol. Teratol. **4:** 331-333.
20. RAPOPORT, J., C. BERG, D. ISMOND, T. ZAHN & A. NEIMS. 1984. Behavioral effects of caffeine in children. Arch. Gen. Psychiatry **41:** 1073-1079.
21. GOLDSTEIN, A., S. KAIZER & O. WHITBY. 1969. Psychotropic effects of caffeine in man. IV. Quantitative and qualitative differences associated with habituation to coffee. Clin. Pharmacol. Ther. **10:** 489-497.
22. TERADA, M. & H. NISHIMURA. 1975. Mitigation of caffeine-induced teratogenicity in mice by prior chronic caffeine ingestion. Teratology **12:** 79-82.
23. SHOROFSKY, M. & R. LAMM. 1977. Caffeine-withdrawal headache and fasting. N. Y. State J. Med. **77:** 217-218.
24. PERLMUTTER, M., C. ADAMS, J. BERRY, M. KAPLAN, D. PERSON & F. VERDONIK. 1987. Aging and memory. Annu. Rev. Gerontol. Geriat. **7:** 57-92.
25. Food and Drug Administration Drug Bulletin. 1980. Caffeine and pregnancy. Vol. **10:** 19-20.

26. COLLINS, T., J. WELSH, T. BLACK & E. COLLINS. 1981. A study of the teratogenic potential of caffeine given by oral intubation to rats. Regul. Toxicol. Pharmacol. 1: 355-378.

27. IKEDA, G., P. SAPIENZA, M. MCGINNIS, L. BRAGG, J. WALSH & T. COLLINS. 1982. Blood levels of caffeine and results of fetal examination after oral administration of caffeine to pregnant rats. J. Appl. Toxicol. 2: 307-314.

28. COLLINS, T., J. WELSH, T. BLACK & D. RUGGLES. 1983. A study of the teratogenic potential of caffeine ingested in drinking water. Food Chem. Toxicol. 21: 763-777.

29. GILBERT, S., K. REUHL, D. RICE & B. STAVRIC. 1988. Chronic caffeine exposure adversely affects reproductive outcome in the monkey. Toxicologist 8: 239 (Abstr. 952).

30. WEATHERSBEE, P., L. OLSEN & J. LODGE. 1977. Caffeine and pregnancy: A retrospective survey. Postgrad. Med. 62: 64-69.

31. STREISSGUTH, A., H. BARR, D. MARTIN & C. HERMAN. 1980. The effects of maternal alcohol, nicotine and caffeine use during pregnancy on infant mental and motor development at eight months. Alcohol. Clin. Exp. Res. 4: 152-164.

32. KURPPA, K., P. HOLMBERG, E. KUOSMA & L. SAXEN. 1982. Coffee consumption during pregnancy (letter). N. Engl. J. Med. 306: 1548.

33. LINN, S., S. SCHOENBAUM, R. MONSON, B. ROSNER, P. STUBBLEFIELD & K. RYAN. 1982. No association between coffee consumption and adverse outcomes of pregnancy. N. Engl. J. Med. 306: 141-145.

34. DAVAL, J. L. & P. VERT. 1986. Effect of chronic exposure to methylxanthines on diazepam cerebral binding in female rats and their offsprings. Dev. Brain Res. 27: 175-180.

35. HUGHES, R. & C. DE'ATH. 1983. Effect of prenatal caffeine on behavior of young rats. IRCS Med. Sci. 11: 504-505.

36. HUGHES, R. & I. BEVERIDGE. 1986. Behavioral effects of prenatal exposure to caffeine in rats. Life Sci. 38: 861-868.

37. SOBOTKA, T., S. SPAID & R. BRODIE. 1979. Neurobehavioral teratology of caffeine exposure in rats. Neurotoxicology 1: 403-416.

38. CONCANNON, J., J. BRAUGHLER & M. SCHECHTER. 1983. Pre- and postnatal effects of caffeine on brain biogenic amines, cyclic nucleotides and behavior in developing rats. J. Pharmacol. Exp. Ther. 226: 673-679.

39. PERUZZI, G., M. ABBRACCHIO, R. CAGIANO, E. COEN, V. CUOMO et al. 1983. Enduring behavioral and biochemical effects of perinatal treatment with caffeine and chlordiazepoxide. In Application of Behavioral Pharmacology in Toxicology. G. Zbinden, V. Cuomo, G. Racagni & B. Weiss, Eds. Raven Press. New York, NY.

40. LOMBARDELLI, G., W. BALDVINI, G. FEDUZZI & F. CATTABENI. 1984. Long lasting tolerance to stimulatory effects of perinatal caffeine treatment. Psychopharmacology 84: 285-286.

41. MARANGOS, P., J.-P. BOULENGER & J. PATEL. 1984. Effects of chronic caffeine on brain adenosine receptors: Regional and ontogenetic studies. Life Sci. 34: 899-907.

42. PERUZZI, G., G. LOMBARDELLI, M. ABBRACCHIO, E. COEN & F. CATTABENI. 1985. Perinatal caffeine treatment: Behavioral and biochemical effect in rats before weaning. Neurobehav. Toxicol. Teratol. 7: 453-460.

43. NAKAMATO, T., A. HARTMAN, H. MILLER, T. TEMPLES & G. QUINBY. 1986. Chronic caffeine intake by rat dams during gestation and lactation affects various parts of the neonatal brain. Biol. Neonate 49: 277-283.

44. SINTON, C., J. VALATX & M. JOUVET. 1981. Gestational caffeine modifies offspring behavior of mice. Psychopharmacology 75: 69-74.

45. GLAVIN, G. & H. KRUEGER. 1985. Effects of prenatal caffeine administration on offspring mortality, open-field behavior and adult gastric ulcer susceptibility. Neurobehav. Toxicol. Teratol. 7: 29-32.

46. HUGHES, R. & I. BEVERIDGE. 1987. Effects of prenatal exposure to chronic caffeine on locomotor and emotional behavior. Psychobiology 15: 179-185.

47. WEST, G., T. SOBOTKA, R. BRODIE, J. BEIER & M. O'DONNELL. 1986. Postnatal neurobehavioral development in rats exposed in utero to caffeine. Neurobehav. Toxicol. Teratol. 8: 29-43.

48. HOLLOWAY, W. 1982. Caffeine: Effects of acute and chronic exposure on the behavior of neonatal rats. Neurobehav. Toxicol. Teratol. 4: 21-32.

49. ENSLEN, M., H. MILON & H. WURZNER. 1980. Brain catecholamines and sleep states in offspring of caffeine treated rats. Experientia **36:** 1105-1106.
50. GILBERT, R. 1976. Caffeine as a drug of abuse. *In* Research Advances in Alcohol and Drug Problems. R. Gibbins, Ed. Vol. **3:** 48-176. John Wiley. New York, NY.
51. BUELKE-SAM, J. 1986. Postnatal functional assessment following CNS stimulant exposure: Amphetamine and caffeine. *In* Handbook of Behavioral Teratology, Chapt. 7. E. Riley & C. Vorhees, Eds. Plenum Press. New York, NY.
52. SNYDER, S., J. KATIMS, Z. ANNAU, R. BRUNS & J. DALY. 1981. Adenosine receptors and behavioral actions of methylxanthines. Proc. Natl. Acad. Sci. **78:** 3260-3264.
53. BOULENGER, J.-P., P. MARANGOS, K. ZANDER & J. HANSON. 1986. Stress and caffeine: Effects on central adenosine receptors. Clin. Neuropharmacol. **9:** 79-83.

Behavioral Teratogenic Effects of Ethanol in Mice

HOWARD C. BECKER, CARRIE L. RANDALL, AND
LAWRENCE D. MIDDAUGH

Veterans Administration Medical Center
and
Department of Psychiatry
Medical University of South Carolina
Charleston, South Carolina 29403

Both clinical and basic research have firmly established the teratogenic properties of ethanol.[1] Furthermore, the deleterious consequences of prenatal ethanol (EtOH) exposure are known to exist on a continuum. At one extreme, *in utero* EtOH exposure can result in abortion or resorption of the fetus, or gross morphological anomalies and severe mental retardation. At the other end of the spectrum, prenatal EtOH exposure can result in more subtle behavioral/cognitive dysfunctions in the absence of any observable physical birth defects. These latter effects have established EtOH as a behavioral teratogen.[2,3]

Although the dysmorphogenic actions of EtOH have been well documented in mice, studies on the behavioral teratogenic effects of EtOH have been conducted primarily with rats. The purpose of this study was to examine the behavioral effects of prenatal EtOH exposure in C57BL mice, a strain known to be highly sensitive to the morphologic teratogenic actions of EtOH. The overall aim of this research was to develop an animal model of Fetal Alcohol Syndrome in which the full range of prenatal EtOH effects may be assessed in the same species.

Pregnant C57BL/6 mice (Charles River Laboratories, Raleigh, NC) were administered a liquid diet containing 25% EtOH-derived calories (EDC) from gestation day 6 to 18 (gestation day 1 = day of plug identification). This level of EtOH exposure is below the threshold for physical birth defects. Control animals were pair-fed an isocaloric 0% EDC diet during the same period of time with sucrose substituted for EtOH. For these groups, the liquid diet constituted their only source of food and fluid. An additional control group was included that was maintained on ad libitum lab chow and water. Offspring were weaned at 22 days. At various ages, different offspring were tested for spontaneous locomotor activity in an open field, and passive and shuttle avoidance performance. No more than two offspring per litter were represented in an experimental group.

The results demonstrate that animals prenatally exposed to EtOH exhibit heightened spontaneous locomotor activity in an electronically-monitored open-field apparatus. With regard to passive avoidance behavior, EtOH-exposed offspring exhibited shorter latencies to enter the shock-associated chamber after receiving a single shock, and required a greater number of trials to reach criterion performance than controls (TABLE 1). Adult mice prenatally exposed to EtOH also exhibited a deficit in the acquisition and performance of a shuttle avoidance task (TABLE 2).

TABLE 1. Passive Avoidance Performance in 25-Day-Old Male C57BL Offspring

Group	N	Trials to Criterion[a]
Ethanol	23	2.22 ± 0.18[b]
Sucrose	24	1.54 ± 0.12
Lab chow	19	1.68 ± 0.20

[a] Mean ± SE.
[b] Significantly greater than sucrose and lab chow controls ($p < 0.01$).

TABLE 2. Shuttle Avoidance Performance in Adult C57BL Offspring

Males			Females		
Group	N	Trials to Criterion[a]	Group	N	Trials to Criterion[a]
Ethanol	9	106.7 ± 22.6[b]	Ethanol	10	158.0 ± 16.0[b]
Sucrose	8	55.0 ± 3.3	Sucrose	9	73.3 ± 16.1
Lab chow	5	78.0 ± 6.6	Lab chow	7	78.6 ± 4.0

[a] Mean ± SE.
[b] Significantly greater than sucrose and lab chow controls ($p < 0.01$).

In summary, the results of this study demonstrate that C57BL mice are sensitive to the behavioral teratogenic effects of EtOH. EtOH-exposed mice exhibited hyperactivity and impaired active and passive avoidance behavior. The deficit in passive avoidance behavior was obtained in young mice while that of shuttle avoidance performance was observed in adult offspring. The fact that prenatal EtOH effects were observed in adult mice suggests relatively permanent functional brain damage. This behavioral profile of mice prenatally exposed to EtOH resembles that obtained with rats.

The development of a mouse model to examine the behavioral effects of prenatal EtOH exposure in C57BL mice is highly desirable, because this mouse strain is also very sensitive to the morphological teratogenic actions of higher doses of EtOH. Thus, depending on the level of prenatal EtOH exposure, it appears this mouse strain is sensitive to a wide range of prenatal EtOH effects and perhaps, as such, provides for an animal model that more closely approximates the clinical condition.

REFERENCES

1. RANDALL, C. L. 1987. Alcohol & Alcoholism Suppl. **1:** 125-312.
2. ABEL, E. L. 1981. Psychol. Bull. **90:** 564-581.
3. MEYER, L. S. & E. P. RILEY. 1986. *In* Handbook of Behavioral Teratology. E. P. Riley & C. V. Vorhees, Eds.: 101-140.

Focusing Prevention of Fetal Alcohol Syndrome on Women at Risk

B. MORSE, L. WEINER, AND P. GARRIDO

Boston University School of Medicine
Fetal Alcohol Education Program
7 Kent Street
Brookline, Massachusetts 02146

Consumption of alcohol during pregnancy is well recognized as a risk factor for a wide range of problems in the developing fetus. Fetal alcohol syndrome (FAS), the most extreme manifestation, includes growth retardation, facial dysmorphology and central nervous system anomalies. Nonspecific morphologic and/or neurologic anomalies may occur even in the absence of the syndrome. While research continues to explore associations between outcome and exposure to various amounts of alcohol, it is clear that alcohol's effects are dose related.[1] Prevention of alcohol-related birth defects requires cessation of drinking by women at the greatest risk: those who drink heavily or abusively.[2]

Although all documented cases of FAS have been born to women who reported abusive levels of drinking, not all heavily drinking women deliver infants with FAS. The difference in susceptibility to alcohol's effects may be due to differences in blood alcohol concentrations, gestational stage, fetal susceptibility, maternal nutrition, ethnicity, parity and chronicity of alcohol abuse.[3,4]

Many public education campaigns have been sponsored by both governmental and private agencies. These campaigns have been effective in increasing general public knowledge, but have not affected the number of heavy drinkers.[5,6] The failure to change behavior among those at highest risk may be linked to the message content (fear and punishment) and the inability of public campaigns to treat addiction. An approach which recognizes the special needs of alcohol addiction is needed to reduce the incidence of alcohol-related birth defects.

Successful intervention with heavily drinking pregnant women is based in secondary or tertiary prevention strategies. Individualized treatment plans focused on redirection and rehabilitation help remove the moral stigma of alcoholism and its attendant guilt. Supportive counseling has been demonstrated to be effective in reducing consumption among women at risk and in improving pregnancy outcome.[7] Heavily drinking women report that physicians and/or other health providers are the best source of information leading to behavioral change.[8]

Since 1984, the Fetal Alcohol Education Program, Boston University School of Medicine, has provided training for more than 7,000 health professionals in Massachusetts, stressing positive, supportive therapeutic techniques. An independent evaluation showed significant increases in the use of systematic drinking histories and in the number of women identified at risk.[9]

Public health strategies must match existing knowledge about alcohol's mechanisms of action with current understandings of behavioral change. Direct intervention focused on changing the drinking patterns of at-risk pregnant women offers one of the best chances to reduce the incidence of alcohol-related birth defects.

REFERENCES

1. U. S. Department of Health and Human Services. 1987. Sixth Special Report to the U.S. Congress on Alcohol and Health.
2. WEINER, L. *et al.* FAS:FAE. Focusing prevention on women at risk. Int. J. Addictions. In press.
3. ROSETT, H. L. & L. WEINER. 1984. Alcohol and the Fetus: A Clinical Perspective. Oxford University Press.
4. ABEL, E. L. & R. J. SOKOL. 1986. Maternal and fetal characteristics affecting alcohol's teratogenicity. Neurobehav. Toxicol. Teratol. **8:** 329.
5. LITTLE, R. E. *et al.* 1984. Preventing fetal alcohol effects: Effectiveness of a demonstration project. *In* Mechanisms of Alcohol Damage in Utero. CIBA.
6. U. S. Department of the Treasury. Bureau of Alcohol, Tobacco and Firearms. 1980.
7. WEINER, L. & G. LARSSON. 1987. Clinical prevention of fetal alcohol effects—a reality. Alcohol Health Res. World.
8. Healthy Mothers/Healthy Babies. 1986. A Compendium of Ideas for Serving Low-Income Women.
9. WEINER, L. *et al.* 1988. A successful inservice training program for healthcare professionals. Subst. Abuse **9**(1): 20-28.

Effects of In-Utero Cocaine Exposure on Sensorineural Reactivity

MICHELLE E. COHEN,[a] ENDLA K. ANDAY,[b] AND
DONALD S. LEITNER[c]

[a] Department of Psychology
Bryn Mawr College
Bryn Mawr, Pennsylvania 19010

[b] Department of Pediatrics
University of Pennsylvania School of Medicine
Philadelphia, Pennsylvania 19104

[c] Department of Psychology
St. Joseph's University
Philadelphia, Pennsylvania 19131

Within the last decade cocaine has evolved from being a "recreational" drug of the upper and middle classes to a major illicit drug among women of child-bearing age in all socioeconomic classes. Research[1,2] suggests that cocaine is teratogenic. Unfortunately, data on the behavioral sequelae in infants born to women who use cocaine during pregnancy are anecdotal or observational at best.[3] Brazelton assessment has shown that infants prenatally exposed to cocaine have a greater degree of tremulousness and more frequent startle responses.[4]

The present study sought to determine if these observed behavioral aberrations merely represent the direct result of cocaine in systemic circulation or are in part the effect of chronic drug exposure on the developing fetus. Previous research with infants revealed that simultaneous presentation of a tone with a tap to the glabella can increase the amplitude of the reflexive eyeblink.[5] Employing this reflex augmentation procedure, results from 19 cocaine-exposed infants were compared to those from 19 healthy matched drug-free infants. Analysis of these data showed the cocaine-exposed infants to be more reactive in general as indicated by a larger glabellar reflex, and more responsive to auditory stimuli as indicated by an increased blink response when the tone accompanied the tap.

Further analysis of 22 of these infants matched for age at time of testing (TABLE 1) showed that whether infants were tested within or after one week of birth, cocaine-exposed infants were more reactive than drug-free infants (FIG. 1).

These data reveal that infants exposed to cocaine in utero show greater behavioral reactivity than infants not exposed. This difference extends beyond the immediate postnatal period, beyond the period wherein cocaine and/or its metabolites may be detected in an infant's urine,[6] and beyond the period of neonatal abstinence syndrome.[7] While infants prenatally exposed to cocaine are a high-risk population, infants in the study presented here were matched with drug-free infants for variables that are known

TABLE 1. Characteristics of Infants in Study Groups[a]

Group	Sex M/F	Apgar Score (1 Min)	Apgar Score (5 Min)	Birth Weight (Gms)	Gestational (Age Wks)	Test Weight (Gms)	Postconceptional Age (Wks)
Cocaine-exposed (n = 11)							
<1 wk (n = 7)	4/3	8.0 ±1.1	8.9 ±.7	2607.1 ±406.7	38.0 ±1.7	2607.1 ±406.7	38.0 ±1.7
>1 wk (n = 4)	2/2	7.0[b] ±2.2	8.5 ±1.0	1347.5[b] ±474.5	30.5[b] ±4.4	1982.5[b] ±253.8	37.75 ±.6
Drug-free (n = 11)							
<1 wk (n = 7)	4/3	8.4 ±.8	9.1 ±.7	2824.3 ±361.2	38.3 ±1.7	2817.4 ±360.6	38.3 ±1.7
>1 wk (n = 4)	2/2	6.0[b] ±2.7	6.7 ±3.2	1475.5[b] ±588.4	30.5[b] ±3.7	2092.5[b] ±386.0	37.5 ±4.3

[a] Values are $\overline{X}$ ± SD.
[b] $p < 0.05$.

to increase neonatal risk and could therefore have an effect on behavioral reactivity and behavioral state. Further, the factors selected for matching were those that may affect the glabellar reflex and its modification. Therefore, the differences in this study are most likely due to the consequences of in-utero cocaine exposure. The data suggest that a central nervous system dysfunction exists in the cocaine-exposed infants that is not a function of the drug in systemic circulation or even a hypersensitive state due to withdrawal.

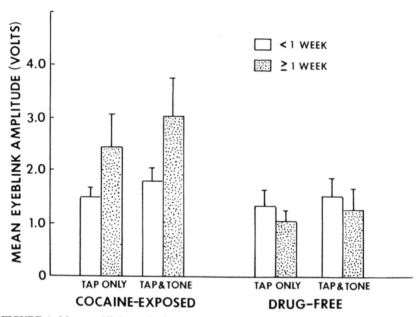

FIGURE 1. Mean eyeblink amplitude averaged across subjects to the tap alone and tap and tone conditions for the drug-free and cocaine-exposed infants tested within one week of birth (*open bar*) or tested one week or more after birth (*filled bar*). A group (cocaine vs drug-free $\times$ time of testing (1 wk vs ≥ 1 wk) $\times$ condition (tap only vs tap and tone) analysis of variance with repeated measures on the last factor showed overall effects of drug exposure ($F(1,18) = 6.26, p < 0.05$) and augmentation ($F(1,18) = 23.73, p < 0.01$) with no effect of time of testing and no interactions.

REFERENCES

1. MAHALIK, M. P., R. F. GAUTIERI & D. E. MANN, JR. 1980. J. Pharm. Sci. **69:** 703-706.
2. BINGOL, N., F. MADGALENA, V. DIAZ, R. K. STONE & D. S. GROMISCH. 1987. J. Pediatr. **110:** 93-96.
3. CHASNOFF, I. F., M. E. BUSSEY, R. SAVISH & C. M. STACK. 1986. J. Pediatr. **108:** 456-459.
4. MOFFENSON, H. C. & T. R. CARACCIO. 1987. Pediatr. Ann. **16:** 864-874.
5. HOFFMAN, H. S., M. E. COHEN & L. M. ENGLISH. 1985. J. Exp. Child Psychol. **139:** 562-579.
6. CHASNOFF, I. J., W. J. BURNS, S. H. SCHNOLL & K. D. BURNS. 1985. N. Engl. J. Med. **313:** 666-669.
7. FINNEGAN, L. P., R. E. KRON, J. F. CONNAUGHTON, JR. & J. P. EMICH, JR. 1975. *In* Basic and Therapeutic Aspects of Perinatal Pharmacology. P. L. Morselli, S. Garattini & F. Sereni, Eds. Raven Press. New York, NY.

Abnormal Hypoxic Arousal Responses in Infants of Cocaine-Abusing Mothers

SALLY L. DAVIDSON WARD,[a] DAISY B. BAUTISTA,[a]
SALLY SCHUETZ,[b] LAURA WACHSMAN,[b] XYLINA
BEAN,[c] AND THOMAS G. KEENS[a]

[a] Division of Neonatology and Pediatric Pulmonology
Childrens Hospital of Los Angeles
4650 Sunset Boulevard, Box 83
Los Angeles, California 90027

[b] Pediatric Pavilion
University of Southern California—Los Angeles
County Medical Center
1129 North State Street
Los Angeles, California 90033

[c] Department of Pediatrics
Martin Luther King, Jr. Medical Center
12021 South Wilmington Avenue
Los Angeles, California 90049

INTRODUCTION

Infants of cocaine-abusing mothers (ICAM) have an increased risk for sudden infant death syndrome (SIDS) and abnormalities of their ventilatory patterns during sleep.[1] Arousal from sleep is an important respiratory defense mechanism for termination of apnea, and normal infants arouse from sleep in response to hypoxia. However, many infants with unexplained apnea, another group of infants at increased risk of SIDS, have an abnormal hypoxic arousal response (HAR) and, therefore, lack this important defense mechanism.[2] We hypothesized that infants of cocaine-abusing mothers have abnormal HAR. We studied 21 ICAM (age 2.1 ± 0.1 [SE] months) and 7 controls (age 1.6 ± 0.3 months; NS). ICAM had intrauterine cocaine exposure documented by positive urine toxicology at birth (maternal and/or infant). Neither ICAM nor controls had a history of prematurity or apnea or a family history of SIDS, and both groups were otherwise healthy and on no medications.

METHODS

Sleep studies were performed during a morning nap, after feeding in a quiet dark room, with an ambient temperature of 24°C. Sedation was not used. Arterial oxygen

347

saturation (SaO_2) by pulse oximetry, the pulse signal from the pulse oximeter, inspired and end-tidal CO_2 and O_2 tensions via a prenasal sensor by mass spectrometry, ECG and heart rate, respirations by chest wall impedence, EOG and EEG were continuously recorded on a strip chart recorder. Infants were observed during sleep for at least 30 minutes prior to HAR. The HAR were performed when the infant was in quiet sleep by the method of van der Hal and co-workers. [2] A plastic hood without a neck seal was placed over the infant's head and room air introduced at a rate sufficient to prevent CO_2 accumulation (10 L/min). The infant was observed under the hood for 3 minutes. The infant was challenged with P_IO_2 80 mm Hg. This was accomplished by blending 100% nitrogen with room air until the P_IO_2 of 80 mm Hg was achieved. The P_IO_2 of 80 mm Hg was maintained until arousal (agitation, body movement, eye opening and crying) occurred or for 3 minutes. Challenges were performed in duplicate when possible. Challenges were stopped and the infant returned to room air if the SaO_2 fell to less than 75% during hypoxia. Challenges were not repeated if the infant developed apnea, periodic breathing or marked desaturation during hypoxia. Informed consents were obtained from parents prior to study. Parents were told that the maximum exposure to hypoxia was equivalent to breathing air at 13,000 feet (3,962 meters) elevation and that the infants would be carefully monitored by a physician throughout the study. The study was approved by the Institutional Review Board of Childrens Hospital of Los Angeles.

RESULTS

Controls aroused in response to hypoxia in 8 of 9 trials (89%), but ICAM aroused in only 6 of 22 trials (27%; $p < 0.01$). Two ICAM HAR were not completed because the infants developed excessive periodic breathing and arterial oxygen desaturation during the first minute of hypoxia. There were no significant differences in the level of inspired oxygen or the lowest oxygen saturation achieved during hypoxic challenge, indicating that failure to arouse was not due to insufficient challenge in either group.

CONCLUSION

Infants of cocaine-abusing mothers have abnormal HAR compared to controls. The abnormal HAR seen in ICAM may be related to their increased risk for SIDS and to their abnormal ventilatory patterns during sleep.

REFERENCES

1. DAVIDSON WARD, S. L., S. SCHUETZ, V. KRISHNA et al. 1986. Abnormal sleeping ventilatory pattern in infants of substance abuse mothers. Am. J. Dis. Child. **140:** 1015-1020.
2. VAN DER HAL, A. L., A. M. RODRIGUEZ, C. W. SARGENT, A. C. G. PLATZKER & T. K. KEENS. 1985. Hypoxia and hypercapneic arousal responses and prediction of subsequent apnea of infancy. Pediatrics **75:** 848-854.

Circulating Catecholamines and Adrenoreceptors in Infants of Cocaine-Abusing Mothers

SALLY L. DAVIDSON WARD,[a] DAISY B. BAUTISTA,[a]
SUE BUCKLEY,[a] SALLY SCHUETZ,[b] LAURA
WACHSMAN,[b] XYLINA BEAN,[c] AND DAVID
WARBURTON[a]

[a] Division of Neonatology and Pediatric Pulmonology
Childrens Hospital of Los Angeles
4650 Sunset Boulevard, Box 83
Los Angeles, California 90027

[b] Los Angeles County—University of Southern California
Medical Center
University of Southern California School of Medicine
1129 North State Street
Los Angeles, California 90033

[c] Martin Luther King, Jr. Medical Center
12021 South Wilmington Avenue
Los Angeles, California 90049

INTRODUCTION

Alterations in catecholamines (CA) and adrenoreceptors (AR) have been demonstrated in animal models of chronic cocaine use and abstinence. [1] Similarly, alterations in CA have been demonstrated in sudden infant death syndrome (SIDS) victims and in some infants at increased risk for SIDS. [2] CA are important in the neurologic control of breathing. Infants of cocaine-abusing mothers (ICAM) have abnormal ventilatory patterns during sleep and have been shown to be at increased risk for SIDS.[3] Therefore, we hypothesized that ICAM have abnormalities in circulating CA and AR. We studied 20 ICAM (age 2.1 ± 0.5 [SE] months) and 8 controls (age 2.4 ± 0.8 months; NS). ICAM had intrauterine cocaine exposure documented by positive urine toxicology at birth (maternal and/or infant). Neither ICAM nor controls had a history of prematurity, or apnea or a family history of SIDS, and both were otherwise healthy and on no medications.

349

METHODS

A venous blood sample was drawn as atraumatically as possible between 0800 and 0900 from the antecubital vein with the infant supine. Plasma epinephrine (E), norepinephrine (NE) and dopamine (D) concentrations were measured by radioenzymatic assay using the method of Passon and Peuler. Lymphocytes were isolated from blood using the method of Boyum *et al.* Beta AR were assayed on intact lymphocytes by the method of Brodd *et al.,* using 125-I-cyanopindolol as the ligand. Maximal binding capacity (Bmax) of beta AR was measured and expressed as binding sites per lymphocyte. Alpha AR were assayed on intact thrombocytes by the method of Motulsky *et al.,* using 3-H-yohimibine as the ligand. Bmax of alpha AR was measured and expressed as binding sites per thrombocyte. Scratchard plots were used for calculation of receptor affinity (K_D) for beta and alpha AR.

RESULTS

Results are shown in TABLES 1 and 2. The mean plasma NE levels in the ICAM group were 2.2-fold higher than those of the control group ($p < 0.025$). Plasma E and D levels and the Bmax and K_D for both alpha and beta AR were not significantly different between ICAM and controls.

CONCLUSIONS

We conclude that ICAM have increased plasma NE concentrations compared to controls at 2 months of age. However, ICAM have normal serum E and D levels. In addition, ICAM have alpha and beta AR which are similar to controls in both Bmax and K_D. We speculate that elevated circulating NE concentrations in ICAM reflect increased sympathetic tone secondary to prenatal cocaine exposure. Contrary to what might have been expected in the face of elevated plasma NE, we did not find decreased or downregulated AR Bmax. We speculate that the absence of AR downregulation

TABLE 1. Comparison of Plasma Epinephrine, Norepinephrine and Dopamine Concentrations between ICAM and Controls[a]

	ICAM (N = 20)	Controls (N = 8)
Epinephrine pg/ml	170 ± 30	128 ± 40
Norepinephrine pg/ml	1064 ± 157	484 ± 112[b]
Dopamine pg/ml	128 ± 42	90 ± 31

[a] Data are expressed as mean ± SEM.
[b] $p < 0.025$ (Student t test).

TABLE 2. Comparison of Alpha and Beta Adrenoreceptors Binding Capacities (Bmax) and Receptor Affinity (K_D) between ICAM and Controls[a]

	ICAM (N = 17)	Controls (N = 8)
Alpha-adrenoreceptors		
Bmax binding site/thrombocyte	238 ± 1	294 ± 34
K_D (nM)	2.9 ± 3.4	1.6 ± 0.4
Beta-adrenoreceptors		
Bmax binding site/lymphocyte	874 ± 53	862 ± 102
K_D (pM)	874 ± 3.4	30 ± 11

[a] Data are expressed as mean ± SEM.

may result in increased sensitivity to CA. These CA and AR abnormalities may be related to the increased risk for SIDS and abnormal ventilatory patterns seen in ICAM. However, these measurements were made on peripheral blood and do not necessarily reflect changes in central neurotransmitters.

REFERENCES

1. POST, R. M., S. R. B. WEISS, A. PERT & T. W. UHDE. 1987. Chronic cocaine administration: sensitization and kindling effects. *In* Cocaine, Clinical and Biomedical Aspects. S. Fisher, A. Raskin & E. Uhlenhuth, Eds.: 109-173. Oxford University Press. New York, NY.
2. RODRIGUEZ, T., D. WARBURTON & T. KEENS. 1987. Elevated catecholamines and absent hypoxic arousal responses in apnea of infancy. Pediatrics **79**: 269-274.
3. WARD DAVIDSON, S. L., S. SCHUETZ, V. KRISHNA *et al.* 1986. Abnormal sleeping ventilatory pattern in infants of substance abuse mothers. Am. J. Dis. Child. **140**: 1015-1020.

Prenatal Exposure to Drugs and Its Influence on Attachment

CAROL RODNING, LEILA BECKWITH, AND JUDY
HOWARD

Department of Pediatrics
University of California, Los Angeles
Los Angeles, California 90024

An increasing number of children are exposed to drugs prenatally and are being reared in substance-abusing families. The long-term effects of prenatal drug exposure on the intellectual, social, and emotional development of children remain undetermined. Preliminary findings in this study suggest effects in the intellectual, social and emotional domains of development.

The impact of prenatal illicit drug exposure on intellectual, social and emotional development was investigated in a sample of 18 18-month-old toddlers who had been prenatally exposed to a variety of drugs including cocaine, heroin, methadone, and PCP. These 18 children lived in a variety of child rearing environments including foster care, extended family care, and biological mothers. In previous studies, poor prenatal care and difficult perinatal events have been implicated in negative developmental outcomes for drug-exposed children. Therefore, the drug-exposed toddlers were compared to a biological high-risk sample of preterm children who weighed less than 2000 grams at birth with the majority experiencing respiratory distress, and a nonrisk sample of fullterm children.

Security and insecurity in the attachment relationship between the child and caregiver was assessed in the laboratory by the standardized paradigm known as the Strange Situation. Developmental scores were determined by the standardized Gesell and Bayley developmental assessment procedures. The content, organization, and quality of the children's spontaneous play activity was assessed in a fifteen-minute laboratory session with a variety of age-appropriate toys in an open floor space area.

The drug-exposed toddlers deviated from the comparison groups in several ways. Only a few of the drug-exposed toddlers displayed the interactive behaviors that are typically expected at this age, such as greeting and moving closer, and seeking close physical contact with the caregiver when she returns after a short separation. The majority of the drug-exposed children did not show the strong feelings of pleasure, anger and distress in relation to novel toys and the caregiver's departure and return that the Strange Situation is designed to elicit. For the most part they remained affectively neutral throughout the procedure. The drug-exposed toddlers showed a higher proportion of insecure attachments than the high-risk preterm or fullterm comparison groups. The highest percentage of insecure drug-exposed toddlers was in the subgroup being raised by their biological mothers. In all cases but one, these mothers continued to abuse drugs. The one mother of the secure drug-exposed toddler stopped using drugs after the child's birth and had a significantly shorter history of drug abuse prior to the birth of her child. In all other cases chronicity of drug abuse

TABLE 1. Developmental Scores and Play in Drug-Exposed Toddlers

	Drug Exposed (N = 19)			High-Risk Preterm (N = 57)			Fullterm[a] (N = 20)		
	M	SD	Range	M	SD	Range	M	SD	Range
Developmental scores at 13 months	97.2	17.3	71.6-142	107.9	15.8	62-142	111.3	5	103-119
Secure	101.4	21.4	76.4-142						
Insecure	94.5	14.7	71.6-117.7						
Fantasy play at 18 to 22 months	4.9	2.8	0-10	14.5	6.5	2-38	10.2	6.1	
Securely attached	6.5	2.2	4-10						
Insecurely attached	3.9	2.7	0-9						

[a] Data from REFERENCE 1.

prior to pregnancy exceeded 4 years. The majority of drug-exposed toddlers reared by extended family members and foster mothers were secure and this percentage of security was not significantly different from the percentage of security in the high-risk group. Security or insecurity of attachment did not depend on the drug abused by the mother. Children who were securely and insecurely attached were prenatally exposed to up to 5 different drugs. Developmental quotients for the drug-exposed toddlers were significantly lower than the high-risk preterm toddlers and the fullterm toddlers. Within the drug-exposed group, the insecure toddlers had significantly lower developmental scores than the secure drug-exposed toddlers. Play for the majority of drug-exposed children was characterized by scattering, batting, and picking-up and putting-down the toys rather than sustained combining of toys, fantasy play, or curious exploration. Fantasy play events, such as combing hair, stirring the pot, and sitting the doll at the table, were significantly less frequent and less varied in the drug-exposed group than the comparison groups. Within the drug-exposed group, the securely attached toddlers showed significantly more fantasy play than the insecurely attached children. See TABLE 1.

Preliminary findings suggest hypotheses for future investigations of the relationships between the physiological and behavioral effects of exposure to drugs. *Prenatal* drug-exposure has an adverse effect on developmental processes. The drug-exposed toddlers were significantly lower in intellectual functioning than the high-risk group with difficult *perinatal* events. The *postnatal* rearing environment is a significant factor in mitigating the prenatal drug exposure to some degree. There appeared to be a pervasive interference with affect as observed in the absence of delight in even the securely attached children. It appeared that the typical inclinations of children in play activity are altered. This may be a complex interaction of cognitive, affective, motor, and environmental variables. The data showed that prenatal drug exposure increased the risk by extending the organic, physiological effects into emotional development in affect regulation, into social development in the organization of relationships, and into cognitive development in the representational and symbolic aspects of children's play.

REFERENCE

1. UNGERER, J. & M. SIGMAN. 1983. Developmental lags in preterm infants from 1 to 3 years of age. Child Dev. **54:** 1217-1228.

Cerebral Sonographic Characteristics and Maternal and Neonatal Risk Factors in Infants of Opiate-Dependent Mothers

M. E. PASTO, S. EHRLICH, K. KALTENBACH,
L. J. GRAZIANI,
A. KURTZ, B. GOLDBERG, AND L. P. FINNEGAN

*Department of Radiology and
Department of Pediatrics
Jefferson Medical College
Thomas Jefferson University
Philadelphia, Pennsylvania 19107*

This longitudinal study sought to evaluate cerebral sonographic characteristics of infants of drug-dependent mothers enrolled in a methadone maintenance program (Family Center, Thomas Jefferson University Hospital). These Family Center infants were compared to a group of control infants. Multiple cerebral measurements were performed sonographically to elaborate possible subtle effects of passive narcotic addiction *in utero*. An analysis of clinical data of both the mothers and infants was also completed to delineate possible risk factors. Subjects included in analysis were those Family Center (46) and control (31) infants who had ultrasound studies at birth, at one month and at six months of age. Clinical data including Apgar scores, birth weight, head circumference, and neonatal complications were tabulated. Sonographic characteristics of the cerebral ventricles (slit-like, *i.e.,* no visible fluid, vs normal) were recorded, as well as transverse measurements of the intracranial hemidiameter (ICHD), right and left lateral ventricles (RLV, LLV), and temporal lobe (TL), and thalamic area measurements (traced in a transaxial view). The percentage of Family Center infants with slit ventricles was statistically significant at all three examinations (FIG. 1). The measurement and clinical data are listed in TABLE 1. Date of Family Center vs control infants are listed, as well as data comparing all slit-like ventricle infants (independent of drug exposure) to all those with normal ventricles at birth. Thalamic areas and temporal lobe measurements were not statistically different at any time. In the Family Center vs control groups, ICHDs at birth and at one month were significantly smaller in the Family Center infants, and the RLVs and head circumferences approached significance. One risk factor identified was maternal age. In the analysis of slit vs normal ventricle infants, LLVs and RLVs were smaller at six months in slit infants, with the ICHDs smaller at all exams. Head circumferences approached significance at birth and at six months. This second grouping showed a greater differential in birth weights than the Family Center vs control group, and further analysis showed mean birth weight to be the lowest among infants with slit ventricles persisting

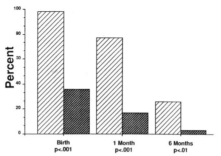

FIGURE 1. Percentage of infants with slit-like ventricles. *Light-hatched columns:* drug-exposed infants (n = 46); *dark-hatched columns:* control infants (n = 31).

to six months of age, along with slightly smaller head circumferences (32.5 vs 33.0 cm). Clinically, the infants had a higher incidence of meconium straining ($p = 0.01$) and transient anemia or bilirubinemia (11% vs 0% in controls). Another interesting finding was a higher percentage of slit-like ventricles among white infants (88%) than black infants (64%) even though groups were comparable in race and relevant socioeconomic factors.

In summary, slit ventricles were strongly associated with narcotic addiction and are slower to resolve in lower birth weight infants. Although gestational age was

TABLE 1. Measurements, Clinical Data, and Maternal Age Factors

	Family Center (N = 46)	Controls (N = 31)	p	Slit (N = 55)	Normal Ventricle (N = 22)	p
Measurements						
Birth weight (gm)	2927.9	3186.3	0.05	2798.5	3091.1	0.04
Head circumference (mm)						
Birth	33.1	34.0	0.03	32.5	33.7	0.02
1 mo	36.2	37.3	0.08	35.4	37.0	0.05
6 mo	42.5	42.8	n.s.	41.8	42.8	0.02
Right lateral ventricle (mm)						
Birth	11.32	12.03	0.02	11.39	12.15	0.031
6 mo	13.16	14.02	n.s.	13.32	14.55	0.001
Left lateral ventricle (mm)						
Birth	11.30	11.89	0.06	11.34	12.0	0.04
6 mo	13.49	13.87	n.s.	13.39	14.42	0.003
Incranial hemidiameter (mm)						
Birth	35.77	37.91	0.01	35.8	38.8	0.001
1 mo	39.57	41.71	0.01	39.5	42.7	0.001
6 mo	48.07	49.99	0.07	47.9	51.4	0.002
Clinical data: Apgar scores						
1 min	7.6	7.9	n.s.	7.7	7.8	n.s.
5 min	8.7	8.9	0.04	8.7	9.0	0.05
Materal age factors	30.1	26.6	0.003	30.0	26.1	0.01
Gravida	4.3	3.7	n.s.	4.3	3.1	n.s.
Parity	2.2	1.6	n.s.	2.2	1.5	n.s.

comparable, Family Center and slit infants were lower in birth weight and head circumferences than drug-free and nonslit infants, respectively. Both affected groups had smaller ICHDs and lateral ventricle measurements, possibly implying slower cortical cerebral growth than their peers. Of the clinical risk factors other than narcotic exposure, Family Center and slit infants had a higher incidence of neonatal complications and were born to older mothers.

REFERENCES

1. PASTO, M. E., L. J. GRAZIANI, B. LEIFER, S. L. TUNIS, T. MATTEUCCI & L. P. FINNEGAN. 1983. Cerebral ventricular changes in newborns exposed to psychoactive agents *in utero.* Pediatr. Res. **17:** 1678.
2. PASTO, M. E., S. M. EHRLICH, J. DEILING & L. P. FINNEGAN. 1986. The effect of narcotics *in utero* on infant brain growth: A cross-sectional study. Pediatr. Res. **20:** 1075.

Cocaine and Pregnancy: Maternal and Infant Outcome

SUSAN LIVESAY, SAUNDRA EHRLICH, LYNN
RYAN, AND LORETTA P. FINNEGAN

Department of Pediatrics
Jefferson Medical College
Thomas Jefferson University
Philadelphia, Pennsylvania 19107

The number of pregnant women using cocaine has grown with the drug's increasing availability, its highly addictive quality, and its persistent image as a socially acceptable and harmless agent. Although the destructive effects of cocaine on the adult user are well known, little has been reported regarding maternal cocaine use and its affect on the perinatal period and the neonate.[1-3] With these concerns in mind, the present study was conducted within Family Center, a treatment program providing pre- and postnatal services for drug-dependent women and their infants.[4] Maternal and infant outcomes for women using cocaine with other drugs were compared to those of drug-dependent women not using cocaine and a group of drug-free women. Subjects included 239 women: 93 cocaine-using, drug-dependent women, 83 noncocaine-using, drug-dependent women, and 63 nondrug-dependent comparison women. The groups were similar in maternal age, socioeconomic status, nicotine use and parity, but differed in race. Emergency cesarean sections, meconium staining and small for gestational age infants occurred more often in the cocaine group. Birth weight, length, head circumference, gestational age, one minute Apgar scores, mean neonatal abstinence scores and incidence of nuchal cords were significantly lower in the infants of the cocaine-using, drug-dependent women. No differences were found in the incidence of intracranial hemorrhage or congenital anomalies. The occurrence of Sudden Infant Death Syndrome and the need for cardiorespiratory monitors was similar for cocaine- and noncocaine-exposed infants of drug-dependent women, but greater than the figures reported in the general population. Abruptio placentae occurred in 9% of cocaine drug-dependent women, 4% of noncocaine drug-dependent women and 2% of drug-free women. More premature deliveries were seen in the cocaine group (20%) than in the noncocaine (11%) and drug-free (3%) groups. The results of this study suggest that maternal and infant outcome are generally poorer when women are drug dependent and use cocaine. A consistent trend is seen in the parameters that define fetal/neonatal and maternal outcome. Drug-free women and their infants have the best outcome, drug-dependent women and their infants a less favorable outcome, and cocaine-abusing women and their infants the least favorable. The life style of drug-dependent women is erratic and hardly conducive to achieving an optimal outcome in pregnancy. The use of cocaine appears to adversely effect this already poor situation. Cocaine has been found to effectively suppress appetite, and it decreases the user's interests in fulfilling bodily needs.[5] Because of the drug's highly addictive quality the search for and use of the drug becomes the most important goal in the user's life.

The "high" it produces is rapid and intense, but is followed by a deep "crash." This leads the user to seek other drugs to come down from the intense stimulation of cocaine and soften the crash. Pregnant women who use cocaine are at high risk because their life styles are dominated by drug-seeking behavior, frequent polydrug abuse, poor nutrition and inadequate prenatal care.

REFERENCES

1. CHASNOFF, I. J., W. J. BURNS, S. H. SCHNOLL & K. A. BURNS. 1985. Cocaine use in pregnancy. N. Engl. Med. **313:** 666-669.
2. AKER, D., B. P. SAKS, K. J. TRACEY & W. E. WISE. 1983. Abruptio placenta associated with cocaine use. Am. J. Obstet. Gynecol. **146:** 220-221.
3. BINGOL, N., M. FUCHS, V. DIAZ, R. K. STONE & D. S. GROMISCH. 1987. Teratogenicity of cocaine in humans. J. Pediatr. **110:** 93-96.
4. FINNEGAN, L., (Ed.) 1987. Drug Dependency in Pregnancy: Clinical Management of Mother and Child. A Manual for Medical Professionals and Para Professionals. Prepared for the National Institute on Drug Abuse, Services Research Branch, Rockville, MD. U.S. Government Printing Office. Washington, DC.
5. GOLD, M. S. 1986. What doctors should know about cocaine abuse. Ann. Intern. Med. **1:** 3,30-31.

Children Exposed to Methadone in Utero

Assessment of Developmental and Cognitive Ability

KAROL KALTENBACH AND
LORETTA P. FINNEGAN

Department of Pediatrics
Jefferson Medical College
Thomas Jefferson University
Philadelphia, Pennsylvania 19107

The consequences of maternal drug abuse on the fetus, newborn and infant have been an area of special concern for more than a decade. Methadone maintenance is often recommended for the care of the pregnant opiate-dependent woman primarily to prevent erratic maternal drug levels so that the fetus is not vulnerable to repeated episodes of withdrawal. However, the reduced medical risks associated with methadone maintenance during pregnancy do not alter the fact that the infant becomes passively addicted in utero and usually undergoes neonatal abstinence at birth. The consequences of such exposure for the neonate and young infant have been widely investigated. Studies have consistently found infants exposed to methadone in utero to be well within the normal range of development by six months of age, as measured by the Bayley Scale of Infant Development.[1] However, there have been few studies to determine if preschool children exposed to methadone in utero have impaired cognitive functioning. The purpose of this study was to evaluate the developmental and cognitive functioning of preschool children born to women maintained on methadone during pregnancy.

Forty-four children (27 methadone-exposed children and 17 nondrug-exposed comparison children) participated in a longitudinal study from birth through five years of age. All of the drug-dependent mothers were enrolled in a comprehensive program for drug-dependent women. Nondrug-dependent mothers were from comparable socioeconomic and racial backgrounds. The mean daily maternal methadone dose during pregnancy was 38.42 mg and 92% of the children required pharmacotherapy for neonatal abstinence. At 6, 12 and 24 months of age infants were evaluated with the Bayley Scale of Mental Development and received a comprehensive neurological exam. At 3 1/2 to 4 1/2 years of age, the children were evaluated with the McCarthy Scale of Children's Abilities and a neurological exam. The results of the Bayley Scale of Mental Development are presented in TABLE 1, and those of the McCarthy Scales of Children's Abilities in TABLE 2. The results of the McCarthy assessments differ from those reported by Wilson *et al.*[2] They found differences between

TABLE 1. Results of the Bayley Scale of Mental Development

	Age					
	6 Months		12 Months		24 Months	
	Mean	SD	Mean	SD	Mean	SD
Methadone-exposed infants (n = 27)	107.9	12.23	102.5	11.38	100.9	18.04
Comparison infants (n = 17)	105.6	7.31	106.53	6.41	103.92	11.49

heroin-exposed children and 3 different comparison groups comprising a Drug Environment Group, a High Risk Group and a Socioeconomic Comparison Group. However our results are consistent with those of Strauss et al.[3] in their investigation of methadone-exposed and comparison children at 5 years of age. They found no difference between groups on the McCarthy General Cognitive Index (GCI) or any of the subscales, although the scores were much lower than those reported here. The inconsistent findings of different studies may reflect the myriad of confounding variables that are present within a population of opiate-dependent women. A large percentage of women maintained on methadone use, in addition, a number of other drugs such as opiates, diazepam, cocaine and barbiturates. They differ in methadone dose, length of methadone maintenance and amount of prenatal care. Pregnant opiate-dependent women also experience a high incidence of medical and obstetrical complications that may compromise the fetus. However, these data suggest that methadone maintenance during pregnancy, when provided within the context of a comprehensive program, does not impair the developmental and general cognitive functioning of the property.

REFERENCES

1. KALTENBACH, K. & L. P. FINNEGAN. 1984. Developmental outcome of children born to methadone maintained women: A review of longitudinal studies. Neurobehav. Toxicol. Teratol. **6:** 271-275.

TABLE 2. Results of McCarthy Scales of Children's Abilities

	Methadone-Exposed Children (n = 27)		Comparison Children (n = 17)		
	Mean	SD	Mean	SD	t
McCarthy General Cogitive Index (GCI)	106.51	12.96	106.05	13.10	0.11
Subscales					
Verbal	53.44	9.13	54.44	7.86	0.33
Perceptual	55.51	9.72	53.00	10.44	0.80
Quantitative	51.33	9.32	53.38	9.98	0.68
Memory	49.51	7.38	52.27	7.74	1.17
Motor	52.29	8.10	50.44	12.00	0.60

2. WILSON, G. S., M. M. DESMOND & R. B. WAIT. 1981. Follow-up of methadone treated women and their infants: Health, developmental, and social implications. J. Pediatr. **98:** 716-722.
3. STRAUSS, M. E., J. K. LESSEN-FIRESTONE, C. J. CHAVEZ & J. C. STRYKER. 1979. Children of methadone treated women at five years of age. Pharmacol. Biochem. Behav. Suppl. **11:** 3-6.

Women at Risk for AIDS and the Effect of Educational Efforts

C. ARENSON AND L. FINNEGAN

Department of Pediatrics
Jefferson Medical College
Thomas Jefferson University
Philadelphia, Pennsylvania 19107

Currently, the IV drug-abusing population is at risk for exposure to the Human Immunodeficiency Virus (HIV) and subsequent development of Acquired Immunodeficiency Syndrome (AIDS).[1,2] Women with AIDS have frequently been IV drug abusers or the sexual partners of IV drug abusers.[3] In addition, women infected with the HIV are at risk for transmitting the virus to their children perinatally.[4] Education in prevention of transmission remains our only weapon to stop the spread of HIV infection. Educational efforts among women at high risk are hampered both by their generally low level of education and socioeconomic class and by the strong denial operative in these women.[5]

In order to evaluate traditional educational efforts in the prevention of HIV infection in at-risk women, 42 drug-dependent pregnant and postpartum women receiving comprehensive treatment were surveyed. Drug use history revealed that 95% were current or past IV drug users with an average of 12 years of needle sharing; 82% of the subjects reported cessation of needle sharing prior to our educational intervention. The women completed questionnaires detailing their sexual and drug-using behaviors over the past 10 years. They then participated in a 30-min workshop covering sexual and parental transmission of HIV, needle cleaning, safe and unsafe sexual practices and the use of a condom, perinatal transmission, and the symptoms of AIDS Related Complex (ARC) and AIDS. Questionnaires covering AIDS knowledge were completed before and two to three weeks after the workshop. Results revealed that 79% were currently engaged in some risk behavior for HIV infection, such as prostitution, lack of condom use and sexual partners who were IV drug users. (TABLE 1). Nearly all the women (97%) knew that AIDS is spread by sharing needles and 88% knew how to effectively clean needles. All women knew that condoms provide protection during intercourse. The women showed concern about AIDS; 71% feared infection, but did not believe that they would catch the disease in spite of their past and/or current high-risk behaviors. AIDS workshops had little influence on the subjects' knowledge and behavior, since differences in pre and post test scores were insignificant. These women were clearly at high risk for exposure to HIV infection, both through sexual and needle-sharing behaviors. Although our survey revealed some cessation of needle-sharing practices, condom use and other safe-sex practices were negligible (FIG. 1). Conventional teaching efforts had a limited effect on increasing knowledge or changing behaviors. These women will clearly remain at high risk for future infection in them and their children until their IV drug use ceases and sexual behaviors change.

TABLE 1. High-Risk Behaviors

1.	Current or part IV drug use	94%
	Average length of drug use	15 years
	Average length of IV use	13 years
	Average length of needle sharing	12 years
2.	IV drug-using sexual partner in the past 5 years	78%
3.	Current high-risk sexual behavior[a]	79%
4.	Prostitution within the past 5 years (n = 34)	24%
5.	Currently prostituting	8%

[a] Prostitution, unprotected sex, partner who is an IV drug user and has shared needles in the past 5 years.

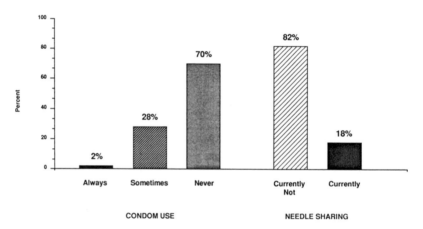

FIGURE 1. Protective behaviors of Philadelphia drug-addicted women in treatment.

REFERENCES

1. BLATTNER, W. A., R. J. BIGGAR, S. H. WEISS, M. MELBYE & J. J. GOEDERT. 1985. Epidemiology of human T-lymphotropic virus type III and the risk of the acquired immunodeficiency syndrome. Ann. Intern. Med. **103:** 665-670.
2. R. E. CHAISSON, A. R. MOSS, R. ONISHI, D. OSMOND & J. R. CARLSON. 1987. Human immunodeficiency virus infection in heterosexual intravenous drug users in San Francisco. Am. J. Public Health **77**(2): 169-172.
3. LEDERMAN, M. M. 1986. Transmission of the acquired immunodeficiency syndrome through heterosexual activity. Ann. Intern. Med. **104:**(1): 115-117.
4. MOK, J. Q., A. DEROSSI, A. E. ADES, C. GIAQUINTO, I. GROSCH-WORNER & C. S. PECKHAM. 1987. Infants born to mothers seropositive for human immunodeficiency virus. Lancet **1:** 1164-1168.
5. WOFSKY, C. B. 1987. Human immunodeficiency virus infection in women. J. Am. Med. Assoc. **257**(15): 2074-2076.

Gender-Identity Variations in Boys Prenatally Exposed to Opiates

O. B. WARD,[a] D. M. KOPERTOWSKI,[a] L. P.
FINNEGAN,[b] AND D. E. SANDBERG[c]

[a] Department of Psychology
Villanova University
Villanova, Pennsylvania 19085

[b] Department of Pediatrics
Jefferson Medical College
Thomas Jefferson University
Philadelphia, Pennsylvania 19107

[c] Department of Psychiatry
Columbia University
722 West 168th Street
New York, New York 10032

A potential consequence of opiate dependence during pregnancy is disruption of gonadal function in male fetuses. In rats, methadone attenuates fetal plasma testosterone titers,[1] and male rat fetuses exposed to morphine show a partial failure of behavioral masculinization, despite normally masculinized external genitals.[2] The present study assessed the effects of prenatal methadone exposure on behaviors that show sex-related variation in 5 to 7 year old children.

Twenty-six boys and 22 girls exposed to opiates *in utero* and 49 matched drug-free controls served as subjects. The drug-exposed children were the offspring of heroin-addicted women who were clients in a methadone maintenance clinic for pregnant women (Thomas Jefferson University Hospital, Philadelphia, PA). The women received an average of 35 mg of methadone daily throughout pregnancy. In addition, the majority continued to use some heroin. Controls were matched on age, sex, socioeconomic status, etc.

We gave two tests widely used in the assessment of gender identity; the Draw-A-Person test and the It Scale for Children. In the It Scale, children play with a stick figure ("It") having no distinct gender cues. The assumption is that the children will project their own sex role preference onto the stick figure. Drug-exposed boys were more likely to view the neuter "It" figure as having feminine characteristics ($p < 0.002$) than were control boys. Regression analyses revealed that drug exposure accounted for a significant portion of the variance among the boys, while being raised without a father figure or by someone other than the biological mother did not. Drug-exposed boys also were more likely to draw a female on the Draw-A-Person test that control boys ($p < 0.01$). It is assumed that the child projects his self image onto the drawing.

We also assessed the development of each child's preference for stereotypically masculine or feminine articles, as reflected in a Playroom Toy Preference Test. Most boys played primarily with masculine toys and most girls played primarily with feminine toys, regardless of drug exposure. However, a larger percentage of the drug-exposed boys showed some brief interest in the feminine toys than did control boys.

Results from both projective-type tests are congruent with the hypothesis that *in utero* exposure to opiates may lead to some feminization of gender identity in boys. However, no profound disturbances in gender identity were found—*i.e.,* no reports of cross dressing, expressing a wish to be a girl, or actually preferring feminine over masculine toys in the playroom test.

REFERENCES

1. SINGH, H. H., V. PUROHIT & B. S. AHLUWALIA. 1980. Effect of methadone treatment during pregnancy on the fetal testes and hypothalamus in rats. Biol. Reprod. **22:** 480-485.
2. WARD, O. B., J. M. ORTH & J. WEISZ. 1983. A possible role of opiates in modifying sexual differentiation. *In* M. Schlumpf & W. Lichtensteiger, Eds., Monographs in Neural Sciences **9:** 194-200. S. Karger. Basel.

Maternal Cigarette Smoking Depresses Placental Amino Acid Transport, Which May Lower the Birthweight of Infants[a]

B. V. RAMA SASTRY,[b] V. E. JANSON,[b] M. AHMED,[c]
J. KNOTS,[c] AND J. S. SCHINFELD[c]

[b] Department of Pharmacology
Vanderbilt University School of Medicine
Nashville, Tennessee 37232
and
[c] The University of Tennessee Center for Health Sciences
Memphis, Tennessee 38163

Maternal tobacco smoking during pregnancy exerts a retarding influence on fetal growth manifested by decreased birth weight and dimensions of the infant. This indicates a common cause for the development of all organs of the fetus.[1] The disparity in growth and development between children of smokers and nonsmokers disappears by the age of eleven, indicating that maternal smoking produces reversible intrauterine fetal growth retardation. One requirement for the growth and maturation of all organs of the fetus is essential amino acids (AA). The fetus is dependent upon the placental transfer of AA from maternal blood to its circulation. The uptake of AA by the human placenta is an active process and is a critical step in the net transfer of AA from the mother to the fetus. This step was depressed by placental hypoxia and several components of tobacco smoke in the isolated placental villus.[2-4] Therefore, placenta and umbilical venous bloods from tobacco cigarette smoking and nonsmoking mothers were collected and the endogenous free AA were analyzed to evaluate the effect of smoking on the placental transport of AA. The experimental protocols were approved by the Institutional Review Boards for Clinical Investigations at both institutions.

METHODS AND RESULTS

The blood-free placental villus samples and umbilical venous plasmas were prepared by well established procedures.[5,6] The AA were extracted with acetonitrile, separated

[a] This work was supported by grants from the Council for Tobacco Research, U.S.A., Inc. and the Smokeless Tobacco Research Council, Inc., and by United States Public Health Service-National Institutes of Health Grants ES-03172 and HD-10607.

by ion exchange chromatography and derivatized using o-phthalaldehyde and 2-mercaptoethanol. The fluorescent derivatives (excitation 340 nm, emission 410 nm) were assayed using a Water HPLC AA system.[5] Concentrations of several essential (val, met, ileu, leu, try, phe, his) and nonessential (glu, gly, ala, arg) AA in placental villi of nonsmoking mothers were significantly higher by about 30–50% than those of smokers (FIG. 1). Concentrations of thr and phe were about 14–15% higher in placental villi of nonsmokers than smokers. Correspondingly, the concentrations of AA in umbilical venous plasma of nonsmokers were higher than those of smokers (FIG. 2). These observations indicate that maternal smoking decreases the uptake of AA by placenta and therefore their net transfer from maternal to fetal circulation.

SUMMARY

Maternal cigarette smoking decreased placental transport of several essential and nonessential AA. Therefore, fetal intrauterine growth retardation in tobacco smokers can be explained partially by fetal undernutrition for AA during gestation.

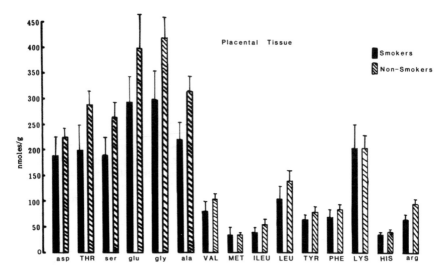

FIGURE 1. Concentrations of primary amino acids in the placental tissues of smoking and nonsmoking mothers. The placental tissues were collected from 16 nonsmoking and 16 smoking mothers. Each bar is a mean + SE. The smoking mothers smoked 17 ± 2 cigarettes per day. The placental weights of the smokers were about 10% higher than those of nonsmokers. The gestation period of all placentas was about 38–40 weeks. The infants of smokers were about 13–14% lighter than those of nonsmokers. The concentrations of aspartic acid, threonine, serine, glutamic acid, alanine, and valine in placentas of smokers were significantly lower than those of nonsmokers as determined by Student $t$test at $p < 0.05$. The concentrations of glycine, methionine, isoleucine, leucine, tyrosine, phenylalanine, lysine, histidine, and arginine in placentas of smokers were significantly lower than those of nonsmokers as determined by sign test at $p < 0.05$.

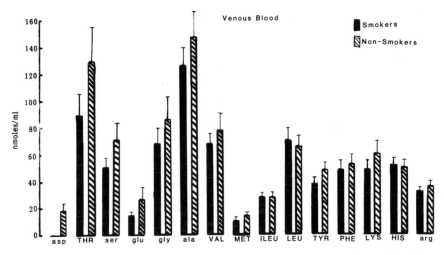

FIGURE 2. Concentrations of primary amino acids in the umbilical venous plasma of smoking and nonsmoking mothers. The blood samples were collected from 16 nonsmoking mothers and 16 smoking mothers. Each bar is a mean + SE. The transport of amino acids from the placental trophoblast cells into umbilical venous blood is by diffusion. Placentas of nonsmokers, which maintain higher concentrations of AA, permit diffusion of larger amounts of AA into umbilical blood than those of smokers. Correspondingly, the concentrations of amino acids in umbilical venous plasmas of smokers were lower than those of nonsmokers.

REFERENCES

1. U. S. Public Health Service. 1979. *In* Smoking and Health: A Report of the Surgeon General. DHEW Publication No. PHS-79-50066, Section 8, 1-93.
2. ROWELL, P. P. & B. V. R. SASTRY. 1978. Toxicol. Appl. Pharmacol. **45:** 79-93.
3. BARNWELL, S. L. & B. V. R. SASTRY. 1979. Toxicol. Appl. Pharmacol. **38:** 856.
4. BARNWELL, S. L. & B. V. R. SASTRY. 1983. Trophoblast Res. **1:** 101-120.
5. SASTRY, B. V. R., V. E. JANSON, M. HORST & C. C. STEPHAN. 1986. J. Liq. Chromatogr. **9**(8): 1689-1710.
6. HORST, M. A. & B. V. R. SASTRY. 1987. Prog. Clin. Biol. Res. **258:** 248-262.

Serum Cotinine Levels in Pregnant Nonsmokers in Relation to Birthweight

J. E. HADDOW, G. J. KNIGHT, G. E. PALOMAKI,
J. E. McCARTHY, AND K. C. FOSS

Foundation for Blood Research
P.O. Box 190
Scarborough, Maine 04074

Traditional methods for judging cigarette smoke exposure have relied heavily on identifying numbers of cigarettes smoked, or, in nonsmokers, hours of exposure to other people's smoke.[1,2] This approach has provided considerable useful information but has been limited by differences in smoking technique, differences in type of cigarette, and differences in ventilation in rooms. Recently it has become possible to determine smoke intake more accurately by measuring cotinine levels in blood, urine, or saliva.[3-5] Cotinine is a metabolic derivative of nicotine with a half-life of one day and allows one to look confidently at active and passive exposure to smoke.

The present study involves measuring serum cotinine levels and relating them to subsequent birthweight in 1,231 nonsmoking white pregnant women consecutively enrolled for second trimester MSAFP screening. Information regarding maternal age, height, weight, gravidity, years of maternal and paternal education, infant sex and birthweight were available for all women in the study. Using an improved RIA technique developed by our laboratory,[6] the lower level of detection for cotinine in serum was 0.5 ng/mL. Women whose level was above 10.0 ng/mL, the cut-off between smoking and nonsmoking, were excluded from the study.

Two thirds of the serum cotinine values fell below 1 ng/mL, and nearly all of the rest fell between 1.0 and 5.0 ng/mL. To avoid the confounding influence in birthweight from known correlated variables,[7] a multivariate regression analysis was applied, including maternal weight, height, age, gravidity, education and infant sex.

Three groups were defined based on cotinine values: (1) <0.5 ng/mL, (2) 0.5-1.0 ng/mL, and (3) 1.1-9.9 ng/mL. When crude birthweights were analyzed, a difference of 107 grams was noted between groups one and three. When multivariate regression analysis was applied, a 108-gram difference was noted. Both of these birthweight differences were significant at a p value of <0.001. This lowering of birthweight indicates a biologic effect to the fetus when the pregnant woman is exposed to cigarette smoke in the environment.

REFERENCES

1. RUBIN, D. H., P. A. KRASILNIKOFF, J. M. LEVENTHAL, B. WEILE & A. BERGET. 1986. Lancet ii: 415-417.

2. MARTIN, T. R. & M. B. BRACKEN. 1986. Am. J. Epidemiol. **124:** 633.
3. WALD, N. J., J. BOREHAM, A. BAILEY, C. RITCHIE, J. E. HADDOW & G. J. KNIGHT. 1984. Lancet **i:** 230-231.
4. LUCK, W. & H. NAU. 1985. J. Pediatr. **107:** 816-820.
5. HADDOW, J. E., G. J. KNIGHT, G. E. PALOMAKI, E. M. KLOZA & N. J. WALD. 1987. Br. J. Obstet. Gynecol. **94**(7): 678-681.
6. KNIGHT, G. J., P. WYLIE, M. S. HOLMAN & J. E. HADDOW. 1985. Clin. Chem. **31**(1): 118-121.
7. DOUGHERTY, C. R. S. & A. D. JONES. 1982. Am. J. Obstet. Gynecol. **144**(2): 190-200.

A New Method for the Rapid Isolation and Detection of Drugs in the Stools (Meconium) of Drug-Dependent Infants

ENRIQUE M. OSTREA, JR., PATRICIA PARKS, AND
MARK BRADY

Department of Pediatrics
Hutzel Hospital
Wayne State University
4707 St. Antoine Boulevard
Detroit, Michigan 48201

The examination of stools (meconium) in newborn infants for the purpose of drug screen has not been done. Instead, urine is routinely screened and the rate of false negative results is high even among infants born to known drug-abusing mothers. We have recently shown that meconium contains significant amount of drugs to which the infant has been chronically exposed, in utero. This report describes our technique for the rapid isolation and quantitation by radioimmunoassay of metabolites of heroin (morphine) and cocaine (benzoylecgonine) in the stools (meconium) of infants of drug-dependent mothers (IDDM).

Stools were collected for the first three days in 10 IDDMs and 5 nondrug-dependent (control) infants. The drug metabolites were not found in the control stools, but were detected in the stools of the IDDM up to the third day of sampling, at concentrations ranging from 0.30 to 10.84 mcg/g stool for cocaine and 0.56 to 12.10 mcg/g stool for morphine. The recovery rate of drug metabolites added to meconium was high with the use of our method; from 84% to 97% for morphine and 70% to 105% for cocaine.

We conclude that drug metabolites (specifically of cocaine and heroin) are detectable in the stools of IDDMs and that the method we describe for their isolation and detection is simple, rapid and accurate.

The Detection of Heroin, Cocaine, and Cannabinoid Metabolites in Meconium of Infants of Drug-Dependent Mothers

Clinical Significance

ENRIQUE M. OSTREA, JR., PATRICIA PARKS, AND
MARK BRADY

Department of Pediatrics
Hutzel Hospital
Wayne State University
4707 St. Antoine Boulevard
Detroit, Michigan 48201

Meconium (first 2-3-day stools) were collected during the first three days from 20 infants of drug-dependent mothers (IDDMs) and 5 nondrug-dependent (control) infants and tested, by radioimmunoassay, for the metabolites of 3 commonly abused drugs: heroin (morphine), cocaine (benzoylecgonine) and cannabinoids (delta 9 THC).

RESULTS

The control stools did not show any drug. Meconium from the IDDMs showed the presence of at least one drug metabolite: 80% of the IDDMs tested (16/20) showed cocaine (range = 0.41-19.91 mcg/g stool); 55% (11/20) showed morphine (range = 0.41-14.97 mcg/g stool) and 60% (12/20) showed cannabinoid (range = 0.05-0.66 mcg/g stool) metabolites. The stools tested positive for drugs up to the third day of sampling although in general, the incidence of positive results and the drug concentrations were highest during the first two days. In contrast, the routine urine drug screen (EMIT) on the infants showed that only 7 out of the 19 IDDMs tested (37%) were positive for drugs. In paired urine and stool specimens analyzed by radioimmunoassay, there were 8 urine samples which tested negative for drugs (predominantly the cannabinoids) despite a positive test in the stools. Likewise the concentration of drugs in the stools was higher than in the urine. We gave to pregnant Wistar rats daily doses of either morphine HCL (50 mg/kg/d), cocaine HCl (50 mg/kg/d) or cannabinoid (25 mg/kg/d). Analysis of drug metabolites in their pups' intestines (mcg/g tissue) showed: 0.47 mcg cocaine, 1.36 mcg morphine or 2.50 mcg cannabinoid in the treated pups.

CONCLUSIONS

Our studies show that meconium is a reservoir of metabolites of drugs which the fetus was exposed to, in utero. Meconium is an ideal specimen to test for drug screen in the suspected neonate: it is easy to collect, it contains drugs which may no longer be detected in the urine, and it contains them for as long as three days after birth.

The Perinatal Clinical Profile of HIV Infection in the Pregnant Addict

ENRIQUE M. OSTREA, JR., ANNA L. RAYMUNDO,
AND FLOSSIE COHEN

Department of Pediatrics
Hutzel Hospital
Wayne State University
4707 St. Antoine Boulevard
Detroit, Michigan 48201

We studied the perinatal clinical profile of HIV (antibody)-positive, drug-dependent, maternal-infant pairs (**Group 1, n = 28**) and compared them to maternal-infant pairs who were HIV-negative, and drug-dependent (**Group 2, n = 58**), and to those who were HIV-negative and nondrug-dependent (**control, n = 400**).

RESULTS

The maternal profile of Group 1 was: maternal age = 29.7 ± 5.4 yr, gravida > 2 = 86%, parity > 2 = 71%, anemia = 14%, other infections = 21%, meconium stained fluid = 22%, multiple births = 25%, PROM = 25%, and abnormal presentation = 7%. The neonatal profile was: LBW = 32%, prematurity = 53%, SGA = 28%, low Apgar = 18%, congenital malformations = 3.6% (although no characteristic dysmorphology was noted), HMD = 11%, jaundice = 18%, transient tachypnea = 10%. The features of Group 1 were significantly increased when compared to Control ($p < 0.01$), but not when compared to Group 2 ($p > 0.05$). Exceptions were the slightly higher rate of prematurity (53% vs 35%), LBW (29% vs 17%) and maternal use of benzodiazepines (4% vs 0.2%) in Group 1 vs Group 2. A 2-year follow-up was completed in 18 HIV-positive infants: 8 (44%) infants developed AIDS.

CONCLUSION

Drug addiction during pregnancy predisposes to a number of perinatal problems, including AIDS. However, superimposed HIV infection in the pregnant addict does not produce a characteristic clinical profile in the mother or infant; thus, detection of HIV infection in this group will still have to rely on routine HIV antibody screening.

Has Cocaine Abuse Increased Perinatal Morbidity in Maternal Drug Addiction?

ENRIQUE M. OSTREA, JR. AND
ANNA L. RAYMUNDO

Department of Pediatrics
Hutzel Hospital
Wayne State University
4707 St. Antoine Boulevard
Detroit, Michigan 48201

Complications from cocaine abuse during pregnancy have been reported; however, to attribute such complications to cocaine alone is difficult since polydrug abuse is common and drug usage by history is generally unreliable. Therefore, to determine cocaine effects on perinatal morbidity, we compared the perinatal outcome of a large population of pregnant addicts who delivered at our hospital in 1973-76 when cocaine was not abused, **Group 1 (n = 830)**; in 1986-87 when cocaine abuse was widespread, **Group 2 (n = 242)**; and in a nondrug-dependent group, **Control (n = 400)**.

RESULTS

Drug addiction, per se, leads to an increase ($p < 0.01$) in perinatal mortality and morbidity (**Group 1 vs Control**): meconium stained fluid (21% vs 14%), maternal anemia (13% vs 8%), PROM (12% vs 8%), maternal hemorrhage (3% vs 1%), prematurity (19% vs 10%), LBW (10% vs 4%), SGA (16% vs 3%), low Apgar (20% vs 10%) neonatal jaundice (13% vs 8%), meconium aspiration (12% vs 2%), transient tachypnea (7% vs 2%), HMD (4% vs 2%), congenital anomalies (5% vs 0.5%), and neonatal mortality (2.7% vs 1%). Cocaine abuse (**Group 2 vs Group 1**) has further increased ($p < 0.01$) the incidence of meconium stained fluid (25% vs 21%), PROM (22% vs 12%), C-section (21% vs 12%), and prematurity (34% vs 18%). Cerebral infarction and cortical atrophy were also noted in two cocaine-exposed neonates.

CONCLUSION

Drug addiction during pregnancy leads to high perinatal mortality and morbidity; cocaine abuse has further increased the overall morbidity.

Developmental, Behavioral, and Structural Effects of Prenatal Opiate Receptor Blockade

NANCY A. SHEPANEK, ROBERT F. SMITH, ZITA
TYER, DAWN ROYALL, AND KAREN ALLEN

George Mason University
Department of Psychology
4400 University Drive
Fairfax, Virginia 22030

The endogenous opiates have been implicated in a number of diverse phenomena such as sexual and social behaviors, locomotor activities and even modulation of tissue growth in the central nervous system (CNS) and elsewhere.[1-4] Furthermore, opiate receptor blockade is now widely used in obstetrical practice to reverse some of the side effects of opiates administered during labor and delivery.[5] Thus, opiate receptor blockade has become an increasingly important tool in both medicine and research. Although there is a paucity of data on the effects of prenatal opiate receptor blockade, Zagon and McLaughlin[3,4] have demonstrated that early *postnatal* exposure produces changes in the normal growth and development of the CNS, with total (24-hour) blockade resulting in enhanced growth in both cerebellum and cortex, while temporary blockade (4 to 6 hours a day) results in a decrease in growth in 21-day-old animals as measured by body weights, morphometric analysis, quantitative analysis of cell number and size, and examination of dendritic branching patterns.

Additionally, recent experiments have revealed that chronic exposure of fetal mouse spinal cord ganglion to naloxone result in increases in Mu type opiate receptor sites.[2] It is clear that the endogenous opiates play a role in growth and development of the CNS.

Since prenatal data on the CNS effects of opiate receptor blockade were extremely limited, and because of the increasing likelihood of the administration of these drugs to pregnant humans, the present study was designed to examine the effects of prenatal exposure to the opiate receptor blocker naloxone on measures of motor development, locomotor behavior, and CNS development.

Pregnant Long-Evans hooded rats were injected with 1 or 5 mg/kg/d from Day 4 to Day 18 of gestation and their offspring were assessed for changes in reflex development, locomotor activity, and learning of a Warden maze. Quantitative neuroanatomical evaluations of three CNS areas related to motor development and spatial learning were also performed. Analyses of variance revealed transient acceleration of development of righting reflex and negative geotaxis for high-dose animals (FIG. 1), and no significant effect on open field activity. Adult females in the low-dose condition exhibited impaired performance in rate of learning on the Warden maze (FIG. 2). Neuroanatomical evaluations also revealed an increased density of granule cells in the ectal limb of the dentate gyrus in these animals, an area associated with spatial learning.

There was also an increased concentration of granule cells in the curvature of the dentate gyrus in the high-dose condition.

These results demonstrate that some neurobehavioral changes are associated with prenatal opiate receptor blockade. Since the endogenous opiates have been implicated in the inhibition of growth and development of the CNS, the direction of these changes was partially predicted by the hypothesis that low doses of opiate receptor blockers might result in increased receptor sites and/or opiate supersensitivity resulting in delays in development. High doses may lead to reduced functional opiates, and enhanced development. Thus, endogenous opiates may have a modulatory effect on growth and development as demonstrated by: accelerated motor reflex development and increased density of granule cells in the dentate gyrus in the high-dose condition; and impaired performance of low-dose females on maze learning. Further study of the extent and mechanisms of the effects of prenatal opiate receptor blockade appear warranted.

REFERENCES

1. COMER, C. R., J. S. GRUNSTEIN, R. J. MASON, S. C. JOHNSTON & M. M. GRUNSTEIN. 1987. Endogenous opioids modulate fetal rabbit lung maturation. J. Appl. Physiol. **62:** 2141-2146.

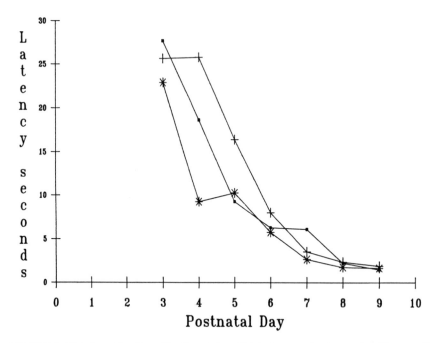

FIGURE 1. Righting reflex. Dose: ■ saline; + low; * high. Drug × day interaction. The overall ANOVA and post hoc tests of simple main effects indicated that development was accelerated in the high-dose group particularly on Postnatal Days 4 and 5. (F(12, 306) = 2.16 p < 0.01.)

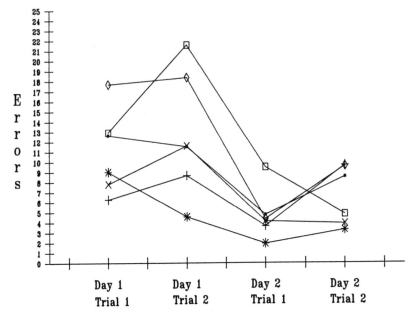

FIGURE 2. Warden maze learning—errors. ■ saline male; + saline female; * low male; □ low female; × high male; ◇ high female; drug × day × sex × trial interaction. The overall ANOVA and tests of simple main and simple interaction effects indicated that the low-dose females committed significantly more errors, particularly on Trial 2, Day 1. ($F(2, 50) = 3.27$, $p < 0.05$).

2. TEMPEL, A., S. M. CRAIN, E. R. PETERSON, E. J. SIMON & R. S. ZUKIN. 1986. Antagonist-induced opiate receptor upregulation in cultures of fetal mouse spinal cord-ganglion explants. Dev. Brain Res. **25:** 287-291.
3. ZAGON, I. S. & P. W. MCLAUGHLIN. 1986. Opioid antagonist modulation of cerebellum development: Histological and morphometric studies. J. Neurosci. **6**(6): 1424-1432.
4. ZAGON, I. S. & P. W. MCLAUGHLIN. 1986. Opioid antagonist-induced modulation of cerebral and hippocampal development: Histological and morphometric studies. Dev. Brain Res. **28:** 233-246.
5. JAFFE, J. H. & W. R. MARTIN. 1980. Opioid antagonists and agonist-antagonists. *In* A. G. Gilman, L. S. Goodman & A. Gilman, Eds. The Pharmacological Basis of Therapeutics. Macmillan. New York, NY.

Attentional Impairment in Rats Exposed to Alcohol Prenatally: Lack of Hypothesized Masking by Food Deprivation

B. J. STRUPP, J. KORAHAIS, D. A. LEVITSKY,
AND S. GINSBERG

Division of Nutritional Sciences and Department of Psychology
Savage Hall
Cornell University
Ithaca, New York 14853-6301

Attentional impairment is a common sequela of neonatal teratogen exposure in humans. This type of cognitive dysfunction may be obscured in animal models of these biological insults due to the frequent use of nutrient deprivation in the assessment of cognitive functioning. This possibility is suggested by the evidence that heightened motivation generally reduces susceptibility to distraction and facilitates sustained attention.[1] The present study was designed to test this hypothesis using prenatal ethanol (PE) exposure as an exemplary case.

On Days 5-20 of gestation, Long-Evans dams were maintained on a liquid diet containing 0 or 35% ethanol-derived calories. Beginning at 42 days of age, female offspring (n = 260) were tested in one of two discrimination tasks. Both tasks were conducted in the animals' homecages and entailed a choice between two distinctive boxes, the "correct" one containing a piece of Froot Loops cereal. In the "Distraction Task" both the boxes and their lids were surfaced with distinctive materials; however, only one of these two sets of cues predicted the location of the reward. For those animals in the Box-Relevant condition, the box cues were predictive and the two lids were randomly associated with reward; for the Lid-Relevant subgroup, the lids were predictive and the box cues "distracting." In contrast, the "Nondistraction task" entailed only predictive cues, located on the lids for half of the animals and on the boxes for the other half. Within each task, half of each treatment group was allowed free access to food; the other half was maintained at 80% of the weight of a matched, nondeprived animal. Assignment of animals to testing and deprivation conditions was random with the stipulation that littermates could not be allocated to the same subgroup.

The PE group required more trials to reach the learning criterion than controls on the Distraction, but not the Nondistraction, Task. This impairment was particularly evident in the Lid-Relevant Distraction Task ($p < 0.016$), due to the greater salience of the box cues relative to those on the lids. Although food restriction, as predicted, significantly facilitated learning in the Distraction Task ($p < 0.04$; FIG. 1), the relative impairment of the PE group was similar under Deprivation and Nondeprivation conditions (FIG. 2).

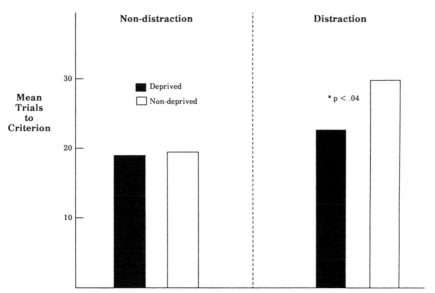

FIGURE 1. Mean trials to criterion on the "Distraction" and "Nondistraction" Tasks for rats maintained under Deprivation and Nondeprivation feeding conditions.

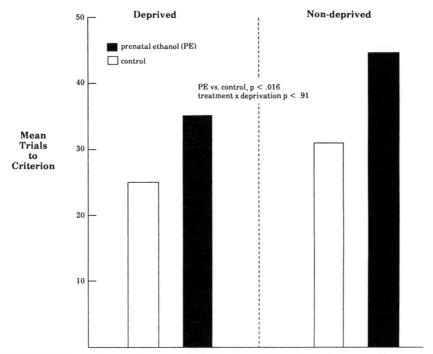

FIGURE 2. Mean trials to criterion on the Lid-Relevant Distraction Task for rats exposed to ethanol prenatally (PE) vs controls, under Deprivation and Nondeprivation feeding conditions.

In summary, rats exposed to ethanol prenatally exhibited a pattern of performance indicative of attentional impairment, the cognitive dysfunction most frequently reported as a result of PE in humans. While the lack of a pair-fed group precludes definitive attribution to the ethanol exposure, demonstration of an attentional deficiency in PE rats has been lacking and is a critical component of an animal model of this syndrome. Although the present results do not support the putative masking of attentional dysfunction by heightened motivation, the fact that clinical experience suggests such an effect necessitates further study of this issue (for discussion, see REF. 2).

REFERENCES

1. EYSENCK, M. 1982. Attention and Arousal: Cognition and Performance. Springer-Verlag. Berlin.
2. STRUPP, B. J. & D. A. LEVITSKY. 1989. An animal model of retarded cognitive development. *In* Advances in Infancy Research. C. Rovee-Collier & L. P. Lipsett, Eds. Vol. 6. Ablex Publishing. Norwood, NJ. In press.

Neurobehavioral Effects of Prenatal Exposure to Cocaine

S. K. SOBRIAN, N. L. ROBINSON,
L. E. BURTON, H. JAMES,
D. L. STOKES, AND L. M. TURNER

Department of Pharmacology
Howard University College of Medicine
Washington, DC 20059

The dramatic increase in cocaine use among young adults of childbearing age has produced a rise in its use during pregnancy,[1] with a subsequent increase in the potential number of fetuses exposed to cocaine. While data concerning the fetal and neonatal consequences of *in utero* cocaine exposure are preliminary and contradictory, intrauterine growth retardation, low birthweight, reduced occipitofrontal head circumference and increased morbidity are consistently reported.[2,3] The possibility that prenatal cocaine alters long-term postnatal development has not been determined and was the focus of the present experiment.

Timed-pregnant Sprague-Dawley rats were injected sc once daily on gestation days (GD) 15-21 with either isotonic saline (control: PS) or 20 mg/kg of cocaine (PC). This dose produced a mean gestational serum level of 621.4 $\pm$ 48.0 ng/ml, which is approximately 1.5-2.5 times higher than values reported after recreational cocaine use in man.[4] Despite appreciable drug levels in the pregnant rat, gestational and birth statistics reflected a lack of maternal toxicity: weight gain during injections (PS: 77.09 $\pm$ 5.44; PC: 78.75 $\pm$ 5.61 g), length of gestation (PS: 22.77 $\pm$ 0.18: PC: 22.92 $\pm$ 0.08 days), and litter size (PS: 12.36 $\pm$ 1.33; PC :13.92 $\pm$ 1.14 pups) were similar in cocaine and saline-treated mothers. Maternal behavior, measured within 4 hours of birth, assessed the possibility that residual cocaine effects could disrupt mother-pup interactions. However, tests of nest building, pup retrieval and nurturing behavior revealed no difference between cocaine and control dams.

In contrast to the mothers, serum cocaine was not detected in pups at birth. Although the incidence of offspring with hematomas was higher in PC litters (83.3%) than in controls (45.0%), gross examination failed to reveal any overt teratogenicity. Consistent with clinical observations, neonates exposed to cocaine *in utero* were smaller at birth than their control counterparts (PS: 6.68 $\pm$ 0.23; PC: 6.27 $\pm$ 0.28 g); this weight difference, was statistically significant from postnatal day (PND) 3 through PND 9. Despite their smaller size, the one-week mortality rate of PC pups was 50% lower than that of PS pups. Differences in body weights were not evident between 9 and 30 days of age.

The appearance of physical features and reflex behaviors, ontogentic landmarks which reflect maturation and integration in the central nervous system (CNS),[5] were monitored every third day from birth to PND 24 (TABLE 1). The development of surface righting, cliff avoidance and startle was accelerated in cocaine-exposed offspring, while acquisition of the learned response required in the test of olfactory

TABLE 1. Development of Reflexes and Physical Features in Prenatal Cocaine (PC) and Prenatal Saline (PS) Offspring[a]

			Postnatal Age (Days)							
	(n)	3	6	9	12	15	18	21	24
Physical development										
Pinna elevation	PS (28)	25	28							
	PC (28)	22	28							
Incisor eruption	PS (28)		0	1	25	28				
	PC (28)		0	1	26	28				
Eye opening	PS (28)				0	27	28			
	PC (28)				0	28	28			
Behavioral development[b]										
Negative geotaxis	PS (20)	3	17	20						
	PC (28)	11	24	28						
Surface righting	PS (20)	15[c]	20							
	PC (28)	28	28							
Olfactory behavior	PS (20)	19	20	20						
(home)	PC (28)	26	28	28						
Cliff avoidance	PS (20)		13[c]	19	20					
	PC (28)		25	27	28					
Startle response	PS (28)				0	13[c]	24	28		
	PC (28)					0	9	27	28	
Free-fall righting	PS (28)					0	6	26	28

[a] Two to 4 pups from each litter were tested repeatedly for the development of physical features, reflexes, and olfactory behavior, which were scored either present or absent. Values listed are the number of animals exhibiting response at each age.

[b] *Negative geotaxis:* pup placed on a 20° slope with its head pointed down the incline, turns around and crawls up the slope. *Surface righting:* pup placed on its back turns over to rest in normal position with all 4 paws on the ground within 30 seconds. *Olfactory behavior:* pup placed at the midpoint of a wire mesh screen suspended over home cage shavings and clean bedding chooses home within 120 seconds. *Cliff avoidance:* pup placed on edge of table top with forepaws and face over the edge backs away from the cliff. *Startle response:* a loud, sharp noise causes a sudden extension of the head and fore- and hindlimbs, which are then withdrawn into a crouching position. *Free-fall righting:* pup dropped dorsal side down from a height of 30 cm lands upright on all 4 paws.

[c] Significantly different from PS pups, $p < 0.05$.

behavior was unaffected. Alteration in the startle reflex[1] and decreased organizational response to environmental stimuli have also been reported in human infants following *in utero* cocaine.[6]

Fetal exposure to CNS depressants can alter the number of receptors for these drugs that develop in the postnatal brain.[7] To indirectly test this hypothesis with respect to cocaine and dopaminergic and noradrenergic receptors, locomotor activity was measured following injections of cocaine or amphetamine (FIG. 1). *In utero* cocaine exposure did not alter the offsprings' postnatal response to stimulants. At PND 15, cocaine (10 mg/kg, sc) significantly increased locomotor activity in both PC and PS offspring; amphetamine (1 mg/kg, sc) had no effect in either group. At PND 30, amphetamine (2 mg/kg, ip) increased motor activity in PC and PS animals and produced equivalent serum amphetamine levels in both groups (PS: 135.0 ± 58.3;

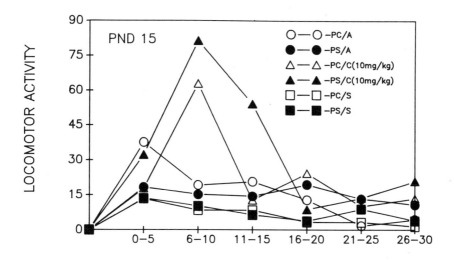

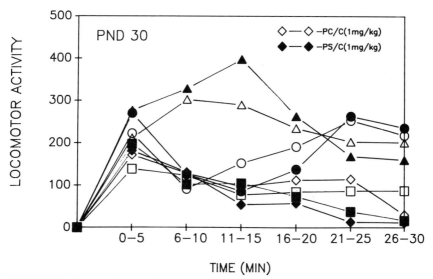

FIGURE 1. Stimulant-induced locomotor activity in offspring exposed prenatally to either cocaine or saline. At PND 15 (*above*) pups received cocaine (10 mg/kg), amphetamine (1 mg/kg) or isotonic saline, sc. At PND 30, (*below*), two doses of cocaine (1.0 and 10 mg/kg, ip) and amphetamine (2 mg/kg, ip) were tested. Following drug injection, locomotor activity was measured for 30 minutes (Automex Activity Meter, Columbus Instruments). Data points represent the mean of 12 offspring; each animal was tested only once.

PC: 170.0 ± 50.7 ng/ml). Cocaine (10 mg/kg, ip) also enhanced activity in both groups at this age. However, serum levels of this drug were higher in animals exposed prenatally to cocaine (PS: 393.3 ± 64.0; PC: 496.7 ± 36.3 ng/ml), suggesting a possible decrease in receptor activity.

These results indicate that in the absence of overt teratogenicity, fetal exposure to cocaine can enhance aspects of neurobehavioral ontogeny. This change, coupled with the apparent decrease in dopamine receptor activity, suggests that brain development is altered by prenatal exposure to cocaine.

REFERENCES

1. CHASNOFF, I. J., W. J. BURNS & S. H. SCHNOLL. 1985. N. Engl. J. Med. **313:** 666-669.
2. ORO, A. S. & S. D. DIXON. 1987. J. Pediatr. **111:** 571-578.
3. SMITH, J. E. & K. V. DEITCH. 1987. J. Pediatr. Health Care **1:** 120-124.
4. MOORE, T. R., J. SORG, L. MILLER, C. KEY & R. RESNIK. 1986. Am. J. Obstet. Gynecol. **155:** 883-888.
5. FOX, W. M. 1965. Anim. Behav. **13:** 234-241.
6. CHASNOFF, I. J., K. A. BURNS & W. J. BURNS. 1987. Neurotoxicol. Teratol. **9:** 291-931.
7. GALLAGER, D. W. & P. MALLORGA. 1980. Science **208:** 64-66.

Index of Contributors